PRAISE FOR *THE CHINA STUDY*

"*The China Study* gives critical, life-saving nutritional information for every health-seeker in America. But it is much more; Dr. Campbell's exposé of the research and medical establishment makes this book a fascinating read and one that could change the future for all of us. Every health care provider and researcher in the world must read it."

—JOEL FUHRMAN, M.D.
Author of the Best-Selling Book, *Eat To Live*

"Backed by well-documented, peer-reviewed studies and overwhelming statistics the case for a vegetarian diet as a foundation for a healthy lifestyle has never been stronger."

—BRADLY SAUL, OrganicAthlete.com

"*The China Study* is the most important book on nutrition and health to come out in the last seventy-five years. Everyone should read it, and it should be the model for all nutrition programs taught at universities. The reading is engrossing if not astounding. The science is conclusive. Dr. Campbell's integrity and commitment to truthful nutrition education shine through."

—DAVID KLEIN, Publisher/Editor
Living Nutrition Magazine

"*The China Study* describes a monumental survey of diet and death rates from cancer in more than 2,400 Chinese counties and the equally monumental efforts to explore its significance and implications for nutrition and health. Dr. Campbell and his son, Thomas, have written a lively, provocative and important book that deserves widespread attention."

—FRANK RHODES, PH.D.
President (1978–1995) Emeritus, Cornell University

"Colin Campbell's *The China Study* is an important book, and a highly readable one. With his son, Tom, Colin studies the relationship between diet and disease, and his conclusions are startling. *The China Study* is a story that needs to be heard."

—ROBERT C. RICHARDSON, PH.D.
Nobel Prize Winner, Professor of Physics
and Vice Provost of Research, Cornell University

"*The China Study* is the account of a ground-breaking research study that provides the answers long sought by physicians, scientists and health-conscious readers. Based on painstaking investigations over many years, it unearths surprising answers to the most important nutritional questions of our time: What really causes cancer? How can we extend our lives? What will turn around the obesity epidemic? *The China Study* quickly and easily dispenses with fad diets, relying on solid and convincing evidence. Clearly and beautifully written by one of the world's most respected nutrition authorities, *The China Study* represents a major turning point in our understanding of health."

—NEAL BARNARD, M.D., President
Physician's Committee for Responsible Medicine

"Everyone in the field of nutrition science stands on the shoulders of T. Colin Campbell, who is one of the giants in the field. This is one of the most important books about nutrition ever written—reading it may save your life."

—DEAN ORNISH, M.D., Founder & President
Preventive Medicine Research Institute Clinical Professor of Medicine,
University of California, San Francisco
Author, *Dr. Dean Ornish's Program for Reversing Heart Disease* and *Love & Survival*

"*The China Study* is the most convincing evidence yet on preventing heart disease, cancer and other Western diseases by dietary means. It is the book of choice both for economically developed countries and for countries undergoing rapid economical transition and lifestyle change."

—JUNSHI CHEN, M.D., PH.D., Senior Research Professor
Institute of Nutrition and Food Safety,
Chinese Center for Disease Control and Prevention

"All concerned with the obesity epidemic, their own health, and the staggering environmental and social impacts of the Western diet will find wise and practical solutions in Dr. Campbell's *The China Study*."

—ROBERT GOODLAND, Lead Advisor on the Environment
The World Bank Group (1978–2001)

"Dr. Campbell's book *The China Study* is a moving and insightful history of the struggle—still ongoing—to understand and explain the vital connection between our health and what we eat. Dr. Campbell knows this subject from the inside: he has pioneered the investigation of the diet-cancer link since the days of the seminal China Study, the NAS report, *Diet, Nutrition and Cancer* and AICR's expert panel report, *Food, Nutrition and the Prevention of Cancer: A Global Perspective*. Consequently, he is able to illuminate every aspect of this question. Today, AICR advocates a *predominantly plant-based diet* for lower cancer risk because of the great work Dr. Campbell and just a few other visionaries began twenty-five years ago."

—Marilyn Gentry, President
American Institute for Cancer Research

"*The China Study* is a well-documented analysis of the fallacies of the modern diet, lifestyle and medicine and the quick fix approach that often fails. The lessons from China provide compelling rationale for a plant-based diet to promote health and reduce the risk of the diseases of affluence."

—Sushma Palmer, Ph.D., Former Executive Director
Food and Nutrition Board, U.S. National Academy of Sciences

"*The China Study* is extraordinarily helpful, superbly written and profoundly important. Dr. Campbell's work is revolutionary in its implications and spectacular in its clarity. I learned an immense amount from this brave and wise book. If you want to eat bacon and eggs for breakfast and then take cholesterol-lowering medication, that's your right. But if you want to truly take charge of your health, read *The China Study* and do it soon! If you heed the counsel of this outstanding guide, your body will thank you every day for the rest of your life."

—John Robbins, Author of the Best-Selling Books
Diet for a New America and *The Food Revolution*

"*The China Study* is a rare treat. Finally, a world-renowned nutritional scholar has explained the truth about diet and health in a way that everyone can easily understand—a startling truth that everyone needs to know. In this superb volume, Dr. Campbell has distilled, with his son Tom, for us the wisdom of his brilliant career. If you feel any confusion about how to find the healthiest path for yourself and your family, you will find precious answers in *The China Study*. Don't miss it!"

—Douglas J. Lisle, Ph.D., & Alan Goldhamer, D.C.
Authors of *The Pleasure Trap: Mastering the Hidden Force
That Undermines Health and Happiness*

"So many diet and health books contain conflicting advice, but most have one thing in common—an agenda to sell something. Dr. Campbell's only agenda is truth. As a distinguished professor at Cornell University, Dr. Campbell is the Einstein of nutrition. *The China Study* is based on hardcore scientific research, not the rank speculation of a Zone, Atkins, SugarBusters or any other current fad. Dr. Campbell lays out his lifetime of research in an accessible, entertaining way. Read this book and you will know why."

—JEFF NELSON, President
VegSource.com (most visited food Web site in the world)

"If you're looking to enhance your health, performance and your success read *The China Study* immediately. Finally, scientifically valid guidance on how much protein we need and where we should get it. The impact of these findings is enormous."

—JOHN ALLEN MOLLENHAUER, Founder
MyTrainer.com and NutrientRich.com

The China Study

THE
China Study

The Most Comprehensive Study
of Nutrition Ever Conducted
and the Startling Implications
for Diet, Weight Loss
and Long-term Health

T. Colin Campbell, Ph.D.
WITH Thomas M. Campbell II

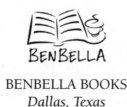

BENBELLA BOOKS
Dallas, Texas

BenBella Books, Inc.
6440 N. Central Expressway
Suite 503
Dallas, TX 75206
www.benbellabooks.com
Send feedback to feedback@benbellabooks.com
www.benbellabooks.com

Printed in the United States of America
20 19

ISBN 978-1932100-66-2

The Library of Congress has cataloged the hardcover edition as follows:

Campbell, T. Colin, 1934–
    The China study : the most comprehensive study of nutrition ever conducted and the startling implications for diet, weight loss, and long-term health / by T. Colin Campbell and Thomas M. Campbell II.
      p. cm.
    ISBN 978-1932100-66-2
    1. Nutrition. 2. Nutritionally induced diseases. 3. Diet in disease.
    I. Campbell, Thomas M. II. Title.
RA784.C235 2004
613.2—dc22
2004007985

Cover design by Melody Cadungog
Text design and composition by John Reinhardt Book Design
Printed by Victor Graphics, Inc.

Distributed by Perseus Distribution
perseusdistribution.com

To place orders through Perseus Distribution:
Tel: 800-343-4499
Fax: 800-351-5073
E-mail: orderentry@perseusbooks.com

To Karen Campbell, whose incredible love and caring made this book possible.

———

And to Thomas McIlwain Campbell and Betty DeMott Campbell for their incredible gifts.

Acknowledgements

This book, from its original conception to its final form, was in the making for many years. But it was the last three that gave the book form. And this happened because Karen, my lifelong love and wife of forty-three years, made it so. I wanted to do it, but she wanted it even more. She said it had to be done for the children of the world. She cajoled, she pushed and she insisted that we keep our nose to the grindstone. She read every word, those kept and those discarded—some several times.

Most importantly, Karen first suggested that I work with Tom, the youngest of our five children. His writing skills, his persistence in keeping integrity with the message and his exceptionally quick learning of the subject matter made the project possible. He wrote several chapters in this book himself and rewrote many more, bringing clarity to my message.

And our other children (Nelson—and wife Kim, LeAnne, Keith, Dan) and grandchildren (Whitney, Colin, Steven, Nelson, Laura) could not have been more encouraging. Their love and support cannot be measured in mere words.

I also am indebted to another family of mine: my many undergraduate honors students, post-graduate doctoral students, post-doctoral research associates and my fellow professorial colleagues who worked in my research group and who were the gems of my career. Regretfully, I could only cite in this book a small sample of their findings, but far, far more could have been included.

Yet more friends, associates and family contributed mightily, through their meticulous reading of various versions of the manuscript and their detailed feedback. Alphabetically, they included Nelson Campbell, Ron Campbell, Kent Carroll, Antonia Demas, Mark Epstein, John and Martha Ferger, Kimberly Kathan, Doug Lisle, John Robbins, Paul Sontrop and Glenn Yeffeth. Advice, support and generous help also came in many other forms from Neal Barnard, Jodi Blanco, Junshi Chen, Robert Goodland, Michael Jacobson, Ted Lange, Howard Lyman,

Bob Mecoy, John Allen Mollenhauer, Jeff Nelson, Sushma Palmer, Jeff Prince, Frank Rhodes, Bob Richardson and Kathy Ward.

Of course, I am grateful to all those at BenBella Books, including Glenn Yeffeth, Shanna Caughey, Meghan Kuckelman, Laura Watkins and Leah Wilson for turning a messy Word document into the book you now have. In addition, Kent Carroll added professionalism, understanding and a clear vision with his valuable editing work.

The heart of this book is the China Study itself. It was not the whole story, of course, but it was the "tipping point" in the development of my ideas. The actual study in China could not have happened without the extraordinary leadership and dedicated hard work of Junshi Chen and Li Junyao in Beijing, Sir Richard Peto and Jillian Boreham at the University of Oxford in England, and Linda Youngman, Martin Root and Banoo Parpia in my own group at Cornell. Dr. Chen directed more than 200 professional workers as they carried out the nationwide study in China. His professional and personal characteristics have been an inspiration to me; it is his kind of work and persona that makes this world a better place.

Similarly, Drs. Caldwell Esselstyn, Jr., and John McDougall (and Ann and Mary, respectively) generously agreed to participate in this book. Their dedication and courage are inspiring.

All of this was possible, of course, because of the exceptional start given to me by my parents, Tom and Betty Campbell, to whom this book is dedicated. Their love and dedication created for me and my siblings more opportunities than they ever dreamed of having.

I must also credit my colleagues who have worked to discredit my ideas and, not infrequently, me personally. They inspire in a different way. They compel me to ask why there is so much unnecessary hostility to ideas that should be part of the scientific debate. In searching for answers, I have gained a wiser, more unique perspective that I could not have considered otherwise.

Lastly, I must thank you, the taxpaying American public. You funded my work for more than four decades, and I hope that in telling you the lessons I've learned, I can begin to repay my debt to you.

—T. Colin Campbell

In addition to all those listed previously, I acknowledge my parents. My involvement in this book was, and still is, a gift from them I shall cherish for the rest of my life. Words cannot describe my good fortune in having parents who are such wonderful teachers, supporters and motivators.

Also, Kimberly Kathan provided support, advice, companionship and passion for this project. She made the lows bearable and the highs exceptional in this great roller coaster of an adventure.

—Thomas M. Campbell, II

Contents

Part IV: Why Haven't You Heard This Before?

Preface

T. COLIN CAMPBELL, at his core, is still a farm boy from northern Virginia. When we spend time together we inevitably share our stories from the farm. Whether it is spreading cow manure, driving tractors or herding cattle, both of us share a rich history in farming.

But from these backgrounds, both he and I went on to other careers. It is for his other career accomplishments that I came to admire Colin. He was involved in the discovery of a chemical later called dioxin, and he went on to direct one of the most important diet and health studies ever conducted, the China Study. In between, he authored hundreds of scientific papers, sat on numerous government expert panels and helped shape national and international diet and health organizations, like the American Institute for Cancer Research/World Cancer Research Fund. As a scientist, he has played an instrumental role in how our country views diet and health.

And yet, as I have gotten to know Colin on a personal level, I have come to respect him for reasons other than just his list of professional accomplishments. I have come to respect him for his courage and integrity.

Colin seriously questions the status quo, and even though the scientific evidence is on his side, going against the grain is never easy. I know this well because I have been a co-defendant with Oprah Winfrey when a group of cattlemen decided to sue her after she stated her intention not to eat beef. I have been in Washington, D.C., lobbying for better agricultural practices and fighting to change the way we raise and grow food in this country. I have taken on some of the most influential, well-funded groups in the country and I know that it's not easy.

Because of our parallel paths, I feel connected to Colin's story. We started on the farm, learning independence, honesty and integrity in small communities, and went on to become established in mainstream careers. Although we both had success (I still remember the first seven-figure check I wrote for my massive cattle operation in Montana), we came to realize that the system we lived in could use some improvements. Challenging the system that provided us with such rewards has demanded an iron will and steadfast integrity. Colin has both, and this book is a brilliant capstone to a long and dignified career. We would do well to learn from Colin, who has reached the top of his profession and then had the courage to reach even higher by demanding change.

Whether you have interest in your personal health or in the wretched state of health in the United States, this book will richly reward you. Read it carefully, absorb its information and apply it to your life.

—Howard Lyman, author of *Mad Cowboy*

Foreword

IF YOU ARE LIKE MOST AMERICANS TODAY, you are surrounded by fast food chain restaurants. You are barraged by ads for junk foods. You see other ads, for weight-loss programs, that say you can eat whatever you want, not exercise and still lose weight. It's easier to find a Snickers bar, a Big Mac or a Coke than it is to find an apple. And your kids eat at a school cafeteria whose idea of a vegetable is the ketchup on the burgers.

You go to your doctor for health tips. In the waiting room, you find a glossy 243-page magazine titled *Family Doctor: Your Essential Guide to Health and Well-being*. Published by the American Academy of Family Physicians and sent free to the offices of all 50,000 family doctors in the United States in 2004, it's full of glossy full-page color ads for McDonald's, Dr Pepper, chocolate pudding and Oreo cookies.

You pick up an issue of *National Geographic Kids*, a magazine published by the National Geographic Society "for ages six and up," expecting to find wholesome reading for youngsters. The pages, however, are filled with ads for Twinkies, M&Ms, Frosted Flakes, Froot Loops, Hostess Cup Cakes and Xtreme Jell-O Pudding Sticks.

This is what scientists and food activists at Yale University call a toxic food environment. It is the environment in which most of us live today.

The inescapable fact is that certain people are making an awful lot of money today selling foods that are unhealthy. They want you to keep eating the foods they sell, even though doing so makes you fat, depletes your vitality and shortens and degrades your life. They want you docile, compliant and ignorant. They do not want you informed, active and passionately alive, and they are quite willing to spend billions of dollars annually to accomplish their goals.

You can acquiesce to all this, you can succumb to the junk food sellers, or you can find a healthier and more life-affirming relationship with your body and the food you eat. If you want to live with radiant health, lean and clear and alive in your body, you'll need an ally in today's environment.

Fortunately, you have in your hand just such an ally. T. Colin Campbell, Ph.D., is widely recognized as a brilliant scholar, a dedicated researcher and a great humanitarian. Having had the pleasure and privilege to be his friend, I can attest to all of that, and I can also add something else. He is also a man of humility and human depth, a man whose love for others guides his every step.

Dr. Campbell's new book—*The China Study*—is a great ray of light in the darkness of our times, illuminating the landscape and the realities of diet and health so clearly, so fully, that you need never again fall prey to those who profit from keeping you misinformed, confused and obediently eating the foods they sell.

One of the many things I appreciate about this book is that Dr. Campbell doesn't just give you his conclusions. He doesn't preach from on high, telling what you should and shouldn't eat, as if you were a child. Instead, like a good and trusted friend who happens to have learned, discovered and done more in his life than most of us could ever imagine, he gently, clearly and skillfully gives you the information and data you need to fully understand what's involved in diet and health today. He empowers you to make informed choices. Sure, he makes recommendations and suggestions, and terrific ones at that. But he always shows you how he has arrived at his conclusions. The data and the truth are what are important. His only agenda is to help you live as informed and healthy a life as possible.

I've read *The China Study* twice already, and each time I've learned an immense amount. This is a brave and wise book. *The China Study* is extraordinarily helpful, superbly written and profoundly important. Dr. Campbell's work is revolutionary in its implications and spectacular in its clarity.

If you want to eat bacon and eggs for breakfast and then take cholesterol-lowering medication, that's your right. But if you want to truly take charge of your health, read *The China Study*, and do it soon! If you heed the counsel of this outstanding guide, your body will thank you every day for the rest of your life.

—John Robbins, author of *Diet for a New America, Reclaiming Our Health* and *The Food Revolution*

Introduction

THE PUBLIC'S HUNGER for nutrition information never ceases to amaze me, even after devoting my entire working life to conducting experimental research into nutrition and health. Diet books are perennial best-sellers. Almost every popular magazine features nutrition advice, newspapers regularly run articles and TV and radio programs constantly discuss diet and health.

Given the barrage of information, are you confident that you know what you should be doing to improve your health?

Should you buy food that is labeled organic to avoid pesticide exposure? Are environmental chemicals a primary cause of cancer? Or is your health "predetermined" by the genes you inherited when you were born? Do carbohydrates really make you fat? Should you be more concerned about the total amount of fat you eat, or just saturated fats and trans-fats? What vitamins, if any, should you be taking? Do you buy foods that are fortified with extra fiber? Should you eat fish, and, if so, how often? Will eating soy foods prevent heart disease?

My guess is that you're not really sure of the answers to these questions. If this is the case, then you aren't alone. Even though information and opinions are plentiful, *very few people truly know what they should be doing to improve their health.*

This isn't because the research hasn't been done. It has. We know an enormous amount about the links between nutrition and health. But the real science has been buried beneath a clutter of irrelevant or even harmful information—junk science, fad diets and food industry propaganda.

1

I want to change that. I want to give you a new framework for understanding nutrition and health, a framework that eliminates confusion, prevents and treats disease and allows you to live a more fulfilling life.

I have been "in the system" for almost fifty years, at the very highest levels, designing and directing large research projects, deciding which research gets funded and translating massive amounts of scientific research into national expert panel reports.

After a long career in research and policy making, I now understand why Americans are so confused. As a taxpayer who foots the bill for research and health policy in America, you deserve to know that many of the common notions you have been told about food, health and disease are wrong:

- Synthetic chemicals in the environment and in your food, as problematic as they may be, are not the main cause of cancer.
- The genes that you inherit from your parents are not the most important factors in determining whether you fall prey to any of the ten leading causes of death.
- The hope that genetic research will eventually lead to drug cures for diseases ignores more powerful solutions that can be employed today.
- Obsessively controlling your intake of any one nutrient, such as carbohydrates, fat, cholesterol or omega-3 fats, will not result in long-term health.
- Vitamins and nutrient supplements do not give you long-term protection against disease.
- Drugs and surgery don't cure the diseases that kill most Americans.
- Your doctor probably does not know what you need to do to be the healthiest you can be.

I propose to do nothing less than redefine what we think of as good nutrition. The provocative results of my four decades of biomedical research, including the findings from a twenty-seven-year laboratory program (funded by the most reputable funding agencies) prove that eating right can save your life.

I will not ask you to believe conclusions based on my personal observations, as some popular authors do. There are over 750 references in this book, and the vast majority of them are primary sources of information, including hundreds of scientific publications from other researchers that point the way to less cancer, less heart disease, fewer strokes, less obesity, less diabetes, less autoimmune disease, less osteoporosis, less Alzheimer's, less kidney stones and less blindness.

Some of the findings, published in the most reputable scientific journals, show that:

- Dietary change can enable diabetic patients to go off their medication.
- Heart disease can be reversed with diet alone.
- Breast cancer is related to levels of female hormones in the blood, which are determined by the food we eat.
- Consuming dairy foods can increase the risk of prostate cancer.
- Antioxidants, found in fruits and vegetables, are linked to better mental performance in old age.
- Kidney stones can be prevented by a healthy diet.
- Type 1 diabetes, one of the most devastating diseases that can befall a child, is convincingly linked to infant feeding practices.

These findings demonstrate that a good diet is the most powerful weapon we have against disease and sickness. An understanding of this scientific evidence is not only important for improving health; it also has profound implications for our entire society. We *must* know why misinformation dominates our society and why we are grossly mistaken in how we investigate diet and disease, how we promote health and how we treat illness.

By any number of measures, America's health is failing. We spend far more, per capita, on health care than any other society in the world, and yet two thirds of Americans are overweight, and over 15 million Americans have diabetes, a number that has been rising rapidly. We fall prey to heart disease as often as we did thirty years ago, and the War on Cancer, launched in the 1970s, has been a miserable failure. Half of Americans have a health problem that requires taking a prescription drug every week, and over 100 million Americans have high cholesterol.

To make matters worse, we are leading our youth down a path of disease earlier and earlier in their lives. One third of the young people in this country are overweight or at risk of becoming overweight. Increasingly, they are falling prey to a form of diabetes that used to be seen only in adults, and these young people now take more prescription drugs than ever before.

These issues all come down to three things: breakfast, lunch and dinner.

More than forty years ago, at the beginning of my career, I would have never guessed that food is so closely related to health problems. For years I never gave much thought to which foods were best to eat. I just ate what everyone else did: what I was told was good food. We all eat what is tasty or what is convenient or what our parents taught us to prefer. Most of us live within cultural boundaries that define our food preferences and habits.

So it was with me. I was raised on a dairy farm where milk was central to our existence. We were told in school that cow's milk made strong, healthy bones and teeth. It was Nature's most perfect food. On our farm, we produced most of our own food in the garden or in the livestock pastures.

I was the first in my family to go to college. I studied pre-veterinary medicine at Penn State and then attended veterinary school at the University of Georgia for a year when Cornell University beckoned with scholarship money for me to do graduate research in "animal nutrition." I transferred, in part, because they were going to pay me to go to school instead of me paying them. There I did a master's degree. I was the last graduate student of Professor Clive McCay, a Cornell professor famed for extending the lives of rats by feeding them much less food than they would otherwise eat. My Ph.D. research at Cornell was devoted to finding better ways to make cows and sheep grow faster. I was attempting to improve on our ability to produce animal protein, the cornerstone of what I was told was "good nutrition."

I was on a trail to promote better health by advocating the consumption of more meat, milk and eggs. It was an obvious sequel to my own life on the farm and I was happy to believe that the American diet was the best in the world. Through these formative years, I encountered a recurring theme: we were supposedly eating the right foods, especially plenty of high-quality animal protein.

Much of my early career was spent working with two of the most toxic chemicals ever discovered, dioxin and aflatoxin. I initially worked at MIT, where I was assigned a chicken feed puzzle. Millions of chicks a year were dying from an unknown toxic chemical in their feed, and I had the responsibility of isolating and determining the structure of this chemical. After two and one-half years, I helped discover dioxin, arguably the most toxic chemical ever found. This chemical has since received widespread attention, especially because it was part of the herbicide 2,4,5-T, or Agent Orange, then being used to defoliate forests in the Vietnam War.

After leaving MIT and taking a faculty position at Virginia Tech, I began coordinating technical assistance for a nationwide project in the Philippines working with malnourished children. Part of the project became an investigation of the unusually high prevalence of liver cancer, usually an adult disease, in Filipino children. It was thought that high consumption of aflatoxin, a mold toxin found in peanuts and corn, caused this problem. Aflatoxin has been called one of the most potent carcinogens ever discovered.

For ten years our primary goal in the Philippines was to improve childhood malnutrition among the poor, a project funded by the U.S. Agency for International Development. Eventually, we established about 110 nutrition "self-help" education centers around the country.

The aim of these efforts in the Philippines was simple: make sure that children were getting as much protein as possible. It was widely thought that much of the childhood malnutrition in the world was caused by a lack of protein, especially from animal-based foods. Universities and governments around the world were working to alleviate a perceived "protein gap" in the developing world.

In this project, however, I uncovered a dark secret. *Children who ate the highest-protein diets were the ones most likely to get liver cancer!* They were the children of the wealthiest families.

I then noticed a research report from India that had some very provocative, relevant findings. Indian researchers had studied two groups of rats. In one group, they administered the cancer-causing aflatoxin, then fed a diet that was composed of 20% protein, a level near what many of us consume in the West. In the other group, they administered the same amount of aflatoxin, but then fed a diet that was only composed of 5% protein. Incredibly, every single animal that consumed the 20% protein diet had evidence of liver cancer, and every single animal that consumed a 5% protein diet avoided liver cancer. It was a 100 to 0 score, leaving no doubt that nutrition trumped chemical carcinogens, even very potent carcinogens, in controlling cancer.

This information countered everything I had been taught. It was heretical to say that protein wasn't healthy, let alone say it promoted cancer. It was a defining moment in my career. Investigating such a provocative question so early in my career was not a very wise choice. Questioning protein and animal-based foods in general ran the risk of my being labeled a heretic, even if it passed the test of "good science."

But I never was much for following directions just for the sake of following directions. When I first learned to drive a team of horses or herd cattle, to hunt animals, to fish our creek or to work in the fields, I came to accept that independent thinking was part of the deal. It had to be. Encountering problems in the field meant that I had to figure out what to do next. It was a great classroom, as any farm boy can tell you. That sense of independence has stayed with me until today.

So, faced with a difficult decision, I decided to start an in-depth laboratory program that would investigate the role of nutrition, especially protein, in the development of cancer. My colleagues and I were cautious in framing our hypotheses, rigorous in our methodology and conservative in interpreting our findings. I chose to do this research at a very basic science level, studying the biochemical details of cancer formation. It was important to understand not only *whether* but also *how* protein might promote cancer. It was the best of all worlds. By carefully following the rules of good science, I was able to study a provocative topic without provoking knee-jerk responses that arise with radical ideas. Eventually, this research became handsomely funded for twenty-seven *years* by the best-reviewed and most competitive funding sources (mostly the National Institutes of Health (NIH), the American Cancer Society and the American Institute for Cancer Research). Then our results were reviewed (a second time) for publication in many of the best scientific journals.

What we found was shocking. Low-protein diets inhibited the initiation of cancer by aflatoxin, regardless of how much of this carcinogen was administered to these animals. After cancer initiation was completed, low-protein diets also dramatically blocked subsequent cancer growth. In other words, the cancer-producing effects of this highly carcinogenic chemical were rendered insignificant by a low-protein diet. *In fact, dietary protein proved to be so powerful in its effect that we could turn on and turn off cancer growth simply by changing the level consumed.*

Furthermore, the amounts of protein being fed were those that we humans routinely consume. We didn't use extraordinary levels, as is so often the case in carcinogen studies.

But that's not all. We found that not all proteins had this effect. What protein consistently and strongly promoted cancer? Casein, which makes up 87% of cow's milk protein, promoted all stages of the cancer process. What type of protein did not promote cancer, even at high levels of intake? The safe proteins were from plants, including wheat and soy. As this picture came into view, it began to challenge and then to shatter some of my most cherished assumptions.

These experimental animal studies didn't end there. I went on to direct the most comprehensive study of diet, lifestyle and disease ever done with humans in the history of biomedical research. It was a massive undertaking jointly arranged through Cornell University, Oxford University and the Chinese Academy of Preventive Medicine. The *New York Times* called it the "Grand Prix of Epidemiology." This project surveyed a vast range of diseases and diet and lifestyle factors in rural China and, more recently, in Taiwan. More commonly known as the China Study, this project eventually produced more than *8,000 statistically significant associations between various dietary factors and disease!*

What made this project especially remarkable is that, among the many associations that are relevant to diet and disease, so many pointed to the same finding: people who ate the most animal-based foods got the most chronic disease. Even relatively small intakes of animal-based food were associated with adverse effects. People who ate the most plant-based foods were the healthiest and tended to avoid chronic disease. These results could not be ignored. From the initial experimental animal studies on animal protein effects to this massive human study on dietary patterns, the findings proved to be consistent. The health implications of consuming either animal or plant-based nutrients were remarkably different.

I could not, and did not, rest on the findings of our animal studies and the massive human study in China, however impressive they may have been. I sought out the findings of other researchers and clinicians. The findings of these individuals have proved to be some of the most exciting findings of the past fifty years.

These findings—the contents of Part II of this book—show that heart disease, diabetes and obesity can be reversed by a healthy diet. Other research shows that various cancers, autoimmune diseases, bone health, kidney health, vision and brain disorders in old age (like cognitive dysfunction and Alzheimer's) are convincingly influenced by diet. Most importantly, the diet that has time and again been shown to reverse and/or prevent these diseases is the same whole foods, plant-based diet that I had found to promote optimal health in my laboratory research and in the China Study. *The findings are consistent.*

Yet, despite the power of this information, despite the hope it generates and despite the urgent need for this understanding of nutrition and health, *people are still confused.* I have friends with heart disease who are resigned and despondent about being at the mercy of what they consider to be an inevitable disease. I've talked with women who are so terrified of breast cancer that they wish to have their own breasts, even their daughters' breasts, surgically removed, as if that's the only way to minimize risk. So many of the people I have met have been led down a path of illness, despondence and confusion about their health and what they can do to protect it.

Americans are confused, and I will tell you why. The answer, discussed in Part IV, has to do with how health information is generated and communicated and who controls such activities. Because I have been behind the scenes generating health information for so long, I have seen what really goes on—and I'm ready to tell the world what is wrong with the system. The distinctions between government, industry, science and medicine have become blurred. The distinctions between making a profit and promoting health have become blurred. The problems with the system do not come in the form of Hollywood-style corruption. The problems are much more subtle, and yet much more dangerous. The result is massive amounts of misinformation, for which average American consumers pay twice. They provide the tax money to do the research, and then they provide the money for their health care to treat their largely preventable diseases.

This story, starting from my personal background and culminating in a new understanding of nutrition and health, is the subject of this book. Six years ago at Cornell University, I organized and taught a new elective course called Vegetarian Nutrition. It was the first such course on an American university campus and has been far more successful than I could have imagined. The course focuses on the health value of a plant-based diet. After spending my time at MIT and Virginia Tech, then coming back to Cornell thirty years ago, I was charged with the task of integrating the concepts and principles of chemistry, biochemistry, physiology and toxicology in an upper-level course in nutrition.

After four decades of scientific research, education and policy making at the highest levels in our society, I now feel I can adequately integrate these disciplines into a cogent story. That's what I have done for my most recent course, and many of my students tell me that their lives are changed for the better by the end of the semester. That's what I intend to do for you; I hope your life will be changed as well.

Part I

THE CHINA STUDY

1
Problems We Face, Solutions We Need

"He who does not know food, how can he understand the diseases of man?"

—Hippocrates, the father of medicine (460–357 B.C.)

ON A GOLDEN MORNING IN 1946, when summer was all tuckered out and fall wanted to be let in, all you could hear on my family's dairy farm was quiet. There was no growl from cars driving by or airplanes burning trails overhead. Just quiet. There were the songbirds, of course, and the cows, and the roosters who would chime in once in a while, but these noises merely filled out the quiet, the peace.

Standing on the second floor of our barn, with the immense brown doors gaping open, allowing the sun to soak through, I was a happy twelve-year-old. I had just finished a big country breakfast of eggs, bacon, sausage, fried potatoes and ham with a couple of glasses of whole milk. My mom had cooked a fantastic meal. I had been working up my appetite since 4:30 A.M., when I had gotten up to milk the cows with my father Tom and my brother Jack.

My father, then forty-five, stood with me in the quiet sun. He opened a fifty-pound sack of alfalfa seed, dumped all the tiny seeds on the

11

wooden barn floor in front of us and then opened a box containing fine black powder. The powder, he explained, was bacteria that would help the alfalfa grow. They would attach themselves to the seeds and become part of the roots of the growing plant throughout its life. Having had only two years of formal education, my father was proud of knowing that the bacteria helped the alfalfa convert nitrogen from the air into protein. The protein, he explained, was good for the cows that would eventually eat it. So our work that morning was to mix the bacteria and the alfalfa seeds before planting. Always curious, I asked my dad why it worked and how. He was glad to explain it, and I was glad to hear it. This was important knowledge for a farm boy.

Seventeen years later, in 1963, my father had his first heart attack. He was sixty-one. At age seventy, he died from a second massive coronary. I was devastated. My father, who had stood with my siblings and me for so many days in the quiet countryside, teaching us the things that I still hold dear in life, was gone.

Now, after decades of doing experimental research on diet and health, I know that the very disease that killed my father, heart disease, can be prevented, even reversed. Vascular (arteries and heart) health is possible without life-threatening surgery and without potentially lethal drugs. I have learned that it can be achieved simply by eating the right food.

This is the story of how food can change our lives. I have spent my career in research and teaching unraveling the complex mystery of why health eludes some and embraces others, and I now know that food primarily determines the outcome. This information could not come at a better time. Our health care system costs too much, it excludes far too many people and it does not promote health and prevent disease. Volumes have been written on how the problem might be solved, but progress has been painfully slow.

SICKNESS, ANYONE?

If you are male in this country, the American Cancer Society says that you have a 47% chance of getting cancer. If you are female, you fare a little better, but you still have a whopping 38% lifetime chance of getting cancer.[1] The rates at which we die from cancer are among the highest in the world, and it has been getting worse (Chart 1.1). Despite thirty years of the massively funded War on Cancer, we have made little progress.

Contrary to what many believe, cancer is not a natural event. Adopting

CHART 1.1: CANCER DEATH RATES (PER 100,000 PEOPLE)[1]

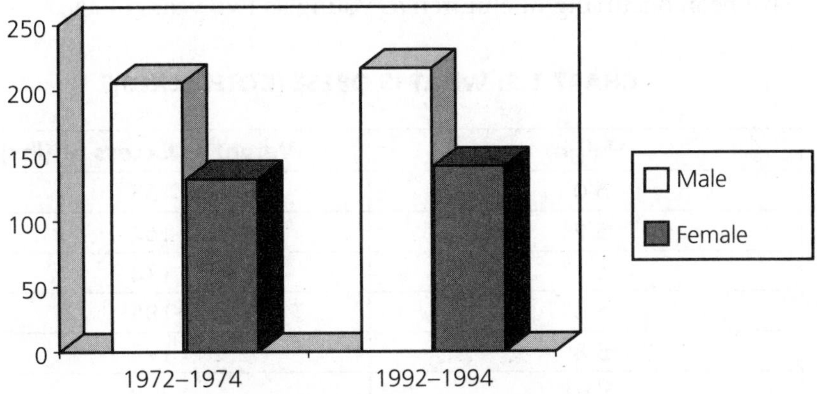

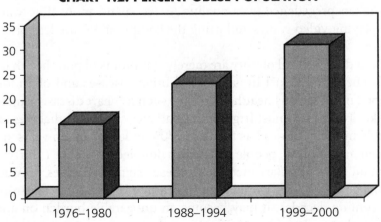

a healthy diet and lifestyle can prevent the majority of cancers in the United States. Old age can and should be graceful and peaceful.

But cancer is only part of a larger picture of disease and death in America. Looking elsewhere, we see that there is an overall pattern of poor health. For example, we are rapidly becoming the heaviest people on earth. Overweight Americans now significantly outnumber those who maintain a healthy weight. As shown in Chart 1.2, our rates of obesity have been skyrocketing over the past several decades.[2]

According to the National Center for Health Statistics, almost a third of the adults twenty years of age and over in this country are obese![3] One is considered obese if he or she is carrying more than a third of a

CHART 1.2: PERCENT OBESE POPULATION[2]

person above and beyond a healthy weight. Similarly frightening trends have been occurring in children as young as two years of age.[3]

CHART 1.3: WHAT IS OBESE (BOTH SEXES)?

Height	Weight in Excess of (lbs)
5'0"	153
5'2"	164
5'4"	174
5'6"	185
5'8"	197
5'10"	209
6'0"	221
6'2"	233

But cancer and obesity are not the only epidemics casting a large shadow over American health. Diabetes has also increased in unprecedented proportions. One out of thirteen Americans now has diabetes, and that ratio continues to rise. If we don't heed the importance of diet, millions of additional Americans will unknowingly develop diabetes and suffer its consequences, including blindness, limb amputation, cardiovascular disease, kidney disease and premature death. Despite this, fast food restaurants that serve nutritionally defunct foods are now fixtures in almost every town. We eat out more than ever[4] and speed has taken precedence over quality. As we spend more time watching TV, playing video games and using the computer, we are less physically active.

Both diabetes and obesity are merely symptoms of poor health in general. They rarely exist in isolation of other diseases and often forecast deeper, more serious health problems, such as heart disease, cancer and stroke. Two of the most frightening statistics show that diabetes among people in their thirties has increased 70% in less than ten years and the percentage of obese people has nearly doubled in the past thirty years. Such an incredibly fast increase in these "signal" diseases in America's young to middle-age population forecasts a health care catastrophe in the coming decades. It may become an unbearable burden on a health system that is already strained in countless ways.

DIABETES STATISTICS

Percent Increase in Incidence from 1990 to 1998[5]:
Age 30–39 (70%)   •   Age 40–49 (40%)   •   Age 50–59 (31%)
Percent of Diabetics Who Aren't Aware of their Illness[5]: 34%
Diabetes Outcomes[6]: Heart Disease and Stroke; Blindness; Kidney Disease; Nervous System Disorders; Dental Disease; Limb Amputation
Annual Economic Cost of Diabetes[7]: $98 Billion

But the most pervasive killer in our culture is not obesity, diabetes or cancer. It is heart disease. Heart disease will kill one out of every three Americans. According to the American Heart Association, over 60 million Americans currently suffer from some form of cardiovascular disease, including high blood pressure, stroke and heart disease.[8] Like me, you undoubtedly have known someone who died of heart disease. But since my own father died from a heart attack over thirty years ago, a great amount of knowledge has been uncovered in understanding this disease. The most dramatic recent finding is that heart disease can be prevented and even reversed by a healthy diet.[9, 10] People who cannot perform the most basic physical activity because of severe angina can find a new life simply by changing their diets. By embracing this revolutionary information, we could collectively defeat the most dangerous disease in this country.

OOPS...WE DIDN'T MEAN TO HAVE THAT HAPPEN!

As increasing numbers of Americans fall victim to chronic diseases, we hope that our hospitals and doctors will do all that they can to help us. Unfortunately, both the newspapers and the courts are filled with stories and cases that tell us that inadequate care has become the norm.

One of the most well regarded voices representing the medical community, the *Journal of the American Medical Association* (JAMA), included a recent article by Barbara Starfield, M.D., stating that physician error, medication error and adverse events from drugs or surgery kill 225,400 people per year (Chart 1.5).[11] That makes our health care system the third leading cause of death in the United States, behind only cancer and heart disease (Chart 1.4).[12]

CHART 1.4: LEADING CAUSES OF DEATH[12]

Cause of Death	Deaths
Diseases of the Heart	710,760
Cancer (Malignant Neoplasms)	553,091
Medical Care[11]	225,400
Stroke (Cerebrovascular Diseases)	167,661
Chronic Lower Respiratory Diseases	122,009
Accidents	97,900
Diabetes Mellitus	69,301
Influenza and Pneumonia	65,313
Alzheimer's Disease	49,558

CHART 1.5: DEATH BY HEALTH CARE[11]

Number of Americans Per Year Who Die From:	
Medication Errors[13]	7,400
Unnecessary Surgery[14]	12,000
Other Preventable Errors in Hospitals[11]	20,000
Hospital Borne Infections[11]	80,000
Adverse Drug Effects[15]	106,000

The last and largest category of deaths in this group are the hospitalized patients who die from the "noxious, unintended and undesired effect of a drug,"[15] which occurs at normal doses.[16] Even with the use of approved medicines and correct medication procedures, over one hundred thousand people die every year from unintended reactions to the "medicine" that is supposed to be reviving their health.[15] Incidentally, this same report, which summarized and analyzed thirty-nine separate studies, found that almost 7% (one out of fifteen) of all hospitalized patients have experienced a serious adverse drug reaction, one that "requires hospitalization, prolongs hospitalization, is permanently disabling or results in death."[15] These are people who took their medicine as directed. This number does not include the tens of thousands of people who suffer from the incorrect administration and use of these drugs. Nor does it include adverse drug events that are labeled "possible" effects, or drugs that do not accomplish their intended goal. In other words, one of fifteen is a conservative number.[15]

If nutrition were better understood, and prevention and natural treatments were more accepted in the medical community, we would not be pouring so many toxic, potentially lethal drugs into our bodies at the last stage of disease. We would not be frantically searching for the new medicine that alleviates the symptoms but often does nothing to address the fundamental causes of our illnesses. We would not be spending our money developing, patenting and commercializing "magic bullet" drugs that often cause additional health problems. The current system has not lived up to its promise. It is time to shift our thinking toward a broader perspective on health, one that includes a proper understanding and use of good nutrition.

As I look back on what I've learned, I am appalled that the circumstances surrounding the way in which Americans die are often unnecessarily early, painful and costly.

AN EXPENSIVE GRAVE

We pay more for our health care than any other country in the world (Chart 1.6).

We spent over a trillion dollars on health care in 1997.[17] In fact, the cost of our "health" is spiraling so far out of control that the Health Care Financing Administration predicted that our system would cost 16 trillion dollars by 2030.[17] Costs have so consistently outpaced inflation that we now spend one out of every seven dollars the economy produces on health care (Chart 1.7). We have seen almost a 300% increase in expenditures, as a percentage of GDP, in less than forty years! What is all the extra financing buying? Is it creating health? I say no, and many serious commentators agree.

Recently the health status of twelve countries including the U.S., Canada, Australia and several Western European countries was compared on the basis of sixteen different indicators of health care efficacy.[19] Other countries spend, on average, only about one-half of what the U.S. spends per capita on health care. Isn't it reasonable, therefore, for us to expect our system to rank above theirs? Unfortunately, among these twelve countries, the U.S. system is consistently among the worst performers.[11] In a separate analysis, the World Health Organization ranked the United States thirty-seventh best in the world according to health care system performance.[20] Our health care system is clearly not the best

CHART 1.6: HEALTH CARE EXPENDITURES PER PERSON, 1997 $US[17]

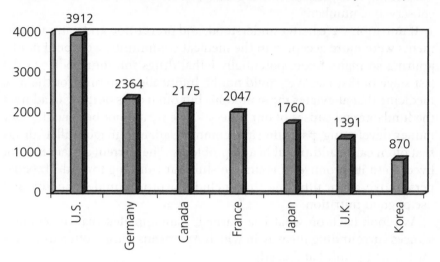

CHART 1.7: PERCENT OF U.S. GDP SPENT ON HEALTH CARE[17, 18]

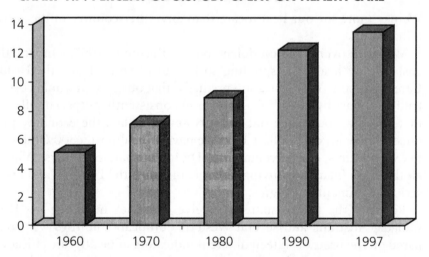

in the world, even though we spend, far and away, the most money on it.

Too often in the United States, a doctor's treatment decisions are made on the basis of money, not health. The consequences of not having health insurance, I suspect, have never been more terrifying, and close to 44 million Americans are uninsured.[21] It's unacceptable to me that we spend more money on health care than any other country on this planet, and we still have tens of millions of people without access to basic care.

From three perspectives—disease prevalence, medical care efficacy and economics—we have a deeply troubled medical system. But I do not do justice to this topic simply by recounting figures and statistics. Many of us have spent awful times in hospitals or in nursing homes watching a loved one succumb to disease. Perhaps you've been a patient yourself and you know firsthand how poorly the system sometimes functions. Isn't it paradoxical that the system that is supposed to heal us too often hurts us?

WORKING TO LESSEN CONFUSION

The American people need to know the truth. They need to know what we have uncovered in our research. People need to know why we are unnecessarily sick, why too many of us die early despite the billions spent on research. The irony is that the solution is simple and inexpensive. The answer to the American health crisis is the food that each of us chooses to put in our mouths each day. It's as simple as that.

Although many of us think we're well informed on nutrition, we're not. We tend to follow one faddish diet after another. We disdain saturated fats, butter or carbohydrates, and then embrace vitamin E, calcium supplements, aspirin or zinc and focus our energy and effort on extremely specific food components, as if this will unlock the secrets of health. All too often, fancy outweighs fact. Perhaps you remember the protein diet fad that gripped the country in the late 1970s. The promise was that you could lose weight by replacing real food with a protein shake. In a very short while, almost sixty women died from the diet. More recently millions have adopted high-protein, high-fat diets based on books such as *Dr. Atkins' New Diet Revolution*, *Protein Power* and *The South Beach Diet*. There is increasing evidence that these modern protein fads continue to inflict a great variety of dangerous health disorders. What we don't know—what we don't understand—about nutrition *can* hurt us.

I've been wrestling with this public confusion for more than two decades. In 1988, I was invited before the U.S. Senate Governmental Affairs Committee, chaired by Senator John Glenn, to give my views on why the public is so confused about diet and nutrition. After examining this issue both before and since that testimony, I can confidently state that one of the major sources of confusion is this: far too often, we scientists focus on details while ignoring the larger context. For example, we pin our efforts and our hopes on one isolated nutrient at a time, whether it is vitamin A to prevent cancer or vitamin E to prevent heart attacks. We oversimplify and disregard the infinite complexity of nature. Often, investigating minute biochemical parts of food and trying to reach broad conclusions about diet and health leads to contradictory results. Contradictory results lead to confused scientists and policy makers, and to an increasingly confused public.

A DIFFERENT KIND OF PRESCRIPTION

Most of the authors of several best-selling "nutrition" books claim to be researchers, but I am not aware that their "research" involves original, professionally developed experimentation. That is, they have not designed and conducted studies under the scrutiny of fellow colleagues or peers. They have few or no publications in peer-reviewed scientific journals; they have virtually no formal training in nutritional science; they belong to no professional research societies; they have not participated as peer reviewers. They do, nonetheless, often develop very lucrative projects and products that put money in their pockets while leaving the reader with yet another short-lived and useless diet fad.

If you are familiar with the "health" books at your nearby bookstore, you have likely heard of *Dr. Atkins' New Diet Revolution, The South Beach Diet, Sugar Busters, The Zone* or *Eat Right for Your Type.* These books have made health information more confusing, more difficult to grasp and ultimately more elusive. If you aren't fatigued, constipated or half-starved by these quick-fix plans, your head is spinning from counting calories and measuring grams of carbohydrates, protein and fat. What's the real problem, anyway? Is it fat? Is it carbohydrates? What's the ratio of nutrients that provides greatest weight loss? Are cruciferous vegetables good for my blood type? Am I taking the right supplements? How much vitamin C do I need every day? Am I in ketosis? How many grams of protein do I need?

You get the picture. This is not health. These are fad diets that embody the worst of medicine, science and the popular media.

If you are only interested in a two-week menu plan to lose weight, then this book is not for you. I am appealing to your intelligence, not to your ability to follow a recipe or menu plan. I want to offer you a more profound and more beneficial way to view health. I have a prescription for maximum health that is simple, easy to follow and offers more benefits than any drug or surgery, without any of the side effects. This prescription isn't merely a menu plan; it doesn't require daily charts or calorie counting; and it doesn't exist to serve my own financial interests. Most importantly, the supporting evidence is overwhelming. This is about changing the way you eat and live and the extraordinary health that will result.

So, what is my prescription for good health? In short, it is about the multiple health benefits of consuming plant-based foods, and the largely unappreciated health dangers of consuming animal-based foods, including all types of meat, dairy and eggs. I did not begin with preconceived ideas, philosophical or otherwise, to prove the worthiness of plant-based diets. I started at the opposite end of the spectrum: as a meat-loving dairy farmer in my personal life and an "establishment" scientist in my professional life. I even used to lament the views of vegetarians as I taught nutritional biochemistry to pre-med students.

My only interest now is to explain the scientific basis for my views in the clearest way possible. Changing dietary practices will only occur and be maintained when people believe the evidence and experience the benefits. People decide what to eat for a number of reasons, health considerations being only one. My task is only to present the scientific evidence in a form that can be understood. The rest is up to you.

The scientific basis for my views is largely empirical, obtained through observation and measurement. It is not illusory, hypothetical or anecdotal; it is from legitimate research findings. It is a type of science originally advocated 2,400 years ago by the Father of Medicine, Hippocrates, who said, "There are, in effect, two things: to know and to believe one knows. To know is science. To believe one knows is ignorance." I plan to show you what I have come to know.

Much of my evidence comes from human studies done by myself and by my students and colleagues in my research group. These studies were diverse both in design and in purpose. They included an investigation of liver cancer in Philippine children and their consumption of a mold toxin, aflatoxin[22, 23]; a nationwide program of self-help nutrition centers for malnourished preschool children in the Philippines[24]; a study of dietary factors affecting bone density and osteoporosis in 800 women in China[25–27]; a study of biomarkers that characterize the emergence of breast cancer[28, 29]; and a nationwide, comprehensive study of dietary and lifestyle factors associated with disease mortality in 170 villages in mainland China and Taiwan (widely known as the China Study).[30–33]

These studies, exceptionally diverse in scope, dealt with diseases

thought to be related to varied dietary practices, thus providing the opportunity to investigate diet and disease associations comprehensively.
The China Study, of which I was director, began in 1983 and is still
ongoing.

In addition to these human studies, I maintained a twenty-seven-year
laboratory research program in experimental animal studies. Begun in
the late 1960s, this National Institutes of Health (NIH)-funded research
investigated the link between diet and cancer in considerable depth.
Our findings, which were published in the highest quality scientific
journals, brought into question the very core principles of cancer causation.

When all was said and done, my colleagues and I were honored to
have received a total of seventy-four grant-years of funding. In other
words, because we had more than one research program being conducted at once, my colleagues and I did seventy-four years' worth of
funded research in less than thirty-five years. From this research I have
authored or co-authored over 350 scientific articles. Numerous awards
were extended to me and to my students and colleagues for this long
series of studies and publications. They included, among others, the
1998 American Institute for Cancer Research award "in recognition
of a lifetime of significant accomplishments in scientific research...in
diet, nutrition and cancer," a 1998 award as one of the "Top 25 Food
Influentials" by *Self* magazine and the 2004 Burton Kallman Scientific
Award by the Natural Nutrition Food Association. Moreover, invitations
to lecture at research and medical institutions in more than forty states
and several foreign countries attested to the interest in these findings
from the professional communities. My appearance before congressional committees and federal and state agencies also indicated substantial
public interest in our findings. Interviews on the *McNeil-Lehrer News
Hour* program, at least twenty-five other TV programs, lead stories in
USA Today, the *New York Times,* and the *Saturday Evening Post* and
widely publicized TV documentaries on our work have also been a part
of our public activities.

THE PROMISE OF THE FUTURE

Through all of this, I have come to see that the benefits produced by eating a plant-based diet are far more diverse and impressive than any drug
or surgery used in medical practice. Heart diseases, cancers, diabetes,
stroke and hypertension, arthritis, cataracts, Alzheimer's disease, impo-

tence and all sorts of other chronic diseases can be largely prevented. These diseases, which generally occur with aging and tissue degeneration, kill the majority of us before our time.

Additionally, impressive evidence now exists to show that advanced heart disease, relatively advanced cancers of certain types, diabetes and a few other degenerative diseases can be reversed by diet. I remember when my superiors were only reluctantly accepting the evidence of nutrition being able to *prevent* heart disease, for example, but vehemently denying its ability to *reverse* such a disease when already advanced. But the evidence can no longer be ignored. Those in science or medicine who shut their minds to such an idea are being more than stubborn; they are being irresponsible.

One of the more exciting benefits of good nutrition is the prevention of diseases that are thought to be due to genetic predisposition. We now know that we can largely avoid these "genetic" diseases even though we may harbor the gene (or genes) that is (are) responsible for the disease. But funding of genetic research continues to spiral upwards in the belief that specific genes account for the occurrence of specific diseases, in the hope that we somehow will be able to "turn off" these nasty genes. Drug company public relations programs now depict a future where each of us will have a personal ID card cataloging all of our good and bad genes. Using this card, we will be expected to go to our doctor, who will prescribe a single pill to suppress our bad genes. I strongly suspect these miracles will never be realized, or if tried they will have serious, unintended consequences. These futuristic pipe dreams obscure the affordable, efficacious health solutions that currently exist: solutions based in nutrition.

In my own laboratory we have shown in experimental animals that cancer growth can be turned on and off by nutrition, despite very strong genetic predisposition. We have studied these effects in great detail and have published our findings in the very best scientific journals. As you will see later, these findings are nothing short of spectacular, and the same effects have been indicated over and over again in humans.

Eating the right way not only prevents disease but also generates health and a sense of well-being, both physically and mentally. Some world-class athletes, such as ironman Dave Scott, track stars Carl Lewis and Edwin Moses, tennis great Martina Navratilova, world champion wrestler Chris Campbell (no relation) and sixty-eight-year-old marathoner Ruth Heidrich have discovered that consuming a low-fat, plant-based diet gives them a significant edge in performance. In the laboratory, we fed experimental rats a diet similar to the usual American fare—rich in animal-based protein—and compared them with other rats fed a diet low in animal-based protein. Guess what happened when both sets of rats had an opportunity to voluntarily use exercise wheels? Those fed the low-animal protein diet exercised substantially more, with less fatigue, than those fed the type of diet that most of us eat. This was the same effect observed by these world-class athletes.

This shouldn't be news to the medical establishment. A century ago, Professor Russell Chittenden, a famous, well established nutrition researcher at Yale University Medical School, investigated whether eating a plant-based diet affected students' physical capacities.[34, 35] He fed some students, fellow faculty and himself a plant-based diet and measured their physical performance tests. He got the same results as our rats almost a century later—and they were equally spectacular.

Then there is the question of our excessive dependence on drugs and surgery to control our health. In its simplest form, eating the right way would largely obviate the enormous costs of using drugs, as well as their side effects. Fewer people would need to wage lengthy, expensive battles with chronic disease in hospitals over their last years of life. Health care costs would drop and medical mistakes would wane as premature death plummeted. In essence, our health care system would finally protect and promote our health as it is meant to do.

SIMPLE BEGINNINGS

As I look back, I often think about life on the farm and how it shaped my thinking in so many ways. My family was immersed in nature every waking moment. In the summer, from sunrise to sunset, we were outdoors planting and harvesting the crops and taking care of the animals. My mother had the best garden in our part of the country and toiled day in and day out during the summer to keep our family well fed with fresh food, all produced on our own farm.

I've had an amazing journey, to be sure. I have been startled time and time again by what I have learned. I wish that my family and others around us had had the same information back in the mid-1900s that we now have about food and health. If we had, my father could have prevented, or reversed, his heart disease. He could have met my youngest son, his namesake, who is collaborating with me on this book. He might have lived for several more years with a higher quality of health.

My journey in science over the past forty-five years has convinced me that it is now more urgent than ever to show how people can avoid these tragedies. The science is there and it must be made known. We cannot let the status quo go unchallenged and watch our loved ones suffer unnecessarily. It is time to stand up, clear the air and take control of our health.

2
A House of Proteins

MY ENTIRE PROFESSIONAL CAREER in biomedical research has centered on protein. Like an invisible leash, protein tethered me wherever I went, from the basic research laboratory to the practical programs of feeding malnourished children in the Philippines to the government boardrooms where our national health policy was being formulated. Protein, often regarded with unsurpassed awe, is the common thread tying together past and present knowledge about nutrition.

The story of protein is part science, part culture and a good dose of mythology. I am reminded of the words of Goethe, first brought to my attention by my friend Howard Lyman, a prominent lecturer, author and former cattle rancher: "We are best at hiding those things which are in plain sight." Nothing has been so well hidden as the untold story of protein. The dogma surrounding protein censures, reproaches and guides, directly or indirectly, almost every thought we have in biomedical research.

Ever since the discovery of this nitrogen-containing chemical in 1839 by the Dutch chemist Gerhard Mulder, protein has loomed as the most sacred of all nutrients. The word protein comes from the Greek word *proteios*, which means "of prime importance."

In the nineteenth century, protein was synonymous with meat, and this connection has stayed with us for well over a hundred years. Many people today still equate protein with animal-based food. If you were to name the first food that comes to mind when I say protein, you might say beef. If you did, you aren't alone.

Confusion reigns on many of the most basic questions about protein:

- What are good sources of protein?
- How much protein should one consume?
- Is plant protein as good as animal protein?
- Is it necessary to combine certain plant foods in a meal to get complete proteins?
- Is it advisable to take protein powders or amino acid supplements, especially for someone who does vigorous exercise or plays sport?
- Should one take protein supplements to build muscle?
- Some protein is considered high quality, some low quality; what does this mean?
- Where do vegetarians get protein?
- Can vegetarian children grow properly without animal protein?

Fundamental to many of these common questions and concerns is the belief that meat is protein and protein is meat. This belief comes from the fact that the "soul" of animal-based foods is protein. In many meat and dairy products, we can selectively remove the fat but we are still left with recognizable meat and dairy products. We do this all the time, with lean cuts of meat and skim milk. But if we selectively remove the protein from animal-based foods, we are left with nothing like the original. A non-protein steak, for example, would be a puddle of water, fat and a small amount of vitamins and minerals. Who would eat that? In brief, for a food to be recognized as an animal-based food, it must have protein. Protein is the core element of animal-based foods.

Early scientists like Carl Voit (1831–1908), a prominent German scientist, were staunch champions of protein. Voit found that "man" needed only 48.5 grams per day, but nonetheless he recommended a whopping 118 grams per day because of the cultural bias of the time. Protein equaled meat, and everyone aspired to have meat on his or her table, just as we aspire to have bigger houses and faster cars. Voit figured you can't get too much of a good thing.

Voit went on to mentor several well-known nutrition researchers of the early 1900s, including Max Rubner (1854–1932) and W.O. Atwater (1844–1907). Both students closely followed the advice of their teacher. Rubner stated that protein intake, meaning meat, was a symbol of civilization itself: "a large protein allowance is the right of civilized man." Atwater went on to organize the first nutrition laboratory at the United States Department of Agriculture (USDA). As director of the USDA, he recommended 125 grams per day (only about fifty-five grams per day is now recommended). Later, we will see how important this early precedent was to this government agency.

A cultural bias had become firmly entrenched. If you were civilized, you ate plenty of protein. If you were rich, you ate meat, and if you were poor, you ate staple plant foods, like potatoes and bread. The lower classes were considered by some to be lazy and inept as a result of not eating enough meat, or protein. Elitism and arrogance dominated much of the burgeoning field of nutrition in the nineteenth century. The entire concept that bigger is better, more civilized and perhaps even more spiritual permeated every thought about protein.

Major McCay, a prominent English physician in the early twentieth century, provided one of the more entertaining, but most unfortunate, moments in this history. Physician McCay was stationed in the English colony of India in 1912 in order to identify good fighting men in the Indian tribes. Among other things, he said that people who consumed less protein were of a "poor physique, and a cringing effeminate disposition is all that can be expected."

PRESSING FOR QUALITY

Protein, fat, carbohydrate and alcohol provide virtually all of the calories that we consume. Fat, carbohydrate and protein, as *macro*nutrients, make up almost all the weight of food, aside from water, with the remaining small amount being the vitamin and mineral *micro*nutrients. The amounts of these latter *micro*nutrients needed for optimum health are tiny (milligrams to micrograms).

Protein, the most sacred of all nutrients, is a vital component of our bodies and there are hundreds of thousands of different kinds. They function as enzymes, hormones, structural tissue and transport molecules, all of which make life possible. Proteins are constructed as long chains of hundreds or thousands of amino acids, of which there are fifteen to twenty different kinds, depending on how they are counted. Proteins wear out on a regular basis and must be replaced. This is accomplished by consuming foods that contain protein. When digested, these proteins give us a whole new supply of amino acid building blocks to use in making new protein replacements for those that wore out. Various food proteins are said to be of different quality, depending on how well they provide the needed amino acids used to replace our body proteins.

This process of disassembling and reassembling the amino acids of proteins is like someone giving us a multicolored string of beads to replace an old string of beads that we lost. However, the colored beads on the string given to us are not in the same order as the string we lost. So, we break the string and collect its beads. Then, we reconstruct our new string so that the colored beads are in the same order as our lost string. But if we are short of blue beads, for example, making our new string is going to be slowed down or stopped until we get more blue beads. This is the same concept as in making new tissue proteins to match our old worn out proteins.

About eight amino acids ("colored beads") that are needed for making our tissue proteins must be provided by the food we eat. They are called "essential" because our bodies cannot make them. If, like our string of beads, our food protein lacks enough of even one of these eight "essential" amino acids, then the synthesis of the new proteins will be slowed down or stopped. This is where the idea of protein quality comes into play. Food proteins of the highest quality are, very simply, those that provide, upon digestion, the right kinds and amounts of amino acids needed to efficiently synthesize our new tissue proteins. This is what that word "quality" really means: it is the ability of food proteins to provide the right kinds and amounts of amino acids to make our new proteins.

Can you guess what food we might eat to most efficiently provide the building blocks for our replacement proteins? The answer is human flesh. Its protein has just the right amount of the needed amino acids. But while our fellow men and women are not for dinner, we do get the next "best" protein by eating other animals. The proteins of other animals are very similar to our proteins because they mostly have the right amounts of each of the needed amino acids. These proteins can be used very efficiently and therefore are called "high quality." Among animal foods, the proteins of milk and eggs represent the best amino acid matches for our proteins, and thus are considered the highest quality. While the "lower quality" plant proteins may be lacking in one or more of the essential amino acids, as a group they do contain all of them.

The concept of quality really means the efficiency with which food proteins are used to promote growth. This would be well and good if the greatest efficiency equaled the greatest health, but it doesn't, and that's why the terms efficiency and quality are misleading. In fact, to give you a taste of what's to come, there is a mountain of compelling research showing that "low-quality" plant protein, which allows for slow but steady synthesis of new proteins, is the healthiest type of protein. Slow but steady wins the race. The quality of protein found in a specific food is determined by seeing how fast animals would grow while consuming it. Some foods, namely those from animals, emerge with a very high protein efficiency ratio and value.[1]

This focus on efficiency of body growth, as if it were good health, encourages the consumption of protein with the highest "quality." As any marketer will tell you, a product that is defined as being high quality instantly earns the trust of consumers. For well over 100 years, we have been captive to this misleading language and have oftentimes made the unfortunate leap to thinking that more quality equals more health.

The basis for this concept of protein quality was not well known among the public, but its impact was—and still is—highly significant. People, for example, who choose to consume a plant-based diet will often ask, even today, "Where do I get my protein?" as if plants don't have protein. Even if it is known that plants have protein, there is still the concern about its perceived poor quality. This has led people to believe that they must meticulously combine proteins from different plant sources during each meal so that they can mutually compensate for each other's amino acid deficits. However, this is overstating the case. We now know that through enormously complex metabolic systems, the human body can derive all the essential amino acids from the natural variety of plant proteins that we encounter every day. It doesn't require eating higher quantities of plant protein or meticulously planning every meal. Unfortunately, the enduring concept of protein quality has greatly obscured this information.

THE PROTEIN GAP

The most important issue in nutrition and agriculture during my early career was figuring out ways to increase the consumption of protein, making sure it was of the highest possible quality. My colleagues and I all believed in this common goal. From my early years on the farm to my graduate education, I accepted this virtual reverence for protein. As a youngster, I remember that the most expensive part of farm animal feed was the protein supplements that we fed to our cows and pigs. Then, at graduate school, I spent three years (1958–1961) doing my Ph.D. research trying to improve the supply of high-quality protein by growing cows and sheep more efficiently so we could eat more of them.[2, 3]

I went all the way through my graduate studies with a profound belief that promoting high-quality protein, as in animal-based foods, was a very important task. My graduate research, although cited a few times over the next decade or so, was only a small part of much larger efforts by other research groups to address a protein situation worldwide. During the 1960s and 1970s, I was to hear over and over again about a so-called "protein gap" in the developing world.[4]

The protein gap stipulated that world hunger and malnutrition among children in the third world was a result of not having enough protein to consume, especially high-quality (i.e. animal) protein.[1, 4, 5] According to this view, those in the third world were especially deficient in "high-quality" protein, or animal protein. Projects were springing up all over the place to address this "protein gap" problem. A prominent MIT professor and his younger colleague concluded in 1976 that "an adequate supply of protein is a central aspect of the world food problem"[5] and further that "unless...desirably [supplemented] by modest amounts of milk, eggs, meat or fish, the predominantly cereal diets [of poor nations] are...deficient in protein for growing children...." To address this dire problem:

- MIT was developing a protein-rich food supplement called INCA-PARINA.
- Purdue University was breeding corn to contain more lysine, the "deficient" amino acid in corn protein.
- The U.S. government was subsidizing the production of dried milk powder to provide high-quality protein for the world's poor.
- Cornell University was providing a wealth of talent to the Philippines to help develop both a high-protein rice variety and a livestock industry.
- Auburn University and MIT were grinding up fish to produce "fish protein concentrate" to feed the world's poor.

The United Nations, the U.S. Government Food for Peace Program, major universities and countless other organizations and universities were taking up the battle cry to eradicate world hunger with high-quality protein. I knew most of the projects firsthand, as well as the individuals who organized and directed them.

The Food and Agriculture Organization (FAO) of the United Nations exerts considerable influence in developing countries through their agriculture development programs. Two of its staffers[6] declared in 1970 that "...by and large, the lack of protein is without question the most serious qualitative deficiency in the nutrition of developing countries. The great mass of the population of these countries subsists mainly on foods derived from plants frequently deficient in protein, which results in poor health and low productivity per man." M. Autret, a very influential man from the FAO, added that "owing to the low-animal protein content of the diet and lack of diversity of supplies [in developing countries], protein quality is unsatisfactory."[4] He reported on a very strong association between consumption of animal-based foods and annual income. Autret strongly advocated increasing the production and consumption of animal protein in order to meet the growing "protein gap" in the world. He also advocated that "all resources of science and technology must be mobilized to create new protein-rich foods or to derive the utmost benefits from hitherto insufficiently utilized resources to feed mankind."[4]

Bruce Stillings at the University of Maryland and the U.S. Department of Commerce, another proponent of consuming animal-based diets, admitted in 1973 that "although there is no requirement for animal protein in the diet *per se*, the quantity of dietary protein from animal sources is usually accepted as being indicative of the overall protein quality of the diet."[1] He went on to say that the "...supply of adequate quantities of animal products is generally recognized as being an ideal way to improve world protein nutrition."

Of course, it's quite correct that a supply of protein can be an important way of improving nutrition in the third world, particularly if populations are getting all of their calories from one plant source. But it's not the only way, and, as we shall see, it isn't necessarily the way most consistent with long-term health.

FEEDING THE CHILDREN

So this was the climate at that time, and I was a part of it as much as anyone else. I left MIT to take a faculty position at Virginia Tech in 1965. Professor Charlie Engel, who was then the head of the Department of Biochemistry and Nutrition at Virginia Tech, had considerable interest in developing an international nutrition program for malnourished children. He was interested in implementing a "mothercraft" self-help project in the Philippines. This project was called "mothercraft" because it focused on educating mothers of malnourished children. The idea was that if mothers were taught that the right kinds of locally grown foods can make their children well, they would not have to rely on scarce medicines and the mostly nonexistent doctors. Engel started the program in 1967 and invited me to be his Campus Coordinator and to come for extended stays in the Philippines while he resided full time in Manila.

Consistent with the emphasis on protein as a means of solving malnutrition, we had to make this nutrient the centerpiece of our educational "mothercraft" centers and thereby help to increase protein consumption. Fish as a source of protein was mostly limited to the seacoast areas. Our own preference was to develop peanuts as a source of protein because this was a crop that could be grown most anywhere. The peanut is a legume, like alfalfa, soybeans, clover, peas and other beans. Like these other nitrogen "fixers," peanuts are rich in protein.

There was, however, a nagging problem with these tasty legumes. Considerable evidence had been emerging, first from England[7-9] and later from MIT (the same lab that I had worked in)[10, 11] to show that peanuts often were contaminated with a fungus-produced toxin called aflatoxin (AF). It was an alarming problem because AF was being shown to cause liver cancer in rats. It was said to be the most potent chemical carcinogen ever discovered.

So we had to tackle two closely related projects: alleviate childhood malnutrition and resolve the AF contamination problem.

Prior to going to the Philippines, I had traveled to Haiti in order to observe a few experimental mothercraft centers organized by my colleagues at Virginia Tech, Professors Ken King and Ryland Webb. It was my first trip to an underdeveloped country, and Haiti certainly fit the bill. Papa Doc Duvalier, president of Haiti, extracted what little resources the country had for his own rich lifestyle. In Haiti at that time 54% of the children were dead before reaching their fifth birthday, largely because of malnutrition.

I subsequently went to the Philippines and encountered more of the same. We decided where mothercraft centers were to be located based on how much malnutrition was present in each village. We focused our efforts on the villages in most need. In a preliminary survey in each village (barrio), children were weighed and their weight for age was compared with a Western reference standard, which was subdivided into first, second and third degree malnutrition. Third degree malnutrition, the worst kind, represented children under the 65th percentile. Keep in mind that a child at the 100th percentile represents only the average for the U.S. Being less than the 65th percentile means near starvation.

In the urban areas of some of the big cities, as many as 15–20% of the children aged three to six years were judged to be third degree. I can so well remember some of my initial observations of these children. A mother, hardly more than a wisp herself, holding her three-year-old twins with bulging eyes, one at eleven pounds, the other at fourteen pounds, trying to get them to open their mouths to eat some porridge. Older children blind from malnutrition, being led around by their younger siblings to seek a handout. Children without legs or arms hoping to get a morsel of food.

A REVELATION TO DIE FOR

Needless to say, those sights gave us ample motivation to press ahead with our project. As I mentioned before, we first had to resolve the problem of AF contamination in peanuts, our preferred protein food.

The first step of investigating AF was to gather some basic information. Who in the Philippines was consuming AF, and who was subject to liver cancer? To answer these questions, I applied for and received a National Institutes of Health (NIH) research grant. We also adopted a second strategy by asking another question: how does AF actually affect liver cancer? We wanted to study this question at the molecular level using laboratory rats. I succeeded in getting a second NIH grant for this in-depth biochemical research. These two grants initiated a two-track research investigation, one basic and one applied, which was to continue for the rest of my career. I found studying questions both from the basic and applied perspectives rewarding because it tells us not only the impact of a food or chemical on health, but also why it has that impact. In so doing, we could better understand not only the biochemical foundation of food and health, but also how it might relate to people in everyday life.

We began with a stepwise series of surveys. First, we wanted to know which foods contained the most AF. We learned that peanuts and corn were the foods most contaminated. All twenty-nine jars of peanut butter we had purchased in the local groceries, for example, were contaminated, with levels of AF as much as 300 times the amount judged to be acceptable in U.S. food. Whole peanuts were much less contaminated; none exceeded the AF amounts allowed in U.S. commodities. This disparity between peanut butter and whole peanuts originated at the peanut factory. The best peanuts, which filled "cocktail" jars, were hand selected from a moving conveyor belt, leaving the worst, moldiest nuts to be delivered to the end of the belt to make peanut butter.

Our second question concerned who was most susceptible to this AF contamination and its cancer-producing effects. We learned that it was children. They were the ones consuming the AF-laced peanut butter. We estimated AF consumption by analyzing the excretion of AF metabolic products in the urine of children living in homes with a partially consumed peanut butter jar.[12] As we gathered this information an interesting pattern emerged: the two areas of the country with the highest rates of liver cancer, the cities of Manila and Cebu, also were the same areas where the most AF was being consumed. Peanut butter was almost exclusively consumed in the Manila area while corn was consumed in Cebu, the second most populated city in the Philippines.

But, as it turned out, there was more to this story. It emerged from my making the acquaintance of a prominent doctor, Dr. Jose Caedo, who was an advisor to President Marcos. He told me that the liver cancer problem in the Philippines was quite serious. What was so devastating was that the disease was claiming the lives of children before the age of ten. Whereas in the West, this disease mostly strikes people only after forty years of age, Caedo told me that he had personally operated on children younger than four years of age for liver cancer!

That alone was incredible, but what he then told me was even more striking. *Namely, the children who got liver cancer were from the best-fed families.* The families with the most money ate what we thought were the healthiest diets, the diets most like our own meaty American diets. *They consumed more protein than anyone else in the country (high quality animal protein, at that), and yet they were the ones getting liver cancer!*

How could this be? Worldwide, liver cancer rates were highest in countries with the lowest average protein intake. It was therefore widely believed that this cancer was the result of a deficiency in protein. Further, the deficiency problem was a major reason we were working in the Philippines: to increase the consumption of protein by as many malnourished children as possible. But now Dr. Caedo and his colleagues were telling me that the most protein-rich children had the highest rates of liver cancer. This seemed strange to me, at first, but over time my own information increasingly confirmed their observations.

At that time, a research paper from India surfaced in an obscure medical journal.[13] It was an experiment involving liver cancer and protein consumption in two groups of laboratory rats. One group was given AF and then fed diets containing 20% protein. The second group was given the same level of AF and then fed diets containing only 5% protein.

Every single rat fed 20% protein got liver cancer or its precursor lesions, but not a single animal fed a 5% protein diet got liver cancer or its precursor lesions. It was not a trivial difference; it was 100% versus 0%. This was very much consistent with my observations for the Philippine children. Those who were most vulnerable to liver cancer were those who consumed diets higher in protein.

No one seemed to accept the report from India. On a flight from Detroit after returning from a presentation at a conference, I traveled with a former but much senior colleague of mine from MIT, Professor Paul Newberne. At the time, Newberne was one of the only people who had given much thought to the role of nutrition in the development of cancer. I told him about my impressions in the Philippines and the paper from India. He summarily dismissed the paper by saying, "They must have gotten the numbers on the animal cages reversed. In no way could a high-protein diet increase the development of cancer."

I realized that I had encountered a provocative idea that stimulated disbelief, even the ire of fellow colleagues. Should I take seriously the observation that protein increased cancer development and run the risk of being thought a fool? Or should I turn my back on this story?

In some ways it seemed that this moment in my career had been foreshadowed by events in my personal life. When I was five years old, my aunt who was living with us was dying of cancer. On several occasions my uncle took my brother Jack and me to see his wife in the hospital. Although I was too young to understand everything that was happening, I do remember being struck by the big "C" word: cancer. I would think, "When I get big, I want to find a cure for cancer."

Many years later, just a few years after getting married, at about the time when I was starting my work in the Philippines, my wife's mother was dying of colon cancer at the young age of fifty-one. At that time, I was becoming aware of a possible diet-cancer connection in our early research. Her case was particularly difficult because she did not receive appropriate medical care due to the fact that she did not have health insurance. My wife Karen was her only daughter and they had a very close relationship. These difficult experiences were making my career choice easy: I would go wherever our research led me to help get a better understanding of this horrific disease.

Looking back on it, this was the beginning of my career focus on diet and cancer. The moment of deciding to investigate protein and cancer was the turning point. If I wanted to stay with this story, there was only one solution: start doing fundamental laboratory research to see not only if, but also how, consuming more protein leads to more cancer. That's exactly what I did. It took me farther than I had ever imagined. The extraordinary findings my colleagues, students and I generated just might make you think twice about your current diet. But even more than that, the findings led to broader questions, questions that would eventually lead to cracks in the very foundations of nutrition and health.

THE NATURE OF SCIENCE—WHAT YOU NEED TO KNOW TO FOLLOW THE RESEARCH

Proof in science is elusive. Even more than in the "core" sciences of biology, chemistry and physics, establishing *absolute* proof in medicine and health is nearly impossible. The primary objective of research investigation is to determine only what is *likely* to be true. This is because research into health is inherently statistical. When you throw a ball in the air, will it come down? Yes, every time. That's physics. If you smoke four packs a day, will you get lung cancer? The answer is maybe. We know that your odds of getting lung cancer are much higher than if you didn't smoke, and we can tell you what those odds (statistics) are, but we can't know with certainty whether you as an individual will get lung cancer.

In nutrition research, untangling the relationship between diet and health is not so straightforward. Humans live all sorts of different ways, have different genetic backgrounds and eat all sorts of different foods. Experimental limitations such as cost restraints, time constraints and measurement error are significant obstacles. Perhaps most importantly, food, lifestyle and health interact through such complex, multifaceted systems that establishing proof for any one factor and any one disease is nearly impossible, even if you had the perfect set of subjects, unlimited time and unlimited financial resources.

Because of these difficulties, we do research using many different strategies. In some cases, we assess whether a hypothetical cause produces a hypothetical effect by *observing* and measuring the differences that already exist between different groups of people. We might *observe* and compare societies who consume different amounts of fat, then *observe* whether these differences correspond to similar differences in the rates of breast cancer or osteoporosis or some other disease condition. We might *observe* and compare the dietary characteristics of people who already have the disease with a comparable group of people who don't have the disease. We might *observe* and compare disease rates in 1950 with disease rates in 1990, then *observe* whether any changes in disease rates correspond to dietary changes.

In addition to *observing* what already exists, we might do an experiment and intentionally *intervene* with a hypothetical treatment to see what happens. We intervene, for example, when testing for the safety and efficacy of drugs. One group of people is given the drug and a second group a placebo (an inactive look-alike substance to please the patient). *Intervening* with diet, however, is far more difficult, especially if people aren't confined to a clinical setting, because then we must rely on everyone to faithfully use the specified diets.

As we do *observational and interventional* research, we begin to amass the findings and weigh the evidence for or against a certain hypothesis. When the weight of the evidence favors an idea so strongly that it can no longer be plausibly denied, we advance the idea as a likely truth. It is in this way that I am advancing an argument for a whole foods, plant-based diet. As you continue reading, realize that those seeking absolute proof of optimal nutrition in one or two studies will be disappointed and confused. However, I am confident that those seeking the truth regarding diet and health by surveying the weight of the evidence from the variety of available studies will be amazed and enlightened. There are several ideas to keep in mind when determining the weight of the evidence, including the following ideas.

CORRELATION VERSUS CAUSATION

In many studies, you will find that the words correlation and association are used to describe a relationship between two factors, perhaps even indicating a cause-and-effect relationship. This idea is featured prominently in the China Study. We observed whether there were patterns of associations for different dietary, lifestyle and disease characteristics within the survey of 65 counties, 130 villages and 6,500 adults and their families. If protein consumption, for example, is higher among populations that have a *high* incidence of liver cancer, we can say that protein is *positively* correlated or associated with liver cancer incidence; as one goes up, the other goes up. If protein intake is higher among populations that have a *low* incidence of liver cancer, we can say that protein is *inversely* associated with liver cancer incidence. In other words, the two factors go in the opposite direction; as one goes up, the other goes down.

In our hypothetical example, if protein is correlated with liver cancer incidence, this does not prove that protein causes or prevents liver cancer. A classic illustration of this difficulty is that countries with more telephone poles often have a higher incidence of heart disease, and many other diseases. Therefore, telephone poles and heart disease are positively correlated. But this does not prove that telephone poles cause heart disease. In effect, correlation does not equal causation.

This does not mean that correlations are useless. When they are properly interpreted, correlations can be effectively used to study nutrition and health relationships. The China Study, for example, has over 8,000 statistically significant correlations, and this is of immense value. When so many correlations like this are available, researchers can begin to identify patterns of relationships between diet, lifestyle and disease. These patterns, in turn, are representative of how diet and health processes, which are unusually complex, truly operate. However, if someone wants proof that a single factor causes a single outcome, a correlation is not good enough.

STATISTICAL SIGNIFICANCE

You might think that deciding whether or not two factors are correlated is obvious—either they are or they aren't. But that isn't the case. When you are looking at a large quantity of data, you have to undertake a statistical analysis to determine if two factors are correlated. The answer isn't yes or no. It's a probability, which we call *statistical significance*. Statistical significance is a measure of whether an observed experimental effect is truly reliable or whether it is merely due to the play of chance. If you flip a coin three times and it lands on heads each time, it's probably chance. If you flip it a hundred times and it lands on heads each time, you can be pretty sure the coin has heads on both sides. That's the concept behind *statistical significance*—it's the odds that the correlation (or other finding) is real, that it isn't just random chance.

A finding is said to be statistically significant when there is less than 5% probability that it is due to chance. This means, for example, that there is a 95% chance that we will get the same result if the study is repeated. This 95% cutoff point is arbitrary, but it is the standard, nonetheless. Another arbitrary cutoff point is 99%. In this case, when the result meets this test, it is said to be *highly statistically significant*. In the discussions of diet and disease research in this book, statistical significance pops up from time to time, and it can be used to help judge the reliability, or "weight," of the evidence.

MECHANISMS OF ACTION

Oftentimes correlations are considered more reliable if other research shows that two correlated factors are biologically related. For example, telephone poles and heart disease are positively correlated, but there is no research that shows how telephone poles are biologically related to heart disease. However, there *is* research that shows the processes by which protein intake and liver cancer might be biologically and causally related (as you will see in chapter three). Knowing the process by which something works in the body means knowing its "mechanism of action." And knowing its mechanism of action strengthens the evidence. Another way of saying this is that the two correlated factors are related in a "biologically plausible" way. If a relationship is biologically plausible, it is considered much more reliable.

METANALYSIS

Finally, we should understand the concept of a metanalysis. A metanalysis tabulates the combined data from multiple studies and analyzes them as one data set. By accumulating and analyzing a large body of combined data, the result can have considerably more weight. Metanalysis findings are therefore more substantial than the findings of single research studies, although, as with everything else, there may be exceptions.

After obtaining the results from a variety of studies, we can then begin to use these tools and concepts to assess the weight of the evidence. Through this effort, we can begin to understand what is most likely to be true, and we can behave accordingly. Alternative hypotheses no longer seem plausible, and we can be very confident in the result. Absolute proof, in the technical sense, is unattainable and unimportant. But common sense proof (99% certainty) is attainable and critical. For example, it was through this process of interpreting research that we formed our beliefs regarding smoking and health. Smoking has never been "100%" proven to cause lung cancer, but the odds that smoking is unrelated to lung cancer are so astronomically low that the matter has long been considered settled.

3
Turning Off Cancer

AMERICANS DREAD CANCER more than any other disease. Slowly and painfully being consumed by cancer for months, even years, before passing away is a terrifying prospect. This is why cancer is perhaps the most feared of the major diseases.

So when the media reports a newly found chemical carcinogen, the public takes notice and reacts quickly. Some carcinogens cause outright panic. Such was the case a few years ago with Alar, a chemical that was routinely sprayed on apples as a growth regulator. Shortly after a report from the Natural Resources Defense Council (NRDC) titled "Intolerable Risk: Pesticides in Our Children's Food,"[1] the television program *60 Minutes* aired a segment on Alar. In February 1989 a representative of NRDC said on CBS's *60 Minutes* that the apple industry chemical was "the most potent carcinogen in the food supply."[2, 3]

The public reaction was swift. One woman called state police to chase down a school bus to confiscate her child's apple.[4] School systems across the country, in New York, Los Angeles, Atlanta and Chicago, among others, stopped serving apples and apple products. According to John Rice, former chairman of the U.S. Apple Association, the apple industry took an economic walloping, losing over $250 million.[5] Finally, in response to the public outcry, the production and use of Alar came to a halt in June of 1989.[3]

The Alar story is not uncommon. Over the past several decades, several chemicals have been identified in the popular press as cancer-causing agents. You may have heard of some:

43

- Aminotriazole (herbicide used on cranberry crops, causing the "cranberry scare'" of 1959)
- DDT (widely known after Rachel Carson's book, *Silent Spring*)
- Nitrites (a meat preservative and color and flavor enhancer used in hot dogs and bacon)
- Red Dye Number 2
- Artificial sweeteners (including cyclamates and saccharin)
- Dioxin (a contaminant of industrial processes and of Agent Orange, a defoliant used during the Vietnam War)
- Aflatoxin (a fungal toxin found on moldy peanuts and corn)

I know these unsavory chemicals quite well. I was a member of the National Academy of Sciences Expert Panel on Saccharin and Food Safety Policy (1978–79), which was charged with evaluating the potential danger of saccharin at a time when the public was up in arms after the FDA proposed banning the artificial sweetener. I was one of the first scientists to isolate dioxin; I have firsthand knowledge of the MIT lab that did the key work on nitrites, and I spent many years researching and publishing on aflatoxin, one of the most carcinogenic chemicals ever discovered—at least for rats.

But while these chemicals are significantly different in their properties, they all have a similar story with regard to cancer. In each and every case, research has demonstrated that these chemicals may increase cancer rates in experimental animals. The case of nitrites serves as an excellent example.

THE HOT DOG MISSILE

If you hazard to call yourself "middle-aged" or older, when I say, "Nitrites, hot dogs and cancer," you might rock back in your chair, nod your head, and say, "Oh yeah, I remember something about that." For the younger folks—well, listen up, because history has a funny way of repeating itself.

The time: the early 1970s. The scene: the Vietnam War was beginning to wind down, Richard Nixon was about to be forever linked to Watergate, the energy crisis was about to create lines at gas stations and nitrite was becoming a headline word.

Sodium Nitrite: A meat preservative used since the 1920s.[6] It kills bacteria and adds a happy pink color and desirable taste to hot dogs, bacon and canned meat.

In 1970, the journal *Nature* reported that the nitrite we consume may be reacting in our bodies to form nitrosamines.[7]

Nitrosamines: A scary family of chemicals. No fewer than seventeen nitrosamines are "reasonably anticipated to be human carcinogens" by the U.S. National Toxicology Program.[8]

Hold on a second. Why are these scary nitrosamines "anticipated to be human carcinogens"? The short answer: animal experiments have shown that as chemical exposure increases, incidence of cancer also increases. But that's not adequate. We need a more complete answer.

Let's look at one nitrosamine, NSAR (N-nitrososarcosine). In one study, twenty rats were divided into two groups, each exposed to a different level of NSAR. The high-dose rats were given twice the amount that the low-dose rats received. Of rats given the lower level of NSAR, just over 35% of them died from throat cancer. Of rats given the higher levels, 100% died of cancer during the second year of the experiment.[9–11]

How much NSAR did the rats get? Both groups of rats were given an incredible amount. Let me translate the "low" dose by giving you a little scenario. Let's say you go over to your friend's house to eat every meal. This friend is sick of you and wants to give you throat cancer by exposing you to NSAR. So he gives you the equivalent of the "low" level given to the rats. You go to his house, and your friend offers you a bologna sandwich that has a whole pound of bologna on it! You eat it. He offers you another, and another, and another.... You'll have to eat 270,000 bologna sandwiches before your friend lets you leave.[9, 12] You better like bologna, because your friend is going to have to feed you this way every day for over thirty years! If he does this, you will have had about as much exposure to NSAR (per body weight) as the rats in the "low"-dose group.

Because higher cancer rates were also seen in mice as well as rats, using a variety of methods of exposure, NSAR is "reasonably anticipated" to be a human carcinogen. Although no human studies were used to make this evaluation, it is likely that a chemical such as this, which consistently causes cancer in both mice and rats, can cause cancer in humans at some level. It is impossible to know, however, what this level of exposure might be, especially because the animal dosages are so astronomical. Nonetheless, animal experiments alone are considered enough to conclude that NSAR is "reasonably anticipated" to be a human carcinogen.[9]

So, in 1970, when an article in the prestigious journal *Nature* concluded that nitrites help to form nitrosamines in the body, thereby implying that they help to cause cancer, people became alarmed. Here was
the official line: "Reduction of human exposure to nitrites and certain
secondary amines, particularly in foods, may result in a decrease in
the incidence of human cancer."[7] Suddenly nitrites became a potential
killer. Because we humans get exposed to nitrites through consumption of processed meat such as hot dogs and bacon, some products
came under fire. Hot dogs were an easy target. Besides containing additives like nitrites, hot dogs can be made out of ground-up lips, snouts,
spleens, tongues, throats and other "variety meats."[13] So as the nitrite/
nitrosamine issue heated up, hot dogs weren't looking so hot. Ralph
Nader had called hot dogs "among America's deadliest missiles."[14] Some
consumer advocacy groups were calling for a nitrite additive ban, and
government officials began a serious review of nitrite's potential health
problems.[3]

The issue jolted forward again in 1978, when a study at the Massachusetts Institute of Technology (MIT) found that nitrite increased lymphatic cancer in rats. The study, as reported in a 1979 issue of *Science*,[15]
found that, on average, rats fed nitrite got lymphatic cancer 10.2% of
the time, while animals not fed nitrite got cancer only 5.4% of the time.
This finding was enough to create a public uproar. Fierce debate ensued
in the government, industry and research communities. When the dust
settled, expert panels made recommendations, industry cut back on nitrite usage and the issue fell out of the spotlight.

To summarize the story: marginal scientific results can make very big
waves in the public when it comes to cancer-causing chemicals. A rise
in cancer incidence from 5% to 10% in rats fed large quantities of nitrite
caused an explosive controversy. Undoubtedly millions of dollars were
spent following the MIT study to investigate and discuss the findings.
And NSAR, a nitrosamine possibly formed from nitrite, was "reasonably
anticipated to be a human carcinogen" after several animal experiments
where exceptionally high levels of chemical were fed to animals for almost half their lifespan.

BACK TO PROTEIN

The point isn't that nitrite is safe. It is the mere possibility, however unlikely it may be, that it could cause cancer that alarms the public. But
what if researchers produced considerably more impressive scientific

results that were far more substantial? What if there was a chemical that experimentally turned on cancer in 100% of the test animals and its relative absence limited cancer to 0% of the animals? Furthermore, what if this chemical were capable of acting in this way at routine levels of intake and not the extraordinary levels used in the NSAR experiments? Finding such a chemical would be the holy grail of cancer research. The implications for human health would be enormous. One would assume that this chemical would be of considerably more concern than nitrite and Alar, and even more significant than aflatoxin, a highly ranked carcinogen.

This is exactly what I saw in the Indian research paper[16] when I was in the Philippines. The chemical was protein, fed to rats at levels that are well within the range of normal consumption. Protein! These results were more than startling. In the Indian study, when all the rats had been predisposed to get liver cancer after being given aflatoxin, only the animals fed 20% protein got the cancer while those fed 5% got none.

Scientists, myself included, tend to be a skeptical bunch, especially when confronted with eye-popping results. In fact, it is our responsibility as researchers to question and explore such provocative findings. We might suspect that this finding was unique to rats exposed to aflatoxin and for no other species, including humans. Maybe there were other unknown nutrients that were affecting the data. Maybe my friend, the distinguished MIT professor, was right; maybe the animal identities in the Indian study got mixed up.

The questions begged for answers. To further study this question, I sought and received the two National Institutes of Health (NIH) research grants that I mentioned earlier. One was for a human study, the other for an experimental animal study. I did not "cry wolf" in either application by suggesting that protein might promote cancer. I had everything to lose and nothing to gain by acting like a heretic. Besides, I wasn't convinced that protein actually might be harmful. In the experimental animal study, I proposed to investigate the "effect of *various factors* [my italics] on aflatoxin metabolism." The human study, mostly focused on aflatoxin's effects on liver cancer in the Philippines, was briefly reviewed in the last chapter and was concluded after three years. It was later renewed in a much more sophisticated study in China (chapter four).

A study of this protein effect on tumor development had to be done extremely well. Anything less would not have convinced anyone, especially my peers who would review my future request for renewed funding! In hindsight, we must have succeeded. The NIH funding for this study continued for the next nineteen years and led to additional funding from other research agencies (American Cancer Society, the American Institute for Cancer Research and the Cancer Research Foundation of America). On these experimental animal findings alone, this project gave rise to more than 100 scientific papers published in some of the best journals, many public presentations and several invitations to participate on expert panels.

ANIMAL RIGHTS

The rest of this chapter concerns experimental animal research, all of which included rodents (rats and mice). I know well that many oppose the use of experimental animals in research. I respect this concern. I respectfully suggest, however, that you consider this: very likely, I would not be advocating a plant-based diet today if it were not for these animal experiments. The findings and the principles derived from these animal studies greatly contributed to my interpretations of my later work, including the China Study, as you will come to see.

One obvious question regarding this issue is whether there was an alternative way to get the same information without using experimental animals. To date, I have found none, even after seeking advice from my "animal rights" colleagues. These experimental animal studies elaborated some very important principles of cancer causation not obtainable in human-based studies. These principles now have enormous potential to benefit all of our fellow creatures, our environment and ourselves.

THREE STAGES OF CANCER

Cancer proceeds through three stages: initiation, promotion and progression. To use a rough analogy, the cancer process is similar to planting a lawn. Initiation is when you put the seeds in the soil, promotion is when the grass starts to grow and progression is when the grass gets completely out of control, invading the driveway, the shrubbery and the sidewalk.

So what is the process that successfully "implants" the grass seed in the soil in the first place, i.e., initiates cancer-prone cells? Chemicals that do this are called carcinogens. These chemicals are most often

CHART 3.1: TUMOR INITIATION BY AFLATOXIN INSIDE A LIVER CELL

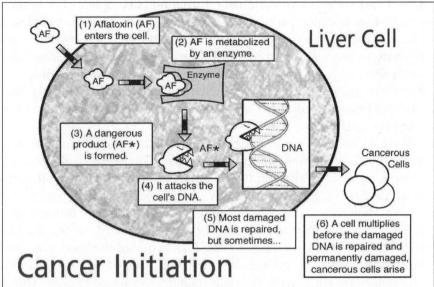

(1) Aflatoxin (AF) enters the cell.

(2) AF is metabolized by an enzyme.

Liver Cell

Enzyme

(3) A dangerous product (AF*) is formed.

AF*

DNA

Cancerous Cells

(4) It attacks the cell's DNA.

(5) Most damaged DNA is repaired, but sometimes...

(6) A cell multiplies before the damaged DNA is repaired and permanently damaged, cancerous cells arise

Cancer Initiation

After entering our cells (Step 1), most carcinogens do not, themselves, initiate the cancer process. They first must be converted to products that are more reactive (Steps 2 & 3), with the help of critically important enzymes. These carcinogen products then bind tightly to the cell's DNA to form carcinogen-DNA complexes, or adducts (Step 4).

Unless repaired or removed, carcinogen-DNA adducts have the potential to create chaos with the genetic workings of the cell. But nature is smart. These adducts can be repaired, and most adducts are repaired fairly quickly (Step 5). However, if they remain in place while cells are dividing to form new "daughter" cells, genetic damage occurs and this new genetic defect (or mutation) is passed on to all new cells formed thereafter (Step 6). [17]

the byproducts of industrial processes, although small amounts may be formed in nature, as is the case with aflatoxin. These carcinogens genetically transform, or mutate, normal cells into cancer-prone cells. A mutation involves permanent alteration of the genes of the cell, with damage to its DNA.

The entire initiation stage (Chart 3.1) can take place in a very short period of time, even minutes. It is the time required for the chemical carcinogen to be consumed, absorbed into the blood, transported into cells, changed into its active product, bonded to DNA and passed on to the daughter cells. When the new daughter cells are formed, the process is complete. These daughter cells and all their progeny will forever be genetically damaged, giving rise to the potential for cancer. Except in rare instances, completion of the initiation phase is considered irreversible.

At this point in our lawn analogy, the grass seeds have been put in the soil and are ready to germinate. Initiation is complete. The second growth stage is called promotion. Like seeds ready to sprout blades of grass and turn into a green lawn, our newly formed cancer-prone cells are ready to grow and multiply until they become a visibly detectable cancer. This stage occurs over a far longer period of time than initiation, often many years for humans. It is when the newly initiated cluster multiplies and grows into larger and larger masses and a clinically visible tumor is formed.

But just like seeds in the soil, the initial cancer cells will not grow and multiply unless the right conditions are met. The seeds in the soil, for example, need a healthy amount of water, sunlight and other nutrients before they make a full lawn. If any of these factors are denied or are missing, the seeds will not grow. If any of these factors are missing after growth starts, the new seedlings will become dormant, while awaiting further supply of the missing factors. This is one of the most profound features of promotion. *Promotion is reversible, depending on whether the early cancer growth is given the right conditions in which to grow.* This is where certain dietary factors become so important. These dietary factors, called promoters, feed cancer growth. Other dietary factors, called anti-promoters, slow cancer growth. Cancer growth flourishes when there are more promoters than anti-promoters; when anti-promoters prevail cancer growth slows or stops. It is a push-pull process. The profound importance of this reversibility cannot be overemphasized.

The third phase, progression, begins when a bunch of advanced cancer cells progress in their growth until they have done their final damage. It is like the fully-grown lawn invading everything around it: the garden, driveway and sidewalk. Similarly, a developing cancer tumor may wander away from its initial site in the body and invade neighboring or distant tissues. When the cancer takes on these deadly properties, it is considered malignant. When it actually breaks away from its initial home and wanders, it is metastasizing. This final stage of cancer results in death.

At the start of our research, the stages of cancer formation were known only in vague outline. But we knew enough about these stages of cancer to be able to structure our research more intelligently. We had no shortage of questions. Could we confirm the findings from India that a low-protein diet represses tumor formation? More importantly, why does protein affect the cancer process? What are the mechanisms; that is, how does protein work? With plenty of questions to be answered, we went about our experimental studies meticulously and in depth in order to obtain results that would withstand the harshest of scrutiny.

PROTEIN AND INITIATION

How does protein intake affect cancer initiation? Our first test was to see whether protein intake affected the enzyme principally responsible for aflatoxin metabolism, the mixed function oxidase (MFO). This enzyme is very complex because it also metabolizes pharmaceuticals and other chemicals, friend or foe to the body. Paradoxically, this enzyme both detoxifies and activates aflatoxin. It is an extraordinary transformation substance.

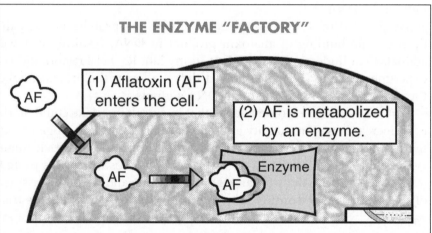

THE ENZYME "FACTORY"

(1) Aflatoxin (AF) enters the cell.

(2) AF is metabolized by an enzyme.

In a simplistic way, the MFO enzyme system can be thought of as a factory within the industrious workings of the cell. Various chemical "raw materials" are fed into the factory, where all the complex reactions are performed. The raw materials may be disassembled or assembled. After a transforming process, the "raw material" chemicals are ready to be shipped out of the factory as mostly normal, safe products. But there also may be byproducts of these complex processes that are exceptionally dangerous. Think of the smokestack at a real-life factory. If someone told you to stick your face down a smokestack and breathe deeply for a couple hours, you'd refuse. Within the cell, the dangerous byproducts, if not held in check, are the highly reactive aflatoxin metabolites that go on to attack the cell's DNA and damage its genetic blueprint.

At the time we started our research, we hypothesized that the protein we consume alters tumor growth by changing how aflatoxin is detoxified by the enzymes present in the liver.

We initially determined whether the amount of protein that we eat could change this enzyme activity. After a series of experiments (Chart 3.2[18]), the answer was clear. Enzyme activity could be easily modified simply by changing the level of protein intake.[18–21]

Decreasing protein intake like that done in the original research in India (20% to 5%) not only greatly decreased enzyme activity, but did so very quickly.[22] What does this mean? Decreasing enzyme activity via low-protein diets implied that less aflatoxin was being transformed into the dangerous aflatoxin metabolite that had the potential to bind and to mutate the DNA.

We decided to test this implication: did a low-protein diet actually decrease the binding of aflatoxin product to DNA, resulting in fewer adducts? An undergraduate student in my lab, Rachel Preston, did the experiment (Chart 3.3) and showed that the lower the protein intake, the lower the amount of aflatoxin-DNA adducts.[23]

We now had impressive evidence that low protein intake could markedly decrease enzyme activity and prevent dangerous carcinogen binding to DNA. These were very impressive findings, to be sure. It might even be enough information to "explain" how consuming less protein leads to less cancer. But we wanted to know more and be doubly assured of this effect, so we continued to look for other explanations. As time passed, we were to learn something really quite remarkable. Almost ev-

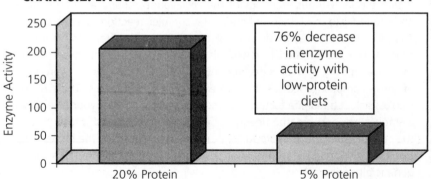

CHART 3.2: EFFECT OF DIETARY PROTEIN ON ENZYME ACTIVITY

76% decrease in enzyme activity with low-protein diets

CHART 3.3: DECREASE IN CARCINOGEN BINDING TO NUCLEUS COMPONENTS CAUSED BY LOW-PROTEIN FEEDING

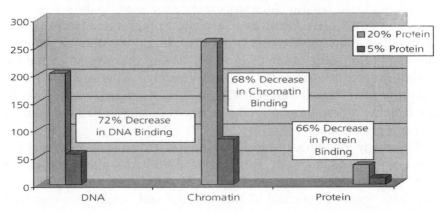

ery time we searched for a way, or mechanism, by which protein works to produce its effects, we found one! For example, we came to discover that low-protein diets, or their equivalents, reduce tumors by the following mechanisms:

- less aflatoxin entered the cell[24–26]
- cells multiplied more slowly[18]
- multiple changes occurred within the enzyme complex to reduce its activity[27]
- the quantity of critical components of the relevant enzymes was reduced[28, 29]
- less aflatoxin-DNA adducts were formed[23, 30]

The fact that we found more than one way (mechanism) that low-protein diets work was eye-opening. It added a great deal of weight to the results of the Indian researchers. It also suggested that biological effects, although often described as operating through single reactions, more likely operate through a large number of varied simultaneous reactions, very likely acting in a highly integrated and concerted manner. Could this mean that the body had lots of backup systems in case one was bypassed in some way? As research unfolded in the subsequent years, the truth of this thesis became increasingly evident.

From our extensive research, one idea seemed to be clear: lower protein intake dramatically decreased tumor initiation. This finding, even though well substantiated, would be enormously provocative for many people.

PROTEIN AND PROMOTION

To go back to the lawn analogy, sowing the grass seeds in the soil was the initiation process. We found, conclusively, through a number of experiments, that a low-protein diet could decrease, at the time of planting, the number of seeds in our "cancerous" lawn. That was an incredible finding, but we needed to do more. We wondered: what happens during the promotion stage of cancer, the all-important reversible stage? Would the benefits of low protein intake achieved during initiation continue through promotion?

Practically speaking, it was difficult to study this stage of cancer because of time and money. It is an expensive study that allows rats to live until they develop full tumors. Each such experiment would take more than two years (the normal lifetime of rats) and would have cost well over $100,000 (even more money today). To answer the many questions that we had, we could not proceed by studying full tumor development; I would still be in the lab, thirty-five years later!

This is when we learned of some exciting work just published by others[31] that showed how to measure tiny clusters of cancer-like cells that appear right after initiation is complete. These little microscopic cell clusters were called foci.

Foci are precursor clusters of cells that grow into tumors. Although most foci do not become full-blown tumor cells, they are predictive of tumor development.

By watching foci develop and measuring how many there are and how big they become,[32] we could learn indirectly how tumors also develop and what effect protein might have. By studying the effects of protein on the promotion of foci instead of tumors we could avoid spending a lifetime and a few million dollars working in the lab.

What we found was truly remarkable. *Foci development was almost entirely dependent on how much protein was consumed, regardless of how much aflatoxin was consumed!*

This was documented in many interesting ways, first done by my graduate students Scott Appleton[33] and George Dunaif[34] (a typical comparison is shown in Chart 3.4). After initiation with aflatoxin, foci grew (were promoted) far more with the 20% protein diet than with the 5% protein diet.[33, 34]

Up to this point, all of the animals were exposed to the same amount of aflatoxin. But what if the initial aflatoxin exposure is varied? Would protein

CHART 3.4: DIETARY PROTEIN AND FOCI FORMATION

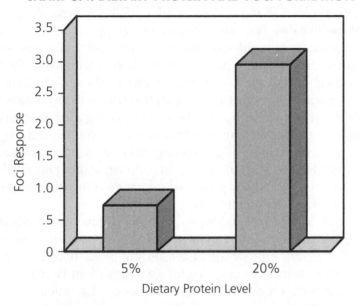

CHART 3.5: CARCINOGEN DOSE VERSUS PROTEIN INTAKE

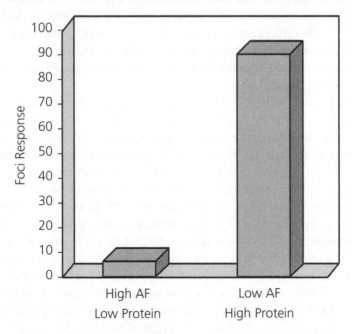

still have an effect? We investigated this question by giving two groups
of rats either a high-aflatoxin dose or a low-aflatoxin dose, along with a
standard baseline diet. Because of this the two groups of rats were starting
the cancer process with different amounts of initiated, cancerous "seeds."
Then, during the promotion phase, we fed a low-protein diet to the high-
aflatoxin dose groups and a high-protein diet to the low-aflatoxin dose
group. We wondered whether the animals that start with lots of cancerous
seeds are able to overcome their predicament by eating a low-protein diet.

Again, the results were remarkable (Chart 3.5). Animals starting with
the most cancer initiation (high-aflatoxin dose) developed *substantially
less foci* when fed the 5% protein diet. In contrast, animals initiated with
a low-aflatoxin dose actually produced *substantially more foci* when subsequently fed the 20% protein diet.

A principle was being established. Foci development, initially determined by the amount of the carcinogen exposure, is actually controlled
far more by dietary protein consumed during promotion. Protein during promotion trumps the carcinogen, regardless of initial exposure.

With this background information we designed a much more substantial experiment. Here is a step-by-step sequence of experiments,
carried out by my graduate student Linda Youngman.[35] All animals were
dosed with the same amount of carcinogen, then alternately fed either
5% or 20% dietary protein during the twelve-week promotion stage.
We divided this twelve-week promotion stage into four periods of three
weeks each. Period 1 represents weeks one to three, period 2 represents
weeks four to six, and so on.

When animals were fed the 20% protein diet during periods 1 and 2
(20-20), foci continued to enlarge, as expected. But when animals were
switched to the low-protein diet at the beginning of period 3 (20-20-
5), there was a sharp decrease in foci development. And, when animals
were subsequently switched back to the 20% protein diet during period
4 (20-20-5-20), foci development was turned on once again.

In another experiment, in animals fed 20% dietary protein during
period 1 but switched to 5% dietary protein during period 2 (20-5), foci
development was sharply decreased. But when these animals were returned to 20% dietary protein during period 3 (20-5-20), we again saw
the dramatic power of dietary protein to promote foci development.

These several experiments, taken together, were quite profound. Foci
growth could be reversed, up and down, by switching the amount of
protein being consumed, and at all stages of foci development.

These experiments also demonstrated that the body could "remember" early carcinogen insults,[35, 36] even though they might then lie dormant with low protein intake. That is, exposure to aflatoxin left a genetic "imprint" that remained dormant with 5% dietary protein until nine weeks later when this imprint reawakened to form foci with 20% dietary protein. In simple terms, the body holds a grudge. It suggests that if we are exposed in the past to a carcinogen that initiates a bit of cancer that remains dormant, this cancer can still be "reawakened" by bad nutrition some time later.

These studies showed that cancer development is modified by relatively modest changes in protein consumption. But how much protein is too much or too little? Using rats, we investigated a range of 4–24% dietary protein (Chart 3.6[37]). Foci did not develop with up to about 10% dietary protein. Beyond 10%, foci development increased dramatically with increases in dietary protein. The results were later repeated a second time in my laboratory by a visiting professor from Japan, Fumiyiki Horio.[38]

CHART 3.6: FOCI PROMOTION BY DIETARY PROTEIN

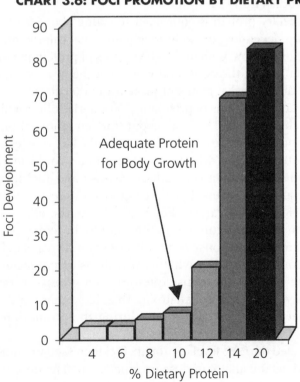

The most significant finding of this experiment was this: foci developed only when the animals met or exceeded the amount of dietary protein (12%) needed to satisfy their body growth rate.[39] That is, when the animals met and surpassed their requirement for protein, disease onset began.

This finding may have considerable relevance for humans even though these were rat studies. I say this because the protein required for growth in young rats and humans as well as the protein required to maintain health for adult rats and humans is remarkably similar.[40, 41]

According to the recommended daily allowance (RDA) for protein consumption, we humans should be getting about 10% of our energy from protein. This is considerably more than the actual amount required. But because requirements may vary from individual to individual, 10% dietary protein is recommended to insure adequate intake for virtually all people. What do most of us routinely consume? Remarkably, it is considerably more than the recommended 10%. The average American consumes 15–16% protein. Does this place us at risk for getting cancer? These animal studies hint that it does.

Ten percent dietary protein is equivalent to eating about 50–60 grams of protein per day, depending on body weight and total calorie intake. The national average of 15–16% is about 70–100 grams of protein per day, with men at the upper part of the range and women at the lower end. In food terms, there are about twelve grams of protein in 100 calories of spinach (fifteen ounces) and five grams of protein in 100 calories of raw chick peas (just over two tablespoons). There are about thirteen grams of protein in 100 calories of porterhouse steak (just over one and a half ounces).

Yet another question was whether protein intake could modify the all-important relationship between aflatoxin dose and foci formation. A chemical is usually not considered a carcinogen unless higher doses yield higher incidences of cancer. For example, as the aflatoxin dose becomes greater, foci and tumor growth should be correspondingly greater. If an increasing response is not observed for a suspect chemical carcinogen, serious doubt arises whether it really is carcinogenic.

To investigate this dose-response question, ten groups of rats were administered increasing doses of aflatoxin, then fed either regular levels (20%) or low levels (5–10%) of protein during the promotion period (Chart 3.7[34]).

In the animals fed the 20% level of protein, foci increased in number and size, as expected, as the aflatoxin dose was increased. The dose-response

CHART 3.7: AFLATOXIN DOSE—FOCI RESPONSE

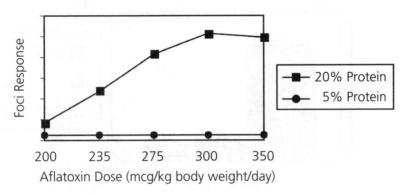

relationship was strong and clear. However, in the animals fed 5% protein, *the dose-response curve completely disappeared.* There was no foci response, even when animals were given the maximum tolerated aflatoxin dose. This was yet another result demonstrating that a low-protein diet could override the cancer-causing effect of a very powerful carcinogen, aflatoxin.

Is it possible that chemical carcinogens, in general, do not cause cancer unless the nutritional conditions are "right"? Is it possible that, for much of our lives, we are being exposed to small amounts of cancer-causing chemicals, but cancer does not occur unless we consume foods that promote and nurture tumor development? Can we control cancer through nutrition?

NOT ALL PROTEINS ARE ALIKE

If you have followed the story so far, you have seen how provocative these findings are. Controlling cancer through nutrition was, and still is, a radical idea. But as if this weren't enough, one more issue would yield explosive information: did it make any difference what type of protein was used in these experiments? For all of these experiments, we were using casein, which makes up 87% of cow's milk protein. So the next logical question was whether plant protein, tested in the same way, has the same effect on cancer promotion as casein. The answer is an astonishing "NO." *In these experiments, plant protein did not promote cancer growth, even at the higher levels of intake.* An undergraduate pre-medical student doing an honors degree with me, David Schulsinger, did the study (Chart 3.8[42]). *Gluten, the protein of wheat, did not produce the same result as casein, even when fed at the same 20% level.*

CHART 3.8: PROTEIN TYPE AND FOCI RESPONSE

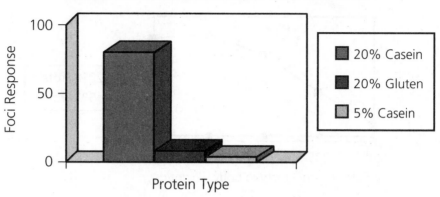

We also examined whether soy protein had the same effect as casein on foci development. *Rats fed 20% soy protein diets did not form early foci, just like the 20% wheat protein diets.* Suddenly protein, milk protein in this case, wasn't looking so good. We had discovered that low protein intake reduces cancer initiation and works in multiple synchronous ways. As if that weren't enough, we were finding that high protein intake, in excess of the amount needed for growth, promotes cancer after initiation. Like flipping a light switch on and off, we could control cancer promotion merely by changing levels of protein, regardless of initial carcinogen exposure. But the cancer-promoting factor in this case was cow's milk protein. It was difficult enough for my colleagues to accept the idea that protein might help cancer grow, but cow's milk protein? Was I crazy?

ADDITIONAL QUESTIONS

For those readers who want to know somewhat more, I've included a few questions in Appendix A.

THE GRAND FINALE

Thus far we had relied on experiments where we measured only the early indicators of tumor development, the early cancer-like foci. Now, it was time to do the big study, the one where we would measure complete tumor formation. We organized a very large study of several hundred rats and examined tumor formation over their lifetimes using several different approaches.[36, 43]

The effects of protein feeding on tumor development were nothing less than spectacular. Rats generally live for about two years, thus the study was 100 weeks in length. All animals that were administered afla-toxin and fed the regular 20% levels of casein either were dead or near death from liver tumors at 100 weeks.[36, 43] All animals administered the same level of aflatoxin but fed the low 5% protein diet were alive, active and thrifty, with sleek hair coats at 100 weeks. This was a virtual 100 to 0 score, something almost never seen in research and almost identical to the original research in India.[16]

In this same experiment,[36] we switched the diets of some rats at either forty or sixty weeks, to again investigate the reversibility of cancer pro-motion. Animals switched from a high-protein to a low-protein diet had significantly less tumor growth (35%–40% less!) than animals fed a high-protein diet. Animals switched from a low-protein diet to a high-protein

CHART 3.9A: TUMOR DEVELOPMENT AT 100 WEEKS

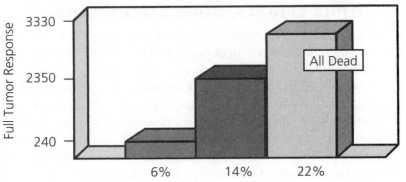

CHART 3.9B: EARLY FOCI, "LIFETIME"

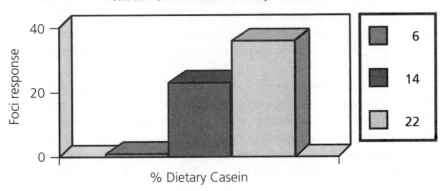

diet halfway through their lifetime started growing tumors again. These findings on full-blown tumors confirmed our earlier findings using foci. Namely, nutritional manipulation can turn cancer "on" and "off."

We also measured early foci in these "lifetime" studies to see if their response to dietary protein was similar to that for tumor response. The correspondence between foci growth and tumor growth could not have been greater (Chart 3.9a).[36, 43]

How much more did we need to find out? I would never have dreamed that our results up to this point would be so incredibly consistent, biologically plausible and statistically significant. We had fully confirmed the original work from India and had done it in exceptional depth.

Let there be no doubt: cow's milk protein is an exceptionally potent cancer promoter in rats dosed with aflatoxin. The fact that this promotion effect occurs at dietary protein levels (10–20%) commonly used both in rodents and humans makes it especially tantalizing—and provocative.

OTHER CANCERS, OTHER CARCINOGENS

Okay, so here's the central question: how does this research apply to human health and human liver cancer in particular? One way to investigate this question is to research other species, other carcinogens and other organs. If casein's effect on cancer is consistent across these categories, it becomes more likely that humans better take note. So our research became broader in scope, to see whether our discoveries would hold up.

While our rat studies were underway, studies were published[44, 45] claiming that chronic infection with hepatitis B virus (HBV) was the major risk factor for human liver cancer. It was thought that people who remained chronically infected with HBV had twenty to forty times the risk of getting liver cancer.

Over the years, considerable research had been done on how this virus causes liver cancer.[46] In effect, a piece of the virus gene inserts itself into the genetic material of the mouse liver where it initiates liver cancer. When this is done experimentally the animals are considered *transgenic*.

Virtually all of the research done in other laboratories on HBV transgenic mice—and there was a lot of it—was done primarily to understand the molecular mechanism by which HBV worked. No attention was given to nutrition and its effect on tumor development. I watched with some amusement for several years how one community of researchers argued for aflatoxin as the key cause of human liver cancer and another community argued for HBV. No one in either community dared to suggest that nutrition had anything to do with this disease.

We wanted to know about the effect of casein on HBV-induced liver cancer in mice. This was a big step. It went beyond aflatoxin as a carcinogen and rats as a species. A brilliant young graduate student from China in my group, Jifan Hu, initiated studies to answer this question and was later joined by Dr. Zhiqiang Cheng. We needed a colony of these transgenic mice. There were two such "breeds" of mice, one living in La Jolla, California, the other in Rockville, Maryland. Each strain had a different piece of HBV gene stuck in the genes of their livers, and each was therefore highly prone to liver cancer. I contacted the responsible researchers and inquired about their helping us to establish our own mouse colony. Both research groups asked what we wanted to do and both were inclined to think that studying the protein effect was foolish. I also sought a research grant to study this question and it was rejected. The reviewers did not take kindly to the idea of a nutritional effect on a virus-induced cancer, especially of a dietary protein effect. I was beginning to wonder: was I now being too explicit in questioning the mythical health value of protein? The reviews of the grant proposal certainly indicated this possibility.

We eventually obtained funding, did the study on both strains of mice *and got essentially the same result as we did with the rats*.[47, 48] You can see the results for yourself. The adjoining picture (Chart 3.10[47]) shows what a cross-section of the mouse livers looks like under a microscope. The dark-colored material is indicative of cancer development (ignore the "hole"; that's only a cross-section of a vein). There is intense early cancer formation in the 22% casein animals (D), much less in the 14% casein animals (C), and none in the 6% casein animals (B); the remaining picture (A) shows a liver having no virus gene (the control).

The adjoining graph (Chart 3.11[47]) shows the expression (activity) of two HBV genes that cause cancer inserted in the mouse liver. Both the picture and the graph show the same thing: the 22% casein diet turned on expression of the viral gene to cause cancer, whereas the 6% casein diet showed almost no such activity.

By this time, we had more than enough information to conclude that casein, that sacred protein of cow's milk, dramatically promotes liver cancer in:

- rats dosed with aflatoxin
- mice infected with HBV

CHART 3.10: DIETARY PROTEIN EFFECT ON GENETICALLY-BASED (HBV) LIVER CANCER (MICE)

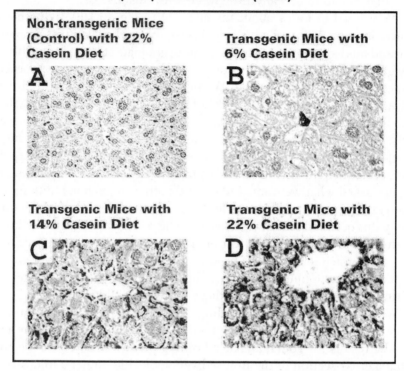

CHART 3.11: DIETARY PROTEIN EFFECT ON GENE EXPRESSION (MICE)

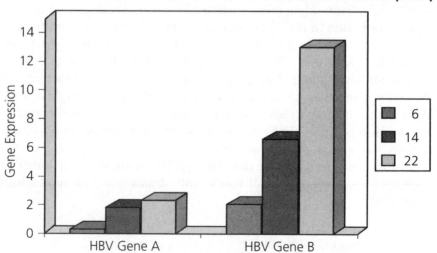

Not only are these effects substantial, but we also discovered a network of complementary ways by which they worked.

Next question: can we generalize these findings to other cancers and to other carcinogens? At the University of Illinois Medical Center in Chicago, another research group was working with mammary (breast) cancer in rats.[49–51] This research showed that increasing intakes of casein promoted the development of mammary (breast) cancer. They found that higher casein intake:

- promotes breast cancer in rats dosed with two experimental carcinogens (7,12-dimethybenz(a)anthracene (DBMA) and N-nitroso-methylurea (NMU))
- operates through a network of reactions that combine to increase cancer
- operates through the same female hormone system that operates in humans

LARGER IMPLICATIONS

An impressively consistent pattern was beginning to emerge. For two different organs, four different carcinogens and two different species, casein promotes cancer growth while using a highly integrated system of mechanisms. It is a powerful, convincing and consistent effect. For example, casein affects the way cells interact with carcinogens, the way DNA reacts with carcinogens and the way cancerous cells grow. The depth and consistency of these findings strongly suggest that they are relevant for humans, for four reasons. First, rats and humans have an almost identical need for protein. Second, protein operates in humans virtually the same way it does in rats. Third, the level of protein intake causing tumor growth is the same level that humans consume. And fourth, in both rodents and humans the initiation stage is far less important than the promotion stage of cancer. This is because we are very likely "dosed" with a certain amount of carcinogens in our everyday lives, but whether they lead to full tumors depends on their promotion, or lack thereof.

Even though I became convinced that increasing casein intake promotes cancer, I still had to be wary of generalizing too much. This was an exceptionally provocative finding that drew fierce skepticism. But these findings nonetheless were a hint of things to come. I wanted to broaden my evidence still more. What effect did other nutrients have on cancer, and how did they interact with different carcinogens and different organs? Might the effects of other nutrients, carcinogens or organs cancel each other, or might there be consistency of effect for nutrients within certain types of food? Would promotion continue to be reversible? If so, cancer might be readily controlled, even reversed, simply by decreasing the intakes of the promoting nutrients and/or increasing the intakes of the anti-promoting nutrients.

We initiated more studies using several different nutrients, including fish protein, dietary fats and the antioxidants known as carotenoids. A couple of excellent graduate students of mine, Tom O'Connor and Youping He, measured the ability of these nutrients to affect liver and pancreatic cancer. *The results of these, and many other studies, showed nutrition to be far more important in controlling cancer promotion than the dose of the initiating carcinogen.* The idea that nutrients primarily affect tumor development during promotion was beginning to appear to be a general property of nutrition and cancer relationships. The *Journal of the National Cancer Institute*, which is the official publication of the U.S. National Cancer Institute, took note of these studies and featured some of our findings on its cover.[52]

Furthermore, a pattern was beginning to emerge: *nutrients from animal-based foods increased tumor development while nutrients from plant-based foods decreased tumor development.* In our large lifetime study of rats with aflatoxin-induced tumors, the pattern was consistent. In mice with hepatitis B virus-altered genes, the pattern was consistent. In studies done by another research group, with breast cancer and different carcinogens, the pattern was consistent. In studies of pancreatic cancer and other nutrients, the pattern was consistent.[52, 53] In studies on carotenoid antioxidants and cancer initiation, the pattern was consistent.[54, 55] From the first stage of cancer initiation to the second stage of cancer promotion, the pattern was consistent. From one mechanism to another, the pattern was consistent.

So much consistency was stunningly impressive, but one aspect of this research demanded that we remain cautious: all this evidence was gathered in experimental animal studies. Although there are strong arguments that these provocative findings are *qualitatively* relevant to human health, we cannot know the *quantitative* relevance. In other words, are these principles regarding animal protein and cancer critically important for all humans in all situations, or are they merely marginally important for a minority of people in fairly unique situations? Are these principles involved in one thousand human cancers every year, one million human cancers every year, or more? We need direct evidence from human research. Ideally, this evidence would be gathered with rigorous methodology and would investigate dietary patterns comprehensively, using large numbers of people who had similar lifestyles, similar genetic backgrounds, and yet had widely varying incidences of disease.

Having the opportunity to do such a study is rare, at best, but by incredibly good luck we were given exactly the opportunity we needed. In 1980 I had the good fortune of welcoming in my laboratory a most personable and professional scientist from mainland China, Dr. Junshi Chen. With this remarkable man, opportunities arose to search for some larger truths. We were given the chance to do a human study that would take all of these principles we had begun to uncover in the lab to the next level. It was time to study the role of nutrition, lifestyle and disease in the most comprehensive manner ever undertaken in the history of medicine. We were on to the China Study.

4
Lessons from China

A SNAPSHOT IN TIME

Have you ever had the sensation of wanting to permanently capture a moment? Such moments can grip you in a way you will never forget. For some people, those moments center on family, close friends or related activities; for others those moments may center on nature, spirituality or religion. For most of us, I suspect, it can be a little of each. They become the personal moments, both happy and sad, which define our memories. It's these moments in which everything just "comes together." They are the snapshots of time that define much of our life experience.

The value of a snapshot of time is not lost on researchers either. We construct experiments, hoping to preserve and analyze the specific details of a certain moment for years to come. I was fortunate enough to be privy to such an opportunity in the early 1980s, after a distinguished senior scientist from China, Dr. Junshi Chen, came to Cornell to work in my lab. He was deputy director of China's premier health research laboratory and one of the first handful of Chinese scholars to visit the U.S. following the establishment of relations between our two countries.

THE CANCER ATLAS

In the early 1970s, the premier of China, Chou EnLai, was dying of cancer. In the grips of this terminal disease, Premier Chou initiated a nationwide survey to collect information about a disease that was not well understood. It was to be a monumental survey of death rates for twelve different kinds of cancer for more than 2,400 Chinese counties and 880 million (96%) of their citizens. The survey was remarkable in many ways. It involved 650,000 workers, the most ambitious biomedical research project ever undertaken. The end result of the survey was a beautiful, color-coded atlas showing where certain types of cancer were high and where they were almost nonexistent.[1]

CHART 4.1: SAMPLE CANCER ATLAS IN CHINA

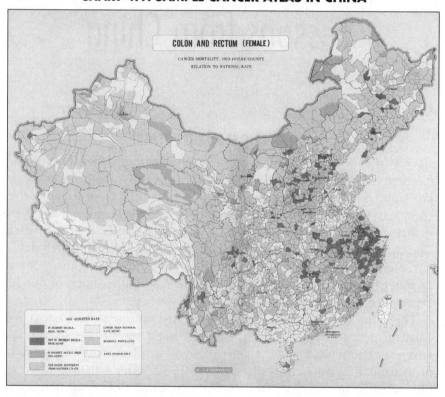

This atlas made it clear that in China cancer was geographically localized. Some cancers were much more common in some places than in others. Earlier studies had set the stage for this idea, showing that cancer incidence also varies widely between different countries.[2-4] But these China data were more remarkable because the geographic variations in cancer rates were much greater (Chart 4.2). They also occurred in a country where 87% of the population is the same ethnic group, the Han people.

CHART 4.2. RANGE OF CANCER RATES IN CHINESE COUNTIES

Cancer Site	Males	Females
All Cancers	35–721	35–491
Nasopharynx	0–75	0–26
Esophagus	1–435	0–286
Stomach	6–386	2–141
Liver	7–248	3–67
Colorectal	2–67	2–61
Lung	3–59	0–26
Breast	—	0–20
*Age-adjusted death rates, representing # cases/100,000 people/year		

Why was there such a massive variation in cancer rates among different counties when genetic backgrounds were similar from place to place? Might it be possible that cancer is largely due to environmental/lifestyle factors, and not genetics? A few prominent scientists had already reached that conclusion. The authors of a major review on diet and cancer, prepared for the U.S. Congress in 1981, estimated that genetics only determines about *2–3% of the total cancer risk.*[4]

The data behind the China cancer atlas were profound. The counties with the highest rates of some cancers were more than 100 times greater than counties with the lowest rates of these cancers. These are truly remarkable figures. By way of comparison, we in the U.S. see, at most, two to three times the cancer rates from one part of the country to another.

In fact, very small and relatively unimportant differences in cancer rates make big news, big money and big politics. There has been a long-standing story in my state of New York about the increased rates of breast cancer in Long Island. Large amounts of money (about $30 million[5]) and years and years of work have been spent examining the issue. What sorts of rates were causing such a furor? Two counties in Long Island had rates of breast cancer only 10–20% higher than the state average. This difference was enough to make front-page news, scare people and move politicians to action. Contrast this with the findings in China where some parts of the country had cancer rates 100 times (10,000%) higher than others.

Because China is relatively homogenous genetically, it was clear that these differences had to be explained by environmental causes. This raised a number of critical questions:

- Why was cancer so high in some rural Chinese counties and not in others?
- Why were these differences so incredibly large?
- Why was overall cancer, in the aggregate, less common in China than in the U.S.?

The more Dr. Chen and I talked, the more we wished that we had a snapshot in time of the dietary and environmental conditions in rural China. If only we could look into these people's lives, note what they eat, how they live, what is in their blood and their urine and how they die. If only we could construct a picture of their experience with unprecedented clarity and detail so that we could study it for years to come. If we could do that, we might be able to offer some answers to our "why" questions.

Occasionally science, politics and financing come together in a way that allows a truly extraordinary study to take place. This happened for us, and we got the opportunity to do everything we wanted, and more. We were able to create the most comprehensive snapshot of diet, lifestyle and disease ever taken.

PULLING IT TOGETHER

We assembled a world-class scientific team. There was Dr. Chen, who was the deputy director of the most significant government diet and health research laboratory in all of China. We enlisted Dr. Junyao Li, one of the authors of the *Cancer Atlas Survey* and a key scientist in China's Academy of Medical Sciences in the Ministry of Health. The third member was Richard Peto of Oxford University. Considered one of the premier epidemiologists in the world, Peto has since been knighted and has received several awards for cancer research. I rounded out the team as the Project Director.

Everything was coming together. It was to be the first major research project between China and the United States. We cleared the necessary funding hurdles, weathering both CIA intrusiveness and Chinese government reticence. We were on our way.

We decided to make the study as comprehensive as possible. From the *Cancer Atlas*, we had access to disease mortality rates on more than four dozen different kinds of disease, including individual cancers, heart diseases and infectious diseases.[6] We gathered data on 367 variables and then compared each variable with every other variable. We went into sixty-five counties across China and administered questionnaires and blood tests on 6,500 adults. We took urine samples, directly measured everything families ate over a three-day period and analyzed food samples from marketplaces around the country.

The sixty-five counties selected for the study were located in rural to semi-rural parts of China. This was intentionally done because we wanted to study people who mostly lived and ate food in the same area for most of their lives. This was a successful strategy, as we were to learn than an average of 90–94% of the adult subjects in each county still lived in the same county where they were born.

When we were done we had *more than 8,000 statistically significant associations* between lifestyle, diet and disease variables. We had a study that was unmatched in terms of comprehensiveness, quality and uniqueness. We had what the *New York Times* termed "the Grand Prix of epidemiology." In short, we had created that revealing snapshot of time that we had originally envisioned.

This was the perfect opportunity to test the principles that we discovered in the animal experiments. Were the findings in the lab going to be consistent with the human experience in the real world? Were our discoveries on aflatoxin-induced liver cancer in rats going to apply to other types of cancer and other types of diseases in humans?

FOR MORE INFORMATION

We take great pride in the comprehensiveness and quality of the China Study. To see why, read Appendix B on page 353. You'll find a more complete discussion of the basic design and characteristics of the study.

THE CHINESE DIETARY EXPERIENCE

Critical to the importance of the China Study was the nature of the diet consumed in rural China. It was a rare opportunity to study health-related effects of a mostly plant-based diet.

In America, 15–16% of our total calories comes from protein and upwards of 80% of this amount comes from animal-based foods. But in rural China only 9–10% of total calories comes from protein and only 10% of the protein comes from animal-based foods. This means that there are major nutritional differences in the Chinese and American diets, as shown in Chart 4.3.

CHART 4.3. CHINESE AND AMERICAN DIETARY INTAKES

Nutrient	China	United States
Calories (kcal/day)[7]	2641	1989
Total fat (% of calories)	14.5	34–38
Dietary fiber (g/day)	33	12
Total protein (g/day)	64	91
Animal protein (% of calories)	0.8	10–11
Total iron (mg/day)	34	18

The findings shown in Chart 4.3 are standardized for a body weight of sixty-five kilograms (143 pounds). This is the standard way that Chinese authorities record such information and it allows us to easily compare different populations. (For an American adult male of seventy-seven kilograms, calorie intake will be about 2,400 calories per day. For an average rural Chinese adult male of seventy-seven kilograms, calorie intake will be about 3,000 calories per day.)

In every category seen above, there are massive dietary differences between the Chinese and American experiences: much higher overall calorie intake, less fat, less protein, much less animal foods, more fiber and much more iron are consumed in China. These dietary differences are supremely important.

While the eating pattern in China is far different from that of the United States, there is still a lot of variation within China. Experimental variation (i.e., a range of values) is essential when we investigate diet and health associations. Fortunately, in the China Study considerable variation existed for most of the measured factors. There was exceptional variation in disease rates (Chart 4.2) and more than adequate variation for clinical measurements and food intakes. For example, blood cholesterol ranged—as county averages—from highest to lowest almost twofold, blood beta-carotene about ninefold, blood lipids about threefold, fat intake about sixfold and fiber intake about fivefold. This was crucial, as we primarily were concerned with comparing each county in China with every other county.

Ours was the first large study that investigated this particular range of dietary experience and its health consequences. In effect, we are comparing, within the Chinese range, diets rich in plant-based foods to diets very rich in plant-based foods. In almost all other studies, all of which are Western, scientists are comparing diets rich in animal-based foods to diets very rich in animal-based foods. The difference between rural Chinese diets and Western diets, and the ensuing disease patterns, is enormous. It was this distinction, as much as any other, that made this study so important.

The media called the China Study a "landmark study." An article in the Saturday Evening Post said the project "should shake up medical and nutrition researchers everywhere."[8] Some in the medical establishment said another study like this could never be done. What I knew was that our study offered an opportunity to investigate many of the most contentious ideas that I was forming about food and health.

Now, I want to show you what we learned from this study and how twenty more years of research, thought and experience have changed not only the way I think about the connection between nutrition and health, but the way my family and I eat as well.

DISEASES OF POVERTY AND AFFLUENCE

It doesn't take a scientist to figure out that the possibility of death has been holding pretty steady at 100% for quite some time. There's only one thing that we have to do in life, and that is to die. I have often met people who use this fact to justify their ambivalence toward health information. But I take a different view. I have never pursued health hoping for immortality. Good health is about being able to fully enjoy the time we do have. It is about being as functional as possible throughout our entire lives and avoiding crippling, painful and lengthy battles with disease. There are many better ways to die, and to live.

Because the China Cancer Atlas had mortality rates for more than four dozen different kinds of disease, we had a rare opportunity to study the many ways that people die. We wondered: do certain diseases tend to group together in certain areas of the country? For example, did colon cancer occur in the same regions as diabetes? If this proved to be the case, we could assume that diabetes and colon cancer (or other diseases that grouped together) shared common causes. These causes could include a variety of possibilities, ranging from the geographic and environmental to the biological. However, because all diseases are biological processes (gone awry), we can assume that whatever "causes" are observed, they will eventually operate through biological events.

When these diseases were cross-listed in a way that allowed every disease rate to be compared with every other disease rate,[9] two groups of diseases emerged: those typically found in more economically developed areas (diseases of affluence) and those typically found in rural agricultural areas (diseases of poverty)[10] (Chart 4.4).

CHART 4.4. DISEASE GROUPINGS OBSERVED IN RURAL CHINA

Diseases of Affluence (Nutritional Extravagance)	Cancer (colon, lung, breast, leukemia, childhood brain, stomach, liver), diabetes, coronary heart disease
Diseases of Poverty (Nutritional inadequacy and poor sanitation)	Pneumonia, intestinal obstruction, peptic ulcer, digestive disease, pulmonary tuberculosis, parasitic disease, rheumatic heart disease, metabolic and endocrine disease other than diabetes, diseases of pregnancy and many others

Chart 4.4 shows that each disease, in either list, tends to associate with diseases in its own list but not in the opposite list. A region in rural China that has a high rate of pneumonia, for example, will not have a high rate of breast cancer, but will have a high rate of a parasitic disease. The disease that kills most Westerners, coronary heart disease, is more common in areas where breast cancer also is more common. Coronary heart disease, by the way, is relatively uncommon in many developing societies of the world. This is not because people die at a younger age, thus avoiding these Western diseases. These comparisons are age-standardized rates, meaning that people of the same age are being compared.

Disease associations of this kind have been known for quite some time. What the China Study added, however, was an unsurpassed amount of data on death rates for many different diseases and a unique range of dietary experience. As expected, certain diseases do cluster together in the same geographic areas, implying that they have shared causes.

These two disease groups have usually been referred to as diseases of affluence and diseases of poverty. As a developing population accumulates wealth, people change their eating habits, lifestyles and sanitation systems. As wealth accumulates, more and more people die from "rich" diseases of affluence than "poor" diseases of poverty. Because these diseases of affluence are so tightly linked to eating habits, diseases of affluence might be better named "diseases of nutritional extravagance." The vast majority of people in the United States and other Western countries die from diseases of affluence. For this reason, these diseases are often referred to as "Western" diseases. Some rural counties had few diseases of affluence while other counties had far more of these diseases. The core question of the China Study was this: is it because of differences in dietary habits?

STATISTICAL SIGNIFICANCE

As I go through this chapter, I will indicate the statistical significance of various observations. Roman numeral one (^{I}) means 95+% certainty; roman numeral two (^{II}) means 99+% certainty; and roman numeral three (^{III}) means 99.9+% certainty. No roman numeral means that the association is something less than 95% certainty.[11] These probabilities also can be described as the probability that an observation is real. A 95% certainty means a 19 in 20 probability that the observation is real; a 99% certainty means a 99 in 100 probability that the observation is real; and a 99.9% certainty means a 999 in 1,000 probability that the observation is real.

BLOOD CHOLESTEROL AND DISEASE

We compared the prevalence of Western diseases in each county with diet and lifestyle variables and, to our surprise, we found that one of the strongest predictors of Western diseases was blood cholesterol.[III]

IN YOUR FOOD—IN YOUR BLOOD

There are two main categories of cholesterol. *Dietary cholesterol* is present in the food we eat. It is a component of food, much like sugar, fat, protein, vitamins and minerals. This cholesterol is found only in animal-based food and is the one we find on food labels. How much dietary cholesterol you consume is *not* something your doctor can know when he or she checks your cholesterol levels. The doctor can't measure dietary cholesterol any more than he or she can measure how many hot dogs and chicken breasts you've been eating. Instead, the doctor measures the amount of cholesterol present in your blood. This second type of cholesterol, *blood cholesterol*, is made in the liver. Blood cholesterol and dietary cholesterol, although chemically identical, do not represent the same thing. A similar situation occurs with fat. Dietary fat is the stuff you eat: the grease on your French fries, for example. Body fat, on the other hand, is the stuff made by your body and is very different from the fat that you spread on your toast in the morning (butter or margarine). Dietary fats and cholesterol don't necessarily turn into body fat and blood cholesterol. The way the body makes body fat and blood cholesterol is extremely complex, involving hundreds of different chemical reactions and dozens of nutrients. Because of this complexity, the health effects of eating dietary fat and dietary cholesterol may be very different from the health effects of having high blood cholesterol (what your doctor measures) or having too much body fat.

As blood cholesterol levels in rural China rose in certain counties, the incidence of "Western" diseases also increased. What made this so surprising was that Chinese levels were far lower than we had expected. The average level of blood cholesterol was only 127 mg/dL, which is almost 100 points less than the American average (215 mg/dL)![12] Some counties had average levels as low as 94 mg/dL. For two groups of about twenty-five women in the inner part of China, average blood cholesterol was at the amazingly low level of 80 mg/dL.

If you know your own cholesterol levels, you'll appreciate how low these values really are. In the U.S., our range is around 170–290 mg/dL. Our low values are near the high values for rural China. Indeed, in the U.S., there was a myth that there might be health problems if cholesterol levels were below 150 mg/dL. If we followed that line of thinking, about 85% of the rural Chinese would appear to be in trouble. But the truth is quite different. *Lower blood cholesterol levels are linked to lower rates of heart disease, cancer and other Western diseases, even at levels far below those considered "safe" in the West.*

At the outset of the China Study, no one could or would have predicted that there would be a relationship between cholesterol and any of the disease rates. What a surprise we got! As blood cholesterol levels decreased from 170 mg/dL to 90 mg/dL, cancers of the liver,[II] rectum,[I] colon,[II] male lung,[I] female lung, breast, childhood leukemia, adult leukemia,[1] childhood brain, adult brain,[1] stomach and esophagus (throat) decreased. As you can see, this is a sizable list. Most Americans know that if you have high cholesterol, you should worry about your heart, but they don't know that you might want to worry about cancer as well.

There are several types of blood cholesterol, including LDL and HDL cholesterol. LDL is the "bad" kind and HDL is the "good" kind. In the China Study higher levels of the bad LDL cholesterol also were associated with Western diseases.

Keep in mind that these diseases, by Western standards, were relatively rare in China and that blood cholesterol levels were quite low by Western standards. Our findings made a convincing case that many Chinese had an advantage at the lower cholesterol levels, even below 170 mg/dL. Now imagine a country where the inhabitants had blood cholesterol levels far higher than the Chinese average. You might expect that these relatively rare diseases, such as heart disease and some cancers, would be prevelant, perhaps even the leading killers!

Of course, this is exactly the case in the West. To give a couple of examples at the time of our study, the death rate from coronary heart disease was *seventeen times higher* among American men than rural Chinese men.[13] The American death rate from breast cancer was *five times higher* than the rural Chinese rate.

Even more remarkable were the extraordinarily low rates of coronary heart disease (CHD) in the southwestern Chinese provinces of Sichuan and Guizhou. During a three-year observation period (1973–1975), there was not one single person who died of CHD before the age of sixty-four, among 246,000 men in a Guizhou county and 181,000 women in a Sichuan county![14]

After these low cholesterol data were made public, I learned from three very prominent heart disease researchers and physicians, Drs. Bill Castelli, Bill Roberts and Caldwell Esselstyn, Jr., that in their long careers they had never seen a heart disease fatality among their patients who had blood cholesterol levels below 150 mg/dL. Dr. Castelli was the long-time director of the famous Framingham Heart Study of NIH; Dr. Esselstyn was a renowned surgeon at the Cleveland Clinic who did a remarkable study reversing heart disease (chapter five); Dr. Roberts has long been editor of the prestigious medical journal *Cardiology.*

BLOOD CHOLESTEROL AND DIET

Blood cholesterol is clearly an important indicator of disease risk. The big question is: how will food affect blood cholesterol? In brief, animal-based foods were correlated with *increasing* blood cholesterol (Chart 4.5). With almost no exceptions, nutrients from plant-based foods were associated with *decreasing* levels of blood cholesterol.

Several studies have now shown, in both experimental animals and in humans, that consuming animal-based protein increases blood cholesterol levels.[15-18] Saturated fat and dietary cholesterol also raise blood cholesterol, although these nutrients are not as effective at doing this as is animal protein. In contrast, plant-based foods contain no cholesterol and, in various other ways, help to decrease the amount of cholesterol made by the body. All of this was consistent with the findings from the China Study.

CHART 4.5. FOODS ASSOCIATED WITH BLOOD CHOLESTEROL

As intakes of meat,[1] milk, eggs, fish,[1-11] fat[1] and animal protein go up . . .	Blood Cholesterol goes up.
As intakes of plant-based foods and nutrients (including plant protein,[1] dietary fiber,[11] cellulose,[11] hemicellulose,[1] soluble carbohydrate,[11] B-vitamins of plants (carotenes, B_2, B_3),[1] legumes, light colored vegetables, fruit, carrots, potatoes and several cereal grains) go up . . .	Blood Cholesterol goes down.

These disease associations with blood cholesterol were remarkable, because blood cholesterol and animal-based food consumption both were so low by American standards. In rural China, animal protein intake (for the same individual) averages only 7.1 g/day whereas Americans average a whopping 70 g/day. To put this into perspective, seven grams of animal protein is found in about three chicken nuggets from McDonald's. We expected that when animal protein consumption and blood cholesterol levels were as low as they are in rural China, there would be no further association with the Western diseases. But we were wrong. Even these small amounts of animal-based food in rural China raised the risk for Western diseases.

We studied dietary effects on the different types of blood cholesterol. The same dramatic effects were seen. Animal protein consumption by men was associated with increasing levels of "bad" blood cholesterol[III] whereas plant protein consumption was associated with decreasing levels of this same cholesterol.[II]

Walk into almost any doctor's office and ask which dietary factors affect blood cholesterol levels and he or she will likely mention saturated fat and dietary cholesterol. In more recent decades, some might also mention the cholesterol-lowering effect of soy or high-fiber bran products, but few will say that animal protein has anything to do with blood cholesterol levels.

It has always been this way. While on sabbatical at the University of Oxford, I attended lectures given to medical students on the dietary causes of heart disease by one of their prominent professors of medicine. He went on and on about the adverse effects of saturated fat and cholesterol intakes on coronary heart disease as if these were the only dietary factors that were important. He was unwilling to concede that animal protein consumption had anything to do with blood cholesterol levels, even though the evidence at that time made it abundantly clear that animal protein was more strongly correlated with blood cholesterol levels than saturated fat and dietary cholesterol.[15] Like too many others, his blind faith in the status quo left him unwilling to be open-minded. As these findings poured in, I was beginning to discover that being open-minded was not a luxury, but a necessity.

FAT AND BREAST CANCER

If there were some sort of nutrition parade, and each nutrient had a float, by far the biggest would belong to fat. So many people, from researchers to educators, from government policy makers to industry representatives, have investigated or made pronouncements on fat for so long. People from a huge number of different communities have been constructing this behemoth for over half a century.

As this strange parade got started on Main Street, USA, the attention of everyone sitting on the sidewalks would inevitably be drawn to the fat float. Most people might see the fat float and say, "I should stay away from that," and then eat a hefty piece of it. Others would climb on the unsaturated half of the float and say that these fats are healthy and only saturated fats are bad. Many scientists would point fingers at the fat float and claim that the heart disease and cancer clowns are hiding inside. Meanwhile, some self-proclaimed diet gurus, like the late Dr. Robert Atkins, might set up shop on the float and start selling books. At the end of the day the average person who gorged on the float would be left scratching his head and feeling queasy, wondering what he should have done and why.

There's good reason for the average consumer to be confused. The unanswered questions on fat remain unanswered, as they have for the past forty years. How much fat can we have in our diets? What kind of fat? Is polyunsaturated fat better than saturated fat? Is monounsaturated fat better than either? What about those special fats like omega-3, omega-6, trans fats and DHA? Should we avoid coconut fat? What about fish oil? Is there something special about flaxseed oil? What's a high-fat diet anyway? A low-fat diet?

This can be confusing, even for trained scientists. The details that underlie these questions, *when considered in isolation*, are very misleading. As you shall see, considering how networks of chemicals behave instead of isolated single chemicals is far more meaningful.

In some ways, however, it is this foolish mania regarding isolated aspects of fat consumption that teaches us the best lessons. Therefore, let's look a little more closely at this story of fat as it has emerged during the past forty years. It illustrates why the public is so confused both about fat and about diet in general.

On average, we consume 35–40% of our total calories as fat.[19] We have been consuming high-fat diets like this since the late nineteenth century, at the onset of our industrial revolution. Because we had more money, we began consuming more meat and dairy, which are relatively high in fat. We were demonstrating our affluence by consuming such foods.

Then came the mid to late twentieth century when scientists began to question the advisability of consuming diets so high in fat. National and international dietary recommendations[20-23] emerged to suggest that we should decrease our fat intake below 30% of calories. That lasted for a couple decades, but now, the fears surrounding high-fat diets are abating. Some authors of popular books even advocate increased fat intake! Some experienced researchers have suggested that it is not necessary to go below 30% fat, as long as we consume the right kind of fat.

The level of 30% fat has become a benchmark, even though there is no evidence to suggest that this is a vital threshold. Let's get some perspective on this figure by considering the fat contents of a few foods, as seen in Chart 4.6.

CHART 4.6: FAT CONTENT OF SAMPLE FOODS

Food	Percent of calories derived from fat
Butter	100%
McDonald's Double Cheeseburger	67%
Whole Cow's Milk	64%
Ham	61%
Hotdog	54%
Soybeans	42%
"Low-Fat" (or 2%) Milk	35%
Chicken	26%
Spinach	14%
Wheaties Breakfast Cereal	8%
Skim Milk	5%
Peas	5%
Carrots	4%
Green Beans	3.5%
Whole Baked Potatoes	1%

With a few exceptions, animal-based foods contain considerably more fat than plant-based foods.[24] This is well illustrated by comparing the amount of fat in the diets of different countries. The correlation between fat intake and animal protein intake is more than 90%.[25] This means that fat intake increases in parallel with animal protein intake. In other words, dietary fat is an indicator of how much animal-based food is in the diet. It is almost a perfect match.

FAT AND A FOCUS ON CANCER

The 1982 National Academy of Sciences (NAS) report on Diet, Nutrition and Cancer, of which I was a co-author, was the first expert panel report that deliberated on the association of dietary fat with cancer. This report was the first to recommend a maximum fat intake of 30% of calories for cancer prevention. Previously, the U.S. Senate Select Committee on Nutrition chaired by Senator George McGovern[26] held widely publicized hearings on diet and heart disease and recommended a maximum intake of 30% dietary fat. Although the McGovern report generated a public discourse on diet and disease, it was the 1982 NAS report that gave momentum to this debate. Its focus on cancer, as opposed to heart disease, increased public interest and concern. It spurred additional research activity and public awareness of the importance of diet in disease prevention.

Many of the reports at the time[20, 27, 28] were centered on the question of how much dietary fat was appropriate for good health. The unique attention given to fat was motivated by international studies showing that the amount of dietary fat consumed was closely associated with the incidence of breast cancer, large bowel cancer and heart disease. These were the diseases that kill the majority of people in Western countries before their time. Clearly, this correlation was destined to attract great public attention. The China Study was begun in the midst of this environment.

The best known study,[29] in my view, was that of the late Ken Carroll, professor at the University of Western Ontario in Canada. His findings showed a very impressive relationship between dietary fat and breast cancer (Chart 4.7).

This finding, which corresponded to the earlier reports of others,[3, 30] became especially intriguing when compared with migrant studies.[31, 32] These studies showed that people who migrated from one area to another and who started eating the typical diet of their new residency assumed the disease risk of the area to which they moved. This strongly

CHART 4.7: TOTAL FAT INTAKE AND BREAST CANCER

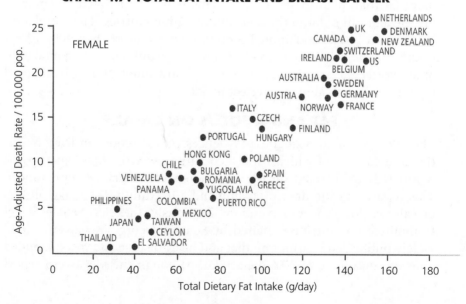

implied that diet and lifestyle were the principle causes of these diseases. It also suggested that genes are not necessarily that important. As noted earlier, a very prominent report by Sir Richard Doll and Sir Richard Peto of the University of Oxford (U.K.) submitted to the U.S. Congress summarized many of these studies and concluded that only 2–3% of all cancers could be attributed to genes.[4]

Do the data from these international and migrant studies mean that we can lower our rate of breast cancer to almost zero if we make perfect lifestyle choices? The information certainly suggests that this could be the case. Concerning the evidence in Chart 4.7, the solution seems obvious: if we eat less fat, then we'll lower our breast cancer risk. Most scientists made this conclusion and some surmised that dietary fat caused breast cancer. But that interpretation was too simple. Other charts prepared by Professor Carroll were largely, almost totally, ignored (Charts 4.8 and 4.9). They show that breast cancer was associated with animal fat intake but not with plant fat.

In rural China, dietary fat intake (at the time of the survey in 1983) was very different from the United States in two ways. First, fat was only 14.5% of calorie intake in China, compared with about 36% in the U.S. Second, the amount of fat in the diets of rural China depended almost entirely on the amount of animal-based food in the diet, just like the

CHART 4.8: ANIMAL FAT INTAKE AND BREAST CANCER

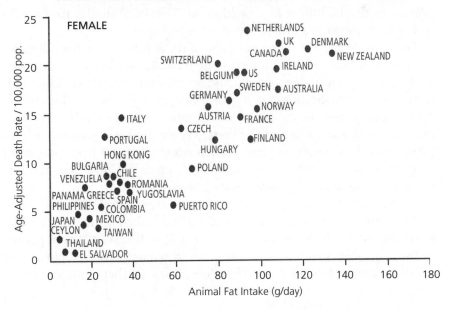

CHART 4.9: PLANT FAT INTAKE AND BREAST CANCER

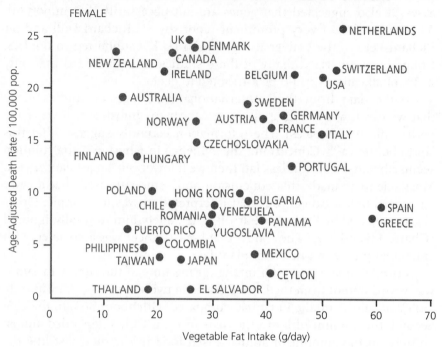

findings in Chart 4.7. The correlation between dietary fat and animal protein in rural China was very high, at 70–84%,[33] similar to the 93% seen when comparing different countries.[25]

This is important because in China and the international studies, fat consumption was only an indication of *animal-based food* consumption. Thus, the association between fat and breast cancer might really be telling us that as consumption of *animal-based foods* goes up, so does breast cancer. This is not the case in the U.S., where we selectively add or remove fat from our foods and our diets. We get as much or more fat from plant-based food (potato chips, French fries) as we get from processed animal-based foods (skim milk, lean cuts of meat). China does not tinker with fat in their food supply as we do here.

At this very low range of dietary fat in China, from 6%–24%, I initially thought that dietary fat would not be linked with diseases like heart disease or the various cancers, as it is in the West. Some people in the U.S.—like many of my colleagues in science and medicine—call a 30% fat diet a "low-fat" diet. Therefore, a low-fat diet containing only

25–30% fat was thought to be low enough to obtain the maximum amount of health benefits. This implied that going lower provided no further benefit. Surprise!

Findings from rural China showed that reducing dietary fat from 24% to 6% was associated with lower breast cancer risk. However, lower dietary fat in rural China meant less consumption not only of fat but, more importantly, of animal-based food.

This connection of breast cancer with dietary fat, thus with animal-based foods, brought into consideration other factors that also place a woman at risk for breast cancer:

- Early age of menarche (age of first menstruation)
- High blood cholesterol
- Late menopause
- High exposure to female hormones

What does the China Study show regarding these risk factors? Higher dietary fat is associated with higher blood cholesterol[1] and both of these factors, along with higher female hormone levels, are associated, in turn, with more breast cancer[1] and earlier age of menarche.[1]

The much later age of menarche in rural China is remarkable. Twenty-five women in each of the 130 villages in the survey were asked when they had their first menstrual period. The range of village averages was fifteen to nineteen years, with an average of seventeen years. The U.S. average is roughly eleven years!

Many studies have shown that earlier menarche leads to higher risk for breast cancer.[34] Menarche is triggered by the growth rate of the girl; the faster the growth, the earlier the age of onset. It also is well established that rapid growth of young girls often leads to greater adult body height and more body weight and body fatness, each of which is associated with higher breast cancer risk. Early age of menarche, both in Chinese and in Western women, also leads to higher levels of blood hormones such as estrogen. These hormone levels remain high throughout the reproductive years if consumption of a diet rich in animal-based food is maintained. Under these conditions, age of menopause is deferred by three to four years,[1] thus extending the reproductive life from beginning to end by about nine to ten years and greatly increasing lifetime exposure to female hormones. Other studies have shown that an increase in years of reproductive life is associated with increased breast cancer risk.[35, 36]

This network of relationships becomes still more impressive. Higher fat consumption is associated with higher blood levels of estrogen during the critical years of thirty-five to forty-four years[III] and higher blood levels of the female hormone prolactin during the later years of fifty-five to sixty-four years.[III] These hormones are highly correlated with animal protein intake[III] and milk[III] and meat.[II] Unfortunately, we could not demonstrate whether these hormone levels were directly related to breast cancer risk in China because the rate of disease is so low.[37]

Nonetheless, when hormone levels among Chinese women were compared with those of British women,[38] Chinese estrogen levels were only about one-half those of the British women, who have an equivalent hormone profile to that of American women. Because the length of the reproductive life of a Chinese woman is only about 75% of that of the British (or American) woman, this means that with lower estrogen levels, the Chinese woman only experiences about 35–40% of the lifetime estrogen exposure of British (and American) women. This corresponds to Chinese breast cancer rates that are only one-fifth of those of Western women.

The strong association of a high-animal protein, high-fat diet with reproductive hormones and early age of menarche, both of which raise the risk of breast cancer, is an important observation. It makes clear that we should not have our children consume diets high in animal-based foods. If you are a woman, would you ever have imagined that eating diets higher in animal-based foods would expand your reproductive life by about nine to ten years? As an aside, an interesting implication of this observation, as noted by Ms. magazine founder Gloria Steinem, is that eating the right foods could reduce teenage pregnancy by delaying the age of menarche.

Beyond the hormone findings, is there a way to show that animal-based food intake relates to overall cancer rates? This is somewhat difficult, but one of the factors we measured was how much cancer there was in each family. Animal protein intake was convincingly associated in the China Study with the prevalence of cancer in families.[III] This association is an impressive and significant observation, considering the unusually low intake of animal protein.

Diet and disease factors such as animal protein consumption or breast cancer incidence lead to changes in the concentrations of certain chemicals in our blood. These chemicals are called biomarkers. As an example, blood cholesterol is a biomarker for heart disease. We measured six blood biomarkers that are associated with animal protein intake.[39] Do they confirm the finding that animal protein intake is associated with cancer in families? Absolutely. Every single animal protein-related blood biomarker is significantly associated with the amount of cancer in a family.[II–III]

In this case, multiple observations, tightly networked into a web, show that animal-based foods are strongly linked to breast cancer. What makes this conclusion especially compelling are two kinds of evidence. First, the individual parts of this web were consistently correlated and, in most cases, were statistically significant. Second, this effect occurred *at unusually low intakes of animal-based foods*.

Our investigation of breast cancer (detailed further in chapter seven) is a perfect example of what makes the China Study so convincing. Rather than a single, simple association of fat and breast cancer,[1] we were able to construct a much more expansive web of information about how diet affects breast cancer risk. We were able to examine in multiple ways the role of diet and cholesterol, age of menarche and female hormone levels, all of which are known risk factors for breast cancer. When each new finding pointed in the same direction, we were able to see a picture that was convincing, consistent and biologically plausible.

THE IMPORTANCE OF FIBER

The late Professor Denis Burkitt, of Trinity College, Dublin, was unusually articulate. His common sense, scientific credibility and sense of humor made quite an impression on me when I first met him at a Cornell seminar. The subject of his work was dietary fiber. He had traveled 10,000 miles in a jeep over rugged countryside to study the dietary habits of Africans.

He asserted that even though fiber was not digested, it was vital for good health. Fiber was able to pull water from the body into the intestines to keep things moving along. These undigested fibers, like stick-um paper, also gather up nasty chemicals that find their way into our intestines and that might be carcinogenic. If we don't consume enough fiber, we are susceptible to constipation-based diseases. According to Burkitt, these include large bowel cancer, diverticulosis, hemorrhoids and varicose veins.

In 1993, Dr. Burkitt was awarded the prestigious Bower Award, the richest award in the world next to the Nobel Prize. He invited me to speak at his award ceremony at the Franklin Institute in Philadelphia, only two months before his unfortunate passing. He offered his opinion that our China Study was the most significant work on diet and health in the world at that time.

Dietary fiber is exclusively found in plant-based foods. This material, which gives rigidity to the cell walls of plants, comes in thousands of different chemical variations. It is mostly made of highly complex carbohydrate molecules. We digest very little or no fiber. Nonetheless, fiber, having few or no calories itself, helps dilute the caloric density of our diets, creates a sense of fullness and helps to shut down appetite, among other things. In doing so, it satisfies our hunger and minimizes the overconsumption of calories.

Average fiber intake (Chart 4.10) is about three times higher in China than in the U.S.[40] These differences are exceptional, especially considering the fact that many county averages were even much higher.

But according to some "experts" in the U.S., there is a dark side to dietary fiber. They contend that if fiber intake is too high our bodies are not able to absorb as much iron and related minerals, which are essential for health. The fiber may bind with these nutrients and carry them through our system before we are able to digest them. They say that the maximum level of fiber intake should be around thirty to thirty-five grams per day, which is only about the average intake of the rural Chinese.

We studied this iron/fiber issue very carefully in the China Study. As it turns out, fiber is not the enemy of iron absorption as so many experts claim it to be. We measured how much iron the Chinese were consuming and how much was in their bodies. Iron was measured in *six* different ways (four blood biomarkers and two estimates of iron intake) and

CHART 4.10: AVERAGE INTAKES OF DIETARY FIBER, GM/DAY

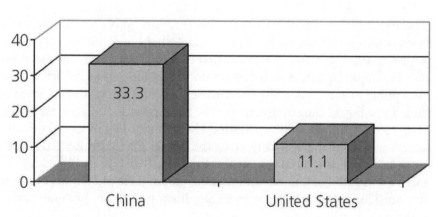

when we compared these measurements with fiber intake, *there was no evidence showing that increasing fiber intake impaired iron absorption in the body.* In fact, we found the opposite effect. A good indicator of how much iron is in the blood, hemoglobin, actually increased with greater intakes of dietary fiber.[1] As it turns out, high-fiber foods, like wheat and corn (but not the polished rice consumed in China) also happen to be high in iron, meaning that the higher the consumption of fiber, the higher the consumption of iron.[III] Iron intake in rural China (34 mg/day) was surprisingly high when compared to the average American intake (18 mg/day) and it was far more associated with plant-based foods than with animal-based foods.[41]

The China findings on dietary fiber and iron, like so many other observations in this study, did not support the common view of Western scientists. People who consume more plant-based foods, thus more dietary fiber, also consume more iron,[III] all of which results in statistically significant higher levels of hemoglobin. Unfortunately, a bit of confusion has arisen over the fact that some people in rural China, including women and children, have low iron levels. This is especially true in areas where parasitic diseases are more common. In areas of rural China where parasitic diseases were more common, iron status was lower.[1] This has given some the opportunity to claim that these people need more meat, but the evidence indicates that the problem would be much better corrected by reducing parasitism in these areas.

Much of the initial interest in dietary fiber arose with Burkitt's travels in Africa and his claim that large bowel cancer is lower among populations who consume high-fiber diets. Burkitt made this claim popular but the story is at least 200 years old. In England during the late eighteenth century and early nineteenth century, it was claimed by some of the leading physicians that constipation, which was associated with less bulky diets (i.e., low-fiber diets), was associated with a higher risk of cancer (usually breast and "intestinal" cancers).

At the beginning of the China Study, this belief that fiber might prevent large bowel cancer was the prevailing view, although the 1982 National Academy of Sciences Committee on Diet, Nutrition and Cancer, "found no conclusive evidence to indicate that dietary fiber...exerts a protective effect against colorectal cancer in humans." The report went on to conclude, "...if there is such an effect, specific components of fiber, rather than total dietary fiber, are more likely to be responsible."[20] In hindsight, our discussion of this issue was inadequate. The question, the review of the research literature and the interpretation of the evidence were too focused on looking for a specific fiber as the responsible cause. Finding none, the fiber hypothesis was dismissed.

It was a mistake. The China Study provided evidence that there is a link with certain cancers. The results showed that high-fiber intake was consistently associated with lower rates of cancers of the rectum and colon. High-fiber intakes also were associated with lower levels of blood cholesterol.[I,II] Of course, high-fiber consumption reflected high plant-based food consumption; foods such as beans, leafy vegetables and whole grains are all high in fiber.

ANTIOXIDANTS, A BEAUTIFUL COLLECTION

One of the more obvious characteristics of plants is their wide range of bright colors. If you admire how food is presented, it's hard to beat a plate of fruits and vegetables. The reds, greens, yellows, purples and oranges of plant foods are tempting and very healthy. This link between nicely colored vegetables and their exceptional health benefits has often been noted. It turns out that there is a beautiful, scientifically sound story behind this color/health link.

The colors of fruits and vegetables are derived from a variety of chemicals called antioxidants. These chemicals are almost exclusively found in plants. They are only present in animal-based foods to the extent that animals eat them and store a small amount in their own tissues.

Living plants illustrate nature's beauty, both in color and in chemistry. They take the energy of the sun and transform it into life through the process of photosynthesis. In this process, the sun's energy is first turned into simple sugars, and then into more complex carbohydrates, fats and proteins.

This complex process amounts to some pretty high-powered activity within the plant, all of which is driven by the exchange of electrons between molecules. Electrons are the medium of energy transfer. The site at which photosynthesis takes place is a bit like a nuclear reactor. The electrons zooming around in the plant that are changing the sunlight into chemical energy must be managed very carefully. If they stray from their rightful places in the process, they may create free radicals, which can wreak havoc in the plant. It would be like the core of a nuclear reactor leaking radioactive materials (free radicals) that can be very dangerous to the surrounding area.

So how does the plant manage these complex reactions and protect against errant electrons and free radicals? It puts up a shield around potentially dangerous reactions that sponges up these highly reactive substances. The shield is made up of antioxidants that intercept and scavenge electrons that might otherwise stray from their course.

Antioxidants are usually colored because the same chemical property that sponges up excess electrons also creates visible colors. Some of these antioxidants are called carotenoids, of which there are hundreds. They vary in color from the yellow color of beta-carotene (squash), to the red color of lycopene (tomatoes), to the orange color of the odd-sounding crytoxanthins (oranges). Other antioxidants may be colorless and these include chemicals such as ascorbic acid (vitamin C) and vitamin E, which act as antioxidants in other parts of plants that need to be protected from the hazards of wayward electrons.

What makes this remarkable process relevant for us animals, however, is that we produce low levels of free radicals throughout our lifetime. Simply being exposed to the sun's rays, to certain industrial pollutants and to improperly balanced nutrient intakes creates a background of unwanted free radical damage. Free radicals are nasty. They can cause our tissues to become rigid and limited in their function. It is a bit like old age, when our bodies become creaky and stiff. To a great extent, this is what aging is. This uncontrolled free radical damage also is part of the processes that give rise to cataracts, to hardening of the arteries, to cancer, to emphysema, to arthritis and many other ailments that become more common with age.

But here's the kicker: we do not naturally build shields to protect ourselves against free radicals. As we are not plants, we do not carry out photosynthesis and therefore do not produce any of our own antioxidants. Fortunately the antioxidants in plants work in our bodies the same way they work in plants. It is a wonderful harmony. The plants make the antioxidant shields, and at the same time make them look incredibly appealing with beautiful, appetizing colors. Then we animals, in turn, are attracted to the plants and eat them and borrow their antioxidant shields for our own health. Whether you believe in God, evolution or just coincidence, you must admit that this is a beautiful, almost spiritual, example of nature's wisdom.

In the China Study, we assessed antioxidant status by recording the intakes of vitamin C and beta-carotene and measuring the blood levels of vitamin C, vitamin E and carotenoids. Among these antioxidant biomarkers, vitamin C provided the most impressive evidence.

The most significant vitamin C association with cancer was its relationship with the number of cancer-prone families in each area.[42]
When levels of vitamin C in the blood were low, these families were
more likely to have a high incidence of cancer.[III] Low vitamin C was
prominently associated with higher risk for esophageal cancer,[III] for
leukemia and cancers of the nasopharynx, breast, stomach, liver,
rectum, colon and lung. It was esophageal cancer that first attracted
NOVA television program producers to report on cancer mortality in
China. It was this television program that spurred our own survey
to see what was behind this story. Vitamin C primarily comes from
fruit, and eating fruit was also inversely associated with esophageal
cancer.[II 43] Cancer rates were five to eight times higher for areas where
fruit intake was lowest. The same vitamin C effect existing for these
cancers also existed for coronary heart disease, hypertensive heart disease and stroke.[II] Vitamin C intake from fruits clearly showed a powerful protective effect against a variety of diseases.

The other measures of antioxidants, blood levels of alpha and beta-
carotene (a vitamin precursor) and alpha and gamma tocopherol (vitamin E) are poor indicators of the effects of antioxidants. These antioxidants are transported in the blood by lipoprotein, which is the carrier of
"bad" cholesterol. So anytime we measured these antioxidants, we were
simultaneously measuring unhealthy biomarkers. This was an experimental compromise that diminished our ability to detect the beneficial
effects of the carotenoids and the tocopherols, even when these benefits
are known to exist.[44] We did, however, find that stomach cancer was
higher when the blood levels of beta-carotene were lower.[45]

Can we say that vitamin C, beta-carotene and dietary fiber are solely
responsible for preventing these cancers? In other words, can a pill containing vitamin C and beta-carotene or a fiber supplement create these
health effects? No. The triumph of health lies not in the individual nutrients, but in the whole foods that contain those nutrients: plant-based
foods. In a bowl of spinach salad, for example, we have fiber, antioxidants and countless other nutrients that are orchestrating a wondrous
symphony of health *as they work in concert* within our bodies. The
message could not be simpler: eat as many whole fruits, vegetables and
whole grains as you can, and you will probably derive all of the benefits
noted above as well as many others.

I have been making this point about the health value of whole plant-
based foods ever since vitamin supplements were introduced on a large

scale in the marketplace. And I have watched in dismay how the industry and the media convinced so many Americans that these products represent the same good nutrition as do whole, plant-based foods. As we shall see in the later chapters, the promised health benefits of taking single-nutrient supplements are proving to be highly questionable. The "take-home message": if you want vitamin C or beta-carotene, don't reach for the pill bottle—reach for the fruit or leafy green vegetables.

THE ATKINS CRISIS

In case you haven't noticed, there is an elephant in the room. It goes by the name "low-carb diet," and it has become very popular. Almost all diet books on store shelves are variations of this one theme: eat as much protein, meat and fat as you want, but stay away from those "fatty" carbs. As you have seen already in this book, my research findings and my point of view show that eating this way is perhaps the single greatest threat to American health we currently face. So what is the story, anyway?

One of the fundamental arguments at the beginning of most low-carbohydrate, high-protein diet books is that America has been wallowing in low-fat mania at the advice of experts for the past twenty years, yet people are fatter than ever. This argument has an intuitive appeal, but there is one inconvenient fact that is consistently ignored: according to a report[46] summarizing government food statistics, "Americans consumed thirteen *pounds* [my emphasis] more [added] fats and oils per person in 1997 than in 1970, up from 52.6 to 65.6 pounds." It is true that we have had a trend to consuming fewer of our total calories as fat, when considered as a percentage, but that's only because we have outpaced our gorging on fat by gorging on sugary junk food. Simply by looking at the numbers, anybody can see that America has not adopted the "low-fat" experiment—not by any stretch of the imagination.

In fact, the claim that the low-fat "brainwashing" experiment has been tried and failed is often the first of many statements of fact in current diet books that can be described either as severe ignorance or opportunistic deceit. It is difficult to know where to begin to refute the maze of misinformation and false promises commonly made by authors completely untrained in nutrition, authors who have never conducted any peer-reviewed, professionally based experimental research. And yet these books are immensely popular. Why? Because people *do lose weight*, at least in the short term.

In one published study[47] funded by the Atkins Center for Complementary Medicine, researchers put fifty-one obese people on the Atkins diet.[48] The forty-one subjects who maintained the diet over the course of six months lost an average of twenty pounds. In addition, average blood cholesterol levels decreased slightly,[47] which was perhaps even more important. Because of these two results, this study was presented in the media as real, scientific proof that the Atkins diet works and is safe. Unfortunately, the media didn't go much deeper than that.

The first sign that all is not rosy is that these obese subjects were severely restricting their calorie intake during the study. The average American consumes about 2,250 calories per day.[49] When the study participants were on the diet, they consumed an average of 1,450 calories per day. That's 35% fewer calories! I don't care if you eat worms and cardboard; if you eat 35% fewer calories, you will lose weight and your cholesterol levels will improve[50] in the short run, but that is not to say that worms and cardboard form a healthy diet. One may argue that those 1,450 calories are so satisfying that people feel full on this diet, but if you compare calorie input and calorie expenditure, it's a matter of simple math that a person cannot sustain this amount of calorie restriction over a period of years or decades without either becoming an invalid or melting away into nothing. People are notoriously unsuccessful at significantly restricting their energy intake over any long period of time, and that is why there has yet to be a long-term study that shows success with the "low-carb" diets. This, however, is only the beginning of the problems.

In this same study, funded by the Atkins group, researchers report, "At some point during the twenty-four weeks, twenty-eight subjects (68%) reported constipation, twenty-six (63%) reported bad breath, twenty-one (51%) reported headache, four (10%) noted hair loss, and one woman (1%) reported increased menstrual bleeding."[47] They also refer to other research, saying, "Adverse effects of this diet in children have included calcium oxalate and urate kidney stones...vomiting, amenorrhea [when a girl misses her period], hypercholesterolemia [high cholesterol] and...vitamin deficiencies (ref. cited)."[47] Additionally, they found that the dieters had a stunning 53% increase in the amount of calcium they excreted in their urine,[47] which may spell disaster for their bone health. The weight loss, some of which is simply initial fluid loss,[51] may come with a very high price.

A different review of low-carbohydrate diets published by researchers in Australia concludes, "Complications such as heart arrhythmias, cardiac contractile function impairment, sudden death, osteoporosis, kidney damage, increased cancer risk, impairment of physical activity and lipid abnormalities can all be linked to long-term restriction of carbohydrates in the diet."[51] One teenage girl recently died suddenly after being on a high-protein diet.[52, 53] In short, most people will be unable to maintain this diet for the rest of their lives, and even if anybody manages to do so, they may be asking for serious health problems down the road. I have heard one doctor call high-protein, high-fat, low-carbohydrate diets "make-yourself-sick" diets, and I think that's an appropriate moniker. You can also lose weight by undergoing chemotherapy or starting a heroin addiction, but I wouldn't recommend those, either.

One final thought: the diet is not all that Atkins recommends. Indeed, most diet books are merely one part of huge food and health empires. In the case of the Atkins diet, Dr. Atkins states that many of his patients require nutrient supplements, some of which are used to combat "common dieters' problems."[54] In one passage, after making unsubstantiated claims about the efficacy of antioxidant supplements that contradict recent studies,[55] he writes, "Add to the [antioxidants] the vita-nutrients known to be useful for each of the myriad medical problems my patients face, and you'll see why many of them take over thirty vitamin pills a day."[56] *Thirty pills a day?*

There are snake oil salesmen, who have no professional research, professional training or professional publications in the field of nutrition, and there are scientists, who have formal training, have conducted research and have reported on their findings in professional forums. Perhaps it is a testament to the power of modern marketing savvy that an obese man with heart disease and high blood pressure[57] became one of the richest snake oil salesmen ever to live, selling a diet that promises to help you lose weight, to keep your heart healthy and to normalize your blood pressure.

THE TRUTH ABOUT CARBOHYDRATES

An unfortunate outcome of the recent popularity of diet books is that people are more confused than ever about the health value of carbohydrates. As you will see in this book, there is a mountain of scientific evidence to show that the healthiest diet you can possibly consume is a *high-carbohydrate* diet. It has been shown to reverse heart disease, reverse diabetes, prevent a plethora of chronic diseases, and yes, it has been shown many times to cause significant weight loss. But it's not quite as simple as that.

At least 99% of the carbohydrates that we consume are derived from fruits, vegetables and grains. When these foods are consumed in the unprocessed, unrefined and natural state, a large proportion of the carbohydrates are in the so-called "complex" form. This means that they are broken down in a controlled, regulated manner during digestion. This category of carbohydrates includes the many forms of dietary fiber, almost all of which remain undigested—but still provide substantial health benefits. In addition, these complex carbohydrates from whole foods are packaged with generous amounts of vitamins, minerals and accessible energy. Fruits, vegetables and whole grains are the healthiest foods you can consume, and they are primarily made of carbohydrates.

On the opposite side of the spectrum, there are highly processed, highly refined carbohydrates that have been stripped of their fiber, vitamins and minerals. Typical simple carbohydrates are found in foods like white bread, processed snack items including crackers and chips made with white flour, sweets including pastries and candy bars and sugar-laden soft drinks. These highly refined carbohydrates originate from grains or sugar plants, like sugar cane or the sugar beet. They are readily broken down during digestion to the simplest form of the carbohydrates, which are absorbed into the body to give blood sugar, or glucose.

Unfortunately, most Americans consume voluminous amounts of simple, refined carbohydrates and paltry amounts of complex carbohydrates. For example, in 1996, 42% of Americans ate cakes, cookies, pastries or pies on any given day, while only 10% ate any dark green vegetables.[46] In another ominous sign, only three vegetables accounted for half of the total vegetable servings in 1996[46]: potatoes, which were mostly consumed as fries and chips; head lettuce, one of the least nutrient-dense vegetables you can consume, and canned tomatoes, which is probably only a reflection of pizza and pasta consumption. Add to that the fact that the average American consumed *thirty-two teaspoons of added sugars per day in 1996,*[46] and it's clear that Americans are gorging almost exclusively on refined, simple carbohydrates, at the exclusion of healthful complex carbohydrates.

This is bad news, and this, in large measure, is why carbohydrates as a whole have gotten such a bad rap; the vast majority of carbohydrates consumed in America are found in junk food or grains so refined that they have to be supplemented with vitamins and minerals. On this point, the popular diet authors and I agree. For example, you could eat a low-fat, high-carbohydrate diet by exclusively eating the following foods: pasta made from refined flour, baked potato chips, soda, sugary cereals and low-fat candy bars. Eating this way is a *bad* idea. You will not derive the health benefits of a plant-based diet eating these foods. In experimental research, the health benefits of a high-carbohydrate diet come from eating the complex carbohydrates found in whole grains, fruits and vegetables. Eat an apple, a zucchini or a plate of brown rice topped with beans and other vegetables.

THE CHINA STUDY WEIGHS IN

With regard to weight loss, there are some surprising findings from the China Study that shed light on the weight loss debate. When we started the China Study, I thought that China had the opposite problem from that of the U.S. I had heard that China could not feed itself, that it was prone to famines and that there was not enough food for people to attain their full adult height. Very simply, there were not enough calories to go around. Although China has, during the last fifty years, had its share of nutritional problems, we were to learn that these views on calorie intake were dead wrong.

We wanted to compare the calorie consumption in China and America, but there was a catch. Chinese are more physically active than Americans, especially in rural areas, where manual labor is the norm. To compare an extremely active laborer with an average American would be misleading. It would be like comparing the amount of energy consumed by a manual laborer at hard work with the amount of energy consumed by an accountant. The vast difference in calorie intake sure to exist between these individuals would tell us nothing of value and only confirm that the manual laborer is more active.

To overcome this problem, we ranked the Chinese into five groups according to their levels of physical activity. After figuring out the calorie intakes of the *least active* Chinese, the equivalent of office workers, we then compared their calorie intake with the *average* American. What we found was astonishing.

Average calorie intake, per kilogram of body weight, was 30% *higher* among the least active Chinese than among average Americans. Yet, body weight was 20% *lower* (Chart 4.11). How can it be that even the least active Chinese consume more calories yet have no overweight problems? What is their secret?

CHART 4.11: CALORIE CONSUMPTION (KCAL/KG) AND BODY WEIGHT

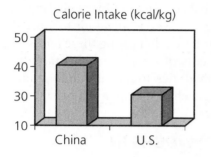

Calorie Intake (kcal/kg)

China   U.S.

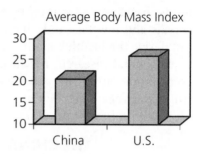

Average Body Mass Index

China   U.S.

There are two possible explanations for this apparent paradox. First, even the Chinese office workers are more physically active than average Americans. Anyone familiar with China knows that many office workers travel on bicycles. Thus, they consume more calories. Even so, we cannot tell how much of the extra calorie consumption was due to physical activity and how much to something else, perhaps their food.

We do know, however, that some people use the calories they consume differently from other people. We often say that "they have a higher rate of metabolism" or "it's in their genes." You know these people. They are the ones who seem to eat all they want and still not gain weight. Then there are most of us, who need to watch our calorie intake—or so we think. This is the simplistic interpretation.

I have a more comprehensive interpretation that is based on our own considerable research and on the studies of others. It goes like this. Provided that we aren't restricting our calorie intake, those of us who consume a high-fat, high-protein diet simply retain more calories than we need. We store these calories as body fat, perhaps weave it into our muscle fibers (we call it "marbling" in beef animals) and perhaps store it in the more obvious places, like our butt, our midsection or around our face and upper thighs.

Here's the clincher: only a small amount of calories needs to be retained by our body to cause significant change in body weight. For example, if we retain only an extra fifty calories per day, this can lead to an extra ten pounds per year. You may not think that this is a lot, but over a period of five years, that's an extra fifty pounds.

Some people would hear this and might be inclined to just eat fifty fewer calories per day. This, theoretically, could make a difference, but it is entirely impractical. It is impossible to keep track of daily calorie intake with such precision. Think about eating a meal at a restaurant. Do you know how many calories each meal has? What about the casserole you might fix? What about the steak you might buy? Do you know the number of calories they contain? Of course not.

The truth is this: despite any short-term caloric restriction regimes we may follow, our body, through many mechanisms, will ultimately choose how many calories to take in and what to do with them. Our attempts to limit calorie intake is short-lived and imprecise, whether we do it by limiting carbohydrates or fat.

The body employs a delicate balancing act and some very intricate mechanisms in deciding how to use the calories being consumed. When we treat our body well by eating the right foods, it knows how to partition the calories away from body fat and into the more desirable functions like keeping the body warm, running the body metabolism, supporting and encouraging physical activity or just disposing of any excess. The body is using multiple intricate mechanisms to decide how calories get used, stored or "burned off."

Consuming diets *high* in protein and fat transfers calories away from their conversion into body heat to their storage form—as body fat (unless severe calorie restriction is causing weight loss). In contrast, diets *low* in protein and fat cause calories to be "lost" as body heat. In research, we say that storing more calories as fat and losing less as heat means being more efficient. I bet that you would rather be a little more inefficient and convert it into body heat rather than body fat, right? Well, simply consuming a diet lower in fat and protein can do this.

This is what our China Study data show. Chinese consume more calories both because they are more physically active and because their consumption of low-fat, low-protein diets shifts conversion of these calories away from body fat to body heat. This is true even for the least physically active Chinese. Remember, it takes very little, only fifty calories a day, to change our storage of body fat and thus change our body weight.[58]

We saw the same phenomenon in our experimental animals fed the low-protein diets. They routinely consumed slightly more calories, gained less weight, disposed of the extra calories as body heat[59] and voluntarily exercised more,[60] while still having far less cancer than animals on standard diets. We found that calories were "burned" at a faster rate and transformed into body heat as more oxygen was consumed.[59]

Understanding that diet can cause small shifts in calorie metabolism that lead to big shifts in body weight is an important and useful concept. It means that there is an orderly process of controlling body weight over time that does work, as opposed to the disorderly process of crash diets that don't work. It also accounts for the frequent observations (discussed in chapter six) that people who consume low-protein, low-fat diets composed of whole plant foods have far less difficulty with weight problems, even if they consume the same, or even slightly more, total calories.

DIET AND BODY SIZE

We now know that eating a low-fat, low-protein diet high in complex carbohydrates from fruits and vegetables will help you lose weight. But what if you want to become bigger? A desire to be as big as possible is pervasive in most cultures. During the colonial period in Asia and Africa, Europeans even considered smaller people to be less civilized. Body size seems to be a mark of prowess, manliness and dominance.

Most people think they can be bigger and stronger by eating protein-rich animal-based foods. This belief stems from the idea that consuming protein (a.k.a. meat) is needed for physical power. This has been a common notion the world over for a long time. The Chinese have even officially recommended a higher-protein diet in order to encourage bigger athletes and to better compete in the Olympics. Animal-based foods have more protein, and this protein is considered to be of "higher quality." Animal protein enjoys the same reputation in a rapidly modernizing China as everywhere else.

There is, however, a problem with the idea that consuming animal-based foods is a good way of becoming bigger. The people who eat the most animal protein have the most heart disease, cancer and diabetes. In the China Study, for example, animal protein consumption was associated with taller and heavier[I] people, but was also associated with higher levels of total and bad cholesterol.[II] Furthermore, body weight, associated with animal protein intake,[I] was associated with more cancer[II-III] and more coronary heart disease.[II] It seems that being bigger, and presumably better, comes with very high costs. But might it be possible for us to achieve our full growth potential, while simultaneously minimizing disease risks?

Childhood growth rates were not measured in the China Study but adult height and weight were. This information proved surprising. Consuming more protein was associated with greater body size ([III] for men and [II] for women).[61] However, this effect was primarily attributed to *plant* protein, because it makes up 90% of the total Chinese protein intake. Animal protein consumption was indeed associated with greater body weight,[I] and consumption of protein-rich milk seemed to be effective as well.[II] But the good news is this: *Greater plant protein intake was closely linked to greater height[II] and body weight.*[II] Body growth is linked to protein in general and both animal and plant proteins are effective!

This means that individuals can achieve their genetic potential for growth and body size by consuming a plant-based diet. So why is it that people in developing nations, who consume little or no animal-based foods, are consistently smaller than Western people? This is because plant-based diets in poor areas of the world usually have insufficient variety, inadequate quantity and quality and are associated with poor public health conditions where childhood diseases are prevalent. Under these conditions, growth is stunted and people do not reach their genetic potential for adult body size. In the China Study, low adult height and weight were strongly associated with areas having high mortality rates for pulmonary tuberculosis,[III] parasitic diseases,[III] pneumonia ([III] for height), "intestinal obstruction"[III] and digestive diseases.[III]

These findings support the idea that body stature can be achieved by consuming a low-fat, plant-based diet, provided that public health conditions effectively control the diseases of poverty. Under these conditions, the diseases of affluence (heart disease, cancers, diabetes, etc.) can be simultaneously minimized.

The same low-animal protein, low-fat diet that helps prevent obesity also allows people to reach their full growth potential while working other wonders as well. It better regulates blood cholesterol and reduces heart disease and a variety of cancers.

What are the odds that all of these associations (and many others) favoring a plant-based diet are due to pure chance? It is extremely unlikely, to say the least. Such consistency of evidence across a broad range of associations is rare in scientific research. It points to a new worldview, a new paradigm. It defies the status quo, promises new health benefits and demands our attention.

CIRCLING BACK

In the beginning of my career, I concentrated on the biochemical processes of liver cancer. Chapter three delineates the decades-long laboratory work we did with experimental animals, work that passed the
requirements to be called "good science." The finding: casein, and very
likely all animal proteins, may be the most relevant cancer-causing substances that we consume. Adjusting the amount of dietary casein has
the power to turn on and turn off cancer growth, and to override the
cancer-producing effects of aflatoxin, a very potent Class IA carcinogen,
but even though these findings were substantially confirmed, they still
applied to experimental animals.

It was therefore with great anticipation that I looked to the China
Study for evidence on the causes of liver cancer in humans.[62]

Liver cancer rates are very high in rural China, exceptionally high in
some areas. Why was this? The primary culprit seemed to be chronic
infection with hepatitis B virus (HBV). On average, about 12–13% of our
study subjects were chronically infected with the virus. In some areas,
one-half of the people were chronically infected! To put this into perspective, only 0.2–0.3% of Americans are chronically infected with this virus.

But there's more. In addition to the virus being a cause of liver cancer
in China, it seems that diet also plays a key role. How do we know? The
blood cholesterol levels provided the main clue. Liver cancer is strongly
associated with increasing blood cholesterol,[III] and we already know
that animal-based foods are responsible for increases in cholesterol.

So, where does HBV fit in? The experimental mice studies gave a
good signal. In mice, HBV initiated the liver cancer but the cancer grew
in response to the feeding of higher levels of casein. In addition, blood
cholesterol also increased. These observations fit perfectly with our human findings. Individuals who are chronically infected with HBV and
who consume animal-based foods have high blood cholesterol and a
high rate of liver cancer. The virus provides the gun, and bad nutrition
pulls the trigger.

A very exciting story was taking shape, at least to my way of thinking. It was a story full of meaning and suggestive of important principles
that might apply to other diet and cancer associations. It also was a
story that had not been told to the public, and yet it was capable of saving lives. Eventually, it was a story that was leading to the idea that our
most powerful weapon against cancer is the food we eat every day.

So there we had it. The years of animal experiments illuminated profound biochemical principles and processes that greatly helped to explain the effect of nutrition on liver cancer. But now we could see that these processes were relevant for humans as well. People chronically infected with hepatitis B virus also had an increased risk of liver cancer. But our findings suggested those who were infected with the virus and who were simultaneously eating more animal-based foods had higher cholesterol levels and more liver cancer than those infected with the virus and not consuming animal-based foods. The experimental animal studies and the human studies made a perfect fit.

PULLING IT TOGETHER

Almost all of us in the United States will die of diseases of affluence. In our China Study, we saw that nutrition has a very strong effect on these diseases. Plant-based foods are linked to lower blood cholesterol; animal-based foods are linked to higher blood cholesterol. Animal-based foods are linked to higher breast cancer rates; plant-based foods are linked to lower rates. Fiber and antioxidants from plants are linked to a lower risk of cancers of the digestive tract. Plant-based diets and active lifestyles result in a healthy weight, yet permit people to become big and strong. Our study was comprehensive in design and comprehensive in its findings. From the labs of Virginia Tech and Cornell University to the far reaches of China, it seemed that science was painting a clear, consistent picture: we can minimize our risk of contracting deadly diseases just by eating the right food.

When we first started this project we encountered significant resistance from some people. One of my colleagues at Cornell, who had been involved in the early planning of the China Study, got quite heated in one of our meetings. I had put forth the idea of investigating how lots of dietary factors, some known but many unknown, work together to cause disease. Thus we had to measure lots of factors, regardless of whether or not they were justified by prior research. If that was what we intended to do, he said he wanted nothing to do with such a "shotgun" approach.

This colleague was expressing a view that was more in line with mainstream scientific thought than with my idea. He and like-minded colleagues think that science is best done when investigating single— mostly known—factors in isolation. An array of largely unspecified factors doesn't show anything, they say. It's okay to measure the specific effect of, say, selenium on breast cancer, but it's not okay to measure multiple nutritional conditions in the same study, in the hope of identifying important dietary patterns.

I prefer the broader picture, for we are investigating the incredible complexities and subtleties of nature itself. I wanted to investigate how dietary patterns related to disease, now the most important point of this book. *Everything in food works together to create health or disease.* The more we think that a single chemical characterizes a whole food, the more we stray into idiocy. As we shall see in Part IV of this book, this way of thinking has generated a lot of poor science.

So I say we need more, not less, of the "shotgun approach." We need more thought about overall dietary patterns and whole foods. Does this mean that I think the shotgun approach is the only way to do research? Of course not. Do I think that the China Study findings constitute absolute scientific proof? Of course not. Does it provide enough information to inform some practical decision-making? Absolutely.

An impressive and informative web of information was emerging from this study. But does every potential strand (or association) in this mammoth study fit perfectly into this web of information? No. Although most statistically significant strands readily fit into the web, there were a few surprises. Most, but not all, have since been explained.

Some associations observed in the China Study, at first glance, were at odds with what might have been expected from Western experience. I've had to use care in separating unusual findings that could be due to chance and experimental insufficiency from those that truly offered new insights into our old ways of thinking. As I mentioned earlier, the range of blood cholesterol levels in rural China was a surprise. At the time when the China Study was begun, a blood cholesterol range of 200–300 milligrams per deciliter (mg/dL) was considered normal, and lower levels were suspect. In fact, some in the scientific and medical communities considered cholesterol levels lower than 150 mg/dL to be dangerous. In fact, my own cholesterol was 260 mg/dL in the late 1970s, not unlike other members of my immediate family. The doctor told me it was "fine, just average."

But when we measured the blood cholesterol levels in China, we were shocked. They ranged from 70–170 mg/dL! Their high was our low, and their low was off the chart you might find in your doctor's office! It became obvious that our idea of "normal" values (or ranges) only applies to Western subjects consuming the Western diet. It so happens, for example, that our "normal" cholesterol levels present a significant risk for heart disease. Sadly, it's also "normal" to have heart disease in America. Over the years, standards have been established that are consistent with what we see in the West. We too often have come to the view that U.S. values are "normal" because we have a tendency to believe that the Western experience is likely to be right.

At the end of the day, the strength and consistency of the majority of the evidence is enough to draw valid conclusions. Namely, whole, plant-based foods are beneficial, and animal-based foods are not. Few other dietary choices, if any, can offer the incredible benefits of looking good, growing tall and avoiding the vast majority or premature diseases in our culture.

The China Study was an important milestone in my thinking. Standing alone, it does not *prove* that diet *causes* disease. Absolute proof in science is nearly unattainable. Instead, a theory is proposed and debated until the weight of the evidence is so overwhelming that everyone commonly accepts that the theory is most likely true. In the case of diet and disease, the China Study adds a lot of weight to the evidence. Its experimental features (multiple diet, disease and lifestyle characteristics, and unusual range of dietary experience, a good means of measuring data quality) provided an unparalleled opportunity to expand our thinking about diet and disease in ways that previously were not available. It was a study that was like a flashlight that illuminated a path that I had never fully seen before.

The results of this study, in addition to a mountain of supporting research, some of it my own and some of it from other scientists, convinced me to turn my dietary lifestyle around. I stopped eating meat fifteen years ago, and I stopped eating almost all animal-based foods, including dairy, within the past six to eight years, except on very rare occasions. My cholesterol has dropped, even as I've aged; I am more physically fit now than when I was twenty-five; and I am forty-five pounds lighter now than I was when I was thirty years old. I am now at an ideal weight for my height. My family has also adopted this way of eating, thanks in large part to my wife Karen, who has managed to create an entire new dietary lifestyle that is attractive, tasty and healthy. This has all been done for health reasons, the result of my research findings telling me to wake up. From a boyhood of drinking at least two quarts of milk a day to an early professional career of scoffing at vegetarians, I have taken an unusual turn in my life.

However, it has been more than my own research that has changed my life. Over the years, I have gone well beyond our own research findings to see what other researchers have found regarding diet and health. As our research findings expanded from the specific to the general, the picture has continued to enlarge. We now can look at the work of other scientists to put my findings into a larger context. As you shall see, it is nothing short of astonishing.

Part II
DISEASES OF AFFLUENCE

HERE IN AMERICA, we are affluent, and we die certain deaths because of it. We eat like feasting kings and queens every day of the week, and it kills us. You probably know people who suffer from heart disease, cancer, stroke, Alzheimer's, obesity or diabetes. There's a good chance that you yourself suffer from one of these problems, or that one of these diseases runs in your family. As we have seen, these diseases are relatively unknown in traditional cultures that subsist mostly on whole plant foods, as in rural China. But these ailments arrive when a traditional culture starts accumulating wealth and starts eating more and more meat, dairy and refined plant products (like crackers, cookies and soda).

In public lectures, I start my presentation by telling the audience my personal story, just as I have done in this book. Invariably, I get a question at the end of the lecture from someone who wants to know more about diet and a specific disease of affluence. Chances are that you yourself also have a question about a specific disease. Chances are, too, that this specific disease is a disease of affluence, because that's what we die of here in America.

You might be surprised to know that the disease that interests you has much in common with other diseases of affluence, especially when it comes to nutrition. There is no such thing as a special diet for cancer and a different, equally special diet for heart disease. The evidence now amassed from researchers around the world shows that the same diet that is good for the prevention of cancer is also good for the prevention of heart disease, as well as obesity, diabetes, cataracts, macular degeneration, Alzheimer's, cognitive dysfunction, multiple sclerosis, osteoporosis and other diseases. Furthermore, this diet can only benefit everyone, regardless of his or her genes or personal dispositions.

All of these diseases, and others, spring forth from the same influence: an unhealthy, largely toxic diet and lifestyle that has an excess of sickness-promoting factors and a deficiency of health-promoting factors. In other words, the Western diet. Conversely, there is one diet to counteract all of these diseases: a whole foods, plant-based diet.

The following chapters are organized by disease, or disease grouping. Each chapter contains evidence showing how food relates to each disease. As you go through each chapter, you will begin to see the breadth and depth of the astonishing scientific argument favoring a whole foods, plant-based diet. For me, the consistency of evidence regarding such a disparate group of diseases has been the most convincing aspect of this argument. When a whole foods, plant-based diet is demonstrably beneficial for such a wide variety of diseases, is it possible that humans were meant to consume any other diet? I say no, and I think you'll agree.

America and most other Western nations have gotten it wrong when it comes to diet and health, and we have paid a grave price. We are sick, overweight and confused. As I have moved on from the laboratory studies and the China Study and encountered the information discussed in Part II, I have become overwhelmed. I have come to realize that some of our most revered conventions are wrong and real health has been grossly obscured. Most unfortunately, the unsuspecting public has paid the ultimate price. In large measure, this book is my effort to right these wrongs. As you will come to see in the following chapters, from heart disease to cancer, and from obesity to blindness, there is a better path to optimal health.

5

Broken Hearts

PUT YOUR HAND on your chest and feel your heart beat. Now put your hand where you can feel your pulse. That pulse is the signature of your being. Your heart, creating that pulse, is working for you every minute of the day, every day of the year, and every year of your entire life. If you live an average lifetime, your heart will beat about 3 billion times.[1]

Now take a moment to realize that during the time it took you to read the above paragraph an artery in the heart of roughly one American clogged up, cut off blood flow and started a rapid process of tissue and cell death. This process is better known, of course, as a heart attack. By the time you finish reading this page, four Americans will have had a heart attack, and another four will have fallen prey to stroke or heart failure.[2] Over the next twenty-four hours, 3,000 Americans will have heart attacks,[2] roughly the same number of people who perished in the terrorist attacks of September 11, 2001.

The heart is the centerpiece of life and, more often than not in America, it is the centerpiece of death. Malfunction of the heart and/or circulation system will kill 40% of Americans,[3] more than those killed by any other injury or ailment, including cancer. Heart disease has been our number one cause of death for almost one hundred years.[4] This disease does not recognize gender or race boundaries; all are affected. If you were to ask most women what disease poses the greatest risk to them, heart disease or breast cancer, many women would undoubtedly say breast cancer. But they would be wrong. Women's death rate from heart disease is *eight times higher* than their death rate from breast cancer.[5, 6]

If there is an "American" game, it is baseball; an "American" dessert, apple pie. If there is an "American" disease, it is heart disease.

EVERYONE'S DOING IT

In 1950, Judy Holliday could be seen on the big screen, Ben Hogan dominated the world of golf, the musical *South Pacific* won big at the Tony Awards and on June 25, North Korea invaded South Korea. The American administration was taken aback but responded quickly. Within days, President Truman sent in troops on the ground and bombers overhead to push back the North Korean army. Three years later, in July of 1953, a formal cease-fire agreement had been signed and the Korean War was over. During this period of time, over 30,000 American soldiers were killed in battle.

At the end of the war, a landmark scientific study was reported in the *Journal of the American Medical Association*. Military medical investigators had examined the hearts of 300 male soldiers killed in action in Korea. The soldiers, at an average age of twenty-two years, had never been diagnosed with heart problems. In dissecting these hearts, researchers found startling evidence of disease in an exceptional number of cases. *Fully 77.3% of the hearts they examined had "gross evidence" of heart disease.*[7] (In this instance, "gross" means large.)

That number, 77.3%, is startling. Coming at a time when our number one killer was still shrouded in mystery, the research clearly demonstrated that heart disease develops over an entire lifetime. Furthermore, almost everyone was susceptible! These soldiers were not couch-potato slouches; they were in top condition in the prime of their physical lives. Since that time, several other studies have confirmed that heart disease is pervasive in young Americans.[8]

THE HEART ATTACK

But what is heart disease? One of the key components is plaque. Plaque is a greasy layer of proteins, fats (including cholesterol), immune system cells and other components that accumulate on the inner walls of the coronary arteries. I have heard one surgeon say that if you wipe your finger on a plaque-covered artery, it has the same feel as wiping your finger across a warm cheesecake. If you have plaque building up in your coronary arteries, you have some degree of heart disease. Of the autopsied soldiers in Korea, one out of twenty diseased men had so much plaque that 90% of an artery was blocked.[7] That's like putting a kink in a garden hose and watering a desperately dry garden with the resulting trickle of water!

Why hadn't these soldiers had a heart attack already? After all, only 10% of the artery was open. How could that be enough? It turns out that if the plaque on the inner wall of the artery accumulates slowly, over several years, blood flow has time to adjust. Think of blood flowing through your artery as a raging river. If you put a few stones on the sides of a river every day over a period of years, like plaque accumulating on the walls of the artery, the water will find another way to get to where it wants to be. Maybe the river will form several smaller streams over the stones. Perhaps the river will go under the stones forming tiny tunnels, or maybe the water will flow through small side streams, taking a new route altogether. These new tiny passageways around or through the stones are called "collaterals." The same thing happens in the heart. If plaque accumulates over a period of several years there will be enough collateral development that blood can still travel throughout the heart. However, too much plaque buildup can cause severe blood restriction, and debilitating chest pain, or angina, can result. But this buildup only rarely leads to heart attacks.[9, 10]

So what leads to heart attacks? It turns out that it's the less severe accumulations of plaque, blocking under 50% of the artery, that often cause heart attacks.[11] These accumulations each have a layer of cells, called the cap, which separates the core of the plaque from the blood flowing by. In the dangerous plaques, the cap is weak and thin. Consequently, as blood rushes by, it can erode the cap until it ruptures. When the cap ruptures, the core contents of the plaque mix with the blood. The blood then begins clotting around the site of rupture. The clot grows and can quickly block off the entire artery. When the artery becomes blocked over such a short period of time, there is little chance for collateral blood flow to develop. When this happens, blood flow downstream of the rupture is severely reduced and the heart muscles don't get the oxygen they require. At this point, as heart muscle cells start to die, heart pumping mechanisms begin to fail, and the person may feel a crushing pain in the chest, or a searing pain down into an arm and up into the neck and jaw. In short, the victim starts to die. This is the process behind most of the 1.1 million heart attacks that occur in America every year. One out of three people who have a heart attack will die from it.[9, 10]

We now know that the small to medium accumulation of plaque, the plaque that blocks less than 50% of the artery, is the most deadly.[11, 12]

So how can we predict the timing of heart attacks? Unfortunately, with existing technologies, we can't. We can't know which plaque will rupture, when, or how severe it might be. What we do know, however, is our relative *risk* for having a heart attack. What once was a mysterious death, which claimed people in their most productive years, has been "demystified" by science. No study has been more influential than that of the Framingham Heart Study.

FRAMINGHAM

After World War II, the National Heart Institute[13] was created with a modest budget[4] and a difficult mission. Scientists knew that the greasy plaques that lined the arteries of diseased hearts were composed of cholesterol, phospholipids and fatty acids,[14] but they didn't know why these lesions developed, how they developed or exactly how they led to heart attacks. In the search for answers, the National Heart Institute decided to follow a population over several years, to keep detailed medical records of everybody in the population and to see who got heart disease and who didn't. The scientists headed to Framingham, Massachusetts.

Located just outside of Boston, Framingham is steeped in American history. European settlers first inhabited the land in the seventeenth century. Over the years the town has had supporting roles in the Revolutionary War, the Salem Witch Trials and the abolition movement. More recently, in 1948, the town assumed its most famous role. Over 5,000 residents of Framingham, both male and female, agreed to be poked and prodded by scientists over the years so that we might learn something about heart disease.

And learn something we did. By watching who got heart disease and who didn't, and comparing their medical records, the Framingham Heart Study developed the concept of risk factors such as cholesterol, blood pressure, physical activity, cigarette smoking and obesity. Because of the Framingham Study, we now know that these risk factors play a prominent role in the causation of heart disease. Doctors have for years used a Framingham prediction model to tell who is at high risk for heart disease and who is not. Over 1,000 scientific papers have been published from this study, and the study continues to this day, having now studied four generations of Framingham residents.

The shining jewel of the Framingham Study is its findings on blood cholesterol. In 1961, they convincingly showed a strong correlation between high blood cholesterol and heart disease. Researchers noted that men with cholesterol levels "over 244 mg/dL (milligrams per deciliter) have more than three times the incidence of CHD (coronary heart disease) as do those with cholesterol levels less than 210 mg/dL."[15] The contentious question of whether blood cholesterol levels could predict heart disease was laid to rest. Cholesterol levels do make a difference. In this same paper, high blood pressure was also demonstrated to be an important risk factor for heart disease.

The importance given to risk factors signaled a conceptual revolution. When this study was started, most doctors believed that heart disease was an inevitable "wearing down" of the body, and we could do little about it. Our hearts were like car engines; as we got older, the parts didn't work as well and sometimes gave out. By demonstrating that we could see the disease in advance by measuring risk factors, the idea of preventing heart disease suddenly had validity. Researchers wrote, " . . . it appears that a preventive program is clearly necessary."[15] Simply lower the risk factors, such as blood cholesterol and blood pressure, and you lower the risk of heart disease.

In modern-day America cholesterol and blood pressure are household terms. We spend over 30 billion dollars a year on drugs to control these risk factors and other aspects of cardiovascular disease.[2] Almost everyone now knows that he or she can work to prevent a heart attack by keeping his or her risk factors at the right levels. This awareness is only about fifty years old and due in large measure to the scientists and subjects of the Framingham Heart Study.

OUTSIDE OUR BORDERS

Framingham is the most well-known heart study ever done, but it is merely one part of an enormous body of research conducted in this country over the past sixty years. Early research led to the alarming conclusion that we have some of the highest rates of heart disease in the world. One study published in 1959 compared the coronary heart disease death rates in twenty different countries (Chart 5.1).[16]

These studies were examining Westernized societies. If we look at more traditional societies, we tend to see even more striking disparities in the incidence of heart disease. The Papua New Guinea Highlanders, for example, pop up in research quite a bit because heart disease is rare in their society.[17] Remember, for example, how low the rate of heart disease was in rural China. American men died from heart disease at a rate almost seventeen times higher than their Chinese counterparts.[18]

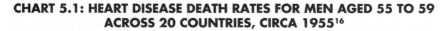

CHART 5.1: HEART DISEASE DEATH RATES FOR MEN AGED 55 TO 59 ACROSS 20 COUNTRIES, CIRCA 1955[16]

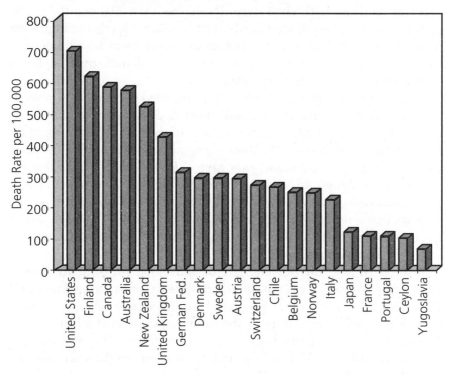

Why were we succumbing to heart disease in the sixties and seventies, when much of the world was relatively unaffected?

Quite simply, it was a case of death by food. The cultures that have lower heart disease rates eat less saturated fat and animal protein and more whole grains, fruits and vegetables. In other words, they subsist mostly on plant foods while we subsist mostly on animal foods.

But might it be that the genetics of one group might just make them more susceptible to heart disease? We know that this is not the case, because within a group with the same genetic heritage, a similar relationship between diet and disease is seen. For example, Japanese men who live in Hawaii or California have a much higher blood cholesterol level and incidence of coronary heart disease than Japanese men living in Japan.[19, 20]

The cause is clearly environmental, as most of these people have the same genetic heritage. Smoking habits are not the cause because men in Japan, who were more likely to smoke, still had less coronary heart disease than the Japanese Americans.[19] The researchers pointed to diet, writing that blood cholesterol increased "with dietary intake of saturated fat, animal protein and dietary cholesterol." On the flip side, blood cholesterol "was negatively associated with complex carbohydrate intake...."[20] In simple terms, animal foods were linked to higher blood cholesterol; plant foods were linked to lower blood cholesterol.

This research clearly implicated diet as one possible cause of heart disease. Furthermore, the early results were painting a consistent picture: the more saturated fat and cholesterol (as indicators of animal food consumption) people eat, the higher their risk for getting heart disease. And as other cultures have come to eat more like us, they also have seen their rates of heart disease skyrocket. In more recent times, several countries have now come to have a higher death rate from heart disease than America.

RESEARCH AHEAD OF ITS TIME

So now we know what heart disease is and what factors determine our risk for it, but what do we do once the disease is upon us? When the Framingham Heart Study was just beginning, there were already doctors who were trying to figure out how to treat heart disease, rather than just prevent it. In many ways, these investigators were ahead of their time because their interventions, which were the most innovative, successful treatment programs at the time, utilized the least advanced technology available: the knife and fork.

These doctors noticed the ongoing research at the time and made some common-sense connections. They realized that[21]:

- excess fat and cholesterol consumption caused atherosclerosis (the hardening of the arteries and the accumulation of plaque) in experimental animals
- eating cholesterol in food caused a rise in cholesterol in the blood
- high blood cholesterol might predict and/or cause heart disease
- most of the world's population didn't have heart disease, and these heart disease-free cultures had radically different dietary patterns, consuming less fat and cholesterol

So they decided to try to alter heart disease in their patients by having them eat less fat and cholesterol.

One of the most progressive doctors was Dr. Lester Morrison of Los

Angeles. He started a study in 1946 (two years before the Framingham Study) to "determine the relationship of dietary fat intake to the incidence of atherosclerosis."[22] In his study he instructed fifty heart attack survivors to maintain their normal diet and fifty different heart attack survivors to consume an experimental diet.

In the experimental diet group he reduced the consumption of fat and cholesterol. One of his published sample menus allowed the patient to have only a small amount of meat two times a day: two ounces of "cold roast lamb, lean, with mint jelly" for lunch, and another two ounces of "lean meats" for dinner.[22] Even if you loved cold roast lamb with mint jelly, you weren't allowed to eat much of it. In fact, the list of prohibited foods in the experimental diet was fairly long and included cream soups, pork, fat meats, animal fats, whole milk, cream, butter, egg yolks and breads and desserts made with butter, whole eggs and whole milk.[22]

Did this progressive diet accomplish anything? After eight years, only twelve of fifty people eating their normal American diet were alive (24%). In the diet group, twenty-eight people were still alive (56%), almost two and one-half times the amount of survivors in the control group. After twelve years, every single patient in the control group was dead. In the diet group, however, nineteen people were still alive, a survival rate of 38%.[22] While it was unfortunate that so many people in the dietary group still died, it was clear that they were staving off their disease by eating moderately less animal foods and moderately more plant foods (see Chart 5.2).

CHART 5.2: SURVIVAL RATE OF DR. MORRISON'S PATIENTS

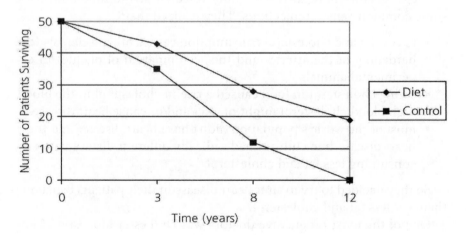

In 1946, when this study began, most scientists believed that heart disease was an inevitable part of aging, and nothing much could be done about it. While Morrison didn't cure heart disease, he proved that something as simple as diet could significantly alter its course, even when the disease is so advanced that it has already caused a heart attack.

Another research group proved much the same thing at about that time. A group of doctors in Northern California took a larger group of patients with advanced heart disease and put them on a low-fat, low-cholesterol diet. These doctors found that the patients who ate the low-fat, low-cholesterol diet died at a rate *four times lower* than patients who didn't follow the diet.[23]

It was now clear that there was hope. Heart disease wasn't the inevitable result of old age, and even when a person had advanced disease, a low-fat, low-cholesterol diet could significantly prolong his or her life. This was a remarkable advance in our understanding of the number one killer in America. Furthermore, this new understanding made diet and other environmental factors the centerpieces of heart disease. Any discussion of diet, however, was narrowly focused on fat and cholesterol. These two isolated food components became the bad guys.

We now know that the attention paid to fat and cholesterol was misguided. The possibility that no one wanted to consider was that fat and cholesterol were merely indicators of animal food intake. For example, look at the relationship between animal protein consumption and heart disease death in men aged fifty-five to fifty-nine across twenty different countries in Chart 5.3.[16]

This study suggests that the more animal protein you eat, the more heart disease you have. In addition, dozens of experimental studies show that feeding rats, rabbits and pigs animal protein (e.g., casein) dramatically raises cholesterol levels, whereas plant protein (e.g., soy protein) dramatically lowers cholesterol levels.[24] Studies in humans not only mirror these findings, but show that eating plant protein has even greater power to lower cholesterol levels than reducing fat or cholesterol intake.[25]

While some of these studies implicating animal protein were conducted in the past thirty years, others were published well over fifty years ago when the health world was first beginning to discuss diet and heart disease. Yet somehow animal protein has remained in the shadows while saturated fat and cholesterol have taken the brunt of the criticism. These three nutrients (fat, animal protein and cholesterol) characterize

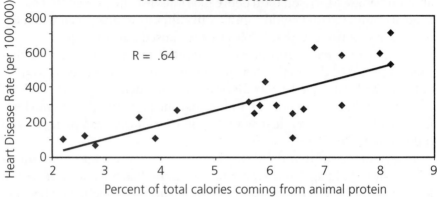

CHART 5.3: HEART DISEASE DEATH RATES FOR MEN AGED 55 TO 59 YEARS AND ANIMAL PROTEIN CONSUMPTION ACROSS 20 COUNTRIES[16]

animal-based food in general. So isn't it perfectly reasonable to wonder whether animal-based food, and not just these isolated nutrients, causes heart disease?

Of course, no one pointed a finger at animal-based foods in general. It would have led immediately to professional isolation and ridicule (for reasons discussed in Part IV). These were contentious times in the nutritional world. A conceptual revolution was taking place, and a lot of people didn't like it. Even talking about diet was too much for many scientists. Preventing heart disease by diet was a threatening idea because it implied that something about the good old meaty American diet was so bad for us that it was destroying our hearts. The status quo boys didn't like it.

One status quo scientist had a good time making fun of people who appeared to have a low risk of heart disease. In 1960, he wrote the following piece of "humor" to mock the then-recent findings[26]:

Thumbnail Sketch of the Man Least Likely to Have Coronary Heart Disease:

An effeminate municipal worker or embalmer, completely lacking in physical and mental alertness and without drive, ambition or competitive spirit who has never attempted to meet a deadline of any kind. A man with poor appetite, subsisting on fruit and vegetables laced with corn and whale oils, detesting tobacco, spurning ownership of radio, TV or motor car, with full head of hair and scrawny and un-athletic in appearance, yet constantly straining his puny muscles by exercise; low in income, B.P. (blood pressure), blood sugar, uric acid and cholesterol, who has been taking nicotinic acid, pyridoxine and long term anticoagulant therapy ever since his prophylactic castration.

The author of this passage might just as well have said, "Only REAL men have heart disease." Also notice how a diet of fruits and vegetables is described as "poor" even though the author suggests that this diet is eaten by those people who are least likely to have heart disease. The unfortunate association of meat with physical ability, general manliness, sexual identity and economic wealth all cloud how the status quo scientists viewed food, regardless of the health evidence. This view had been passed down from the early protein pioneers described in chapter two.

Perhaps this author should have met a friend of mine, Chris Campbell (no relation). Chris is a two-time NCAA Division 1 wrestling champion, three-time U.S. Senior wrestling champion, two-time Olympic wrestler and Cornell Law School graduate. At the age of thirty-seven he became the oldest American ever to win an Olympic medal in wrestling, weighing in at 198 pounds. Chris Campbell is a vegetarian. As a man not likely to have heart disease, I think he might disagree with the characterization above.

The battle between the status quo and the dietary prevention camp was intense. I remember attending a lecture at Cornell University during the late 1950s when a famous researcher, Ancel Keys, came to talk about preventing heart disease by diet. Some scientists in the audience just shook their heads in disbelief, saying diet can't possibly affect heart disease. In those first decades of heart disease research, a heated, personal battle flared, and open-mindedness was the first casualty.

RECENT HISTORY

Today, this epic battle between defenders of the status quo and advocates of diet is as strong as ever. But there have been significant changes in the landscape of heart disease. How far have we come, and how have we proceeded to fight this disease? Mostly, the status quo has been protected. Despite the potential of diet and disease prevention, most of the attention given to heart disease has been on mechanical and chemical intervention for those people who have advanced disease. Diet has been pushed aside. Surgery, drugs, electronic devices and new diagnostic tools have stolen the spotlight.

We now have coronary bypass surgery, where a healthy artery is "pasted" over a diseased artery, thereby bypassing the most dangerous plaque on the artery. The ultimate surgery, of course, is the heart transplant, which even utilizes an artificial heart on occasion. We also have a procedure that doesn't require cracking the chest plate open, called coronary angioplasty, where a small balloon is inflated in a narrowed, diseased artery, squishing the plaque back against the wall, opening up the passage for increased blood flow. We have defibrillators to revive hearts, pacemakers and precise imaging techniques so that we can observe individual arteries without having to expose the heart.

The past fifty years have truly been a celebration of chemicals and technology (as opposed to diet and prevention). In summarizing the initial widespread research on heart disease, one doctor recently highlighted the mechanical:

> It was hoped that the strength of science and engineering developed after World War II could be applied to this battle [against heart disease].... The enormous advances in mechanical engineering and electronics that had been stimulated by the war seemed to lend themselves particularly well to the study of the cardiovascular system....[4]

Some great advances have been made, to be sure, which may account for the fact that our death rate from heart disease is a full 58% lower than what it was in 1950.[2] A 58% reduction in the death rate seems a great victory for chemicals and technology. One of the greatest strides has come from better emergency room treatment of heart attack victims. In 1970, if you were older than sixty-five years, had a heart attack and were lucky enough to make it to the hospital alive, you had a 38% chance of dying. Today, if you make it to the hospital alive, you only have a 15% chance of dying. The hospital's emergency response is much better, and consequently huge numbers of lives are being spared.[2]

In addition, the number of people smoking has steadily been decreasing,[27, 28] which in turn lowers our death rate from heart disease. Between hospital advances, mechanical devices, drug discoveries, lower smoking rates and more surgical options, there clearly seems to be much to cheer about. We've made progress, so it seems.

Or have we?

After all, heart disease is still our number one cause of death. Every twenty-four hours, almost 2,000 Americans will die from this disease.[2] For all the advances, there are a huge number of people still succumbing to broken hearts.

In fact, the incidence rate (not death rate) for heart disease[29] is about the same as it was in the early 1970s.[2] In other words, while we don't die as much from heart disease, we still get it as often as we used to. It seems that we simply have gotten slightly better at postponing death from heart disease, but *we have done nothing to stop the rate at which our hearts become diseased.*

SURGERY: THE PHANTOM SAVIOR

The mechanical interventions that we use in this country are much less effective than most people realize. Bypass surgery has become particularly popular. As many as 380,000 bypass operations were performed in 1990,[30] meaning that about 1 out of 750 Americans underwent this extreme surgery. During the operation, the patient's chest is split open, blood flow is rerouted by a series of clamps, pumps and machines, and a leg vein or chest artery is cut out and sewn over a diseased part of the heart, thereby allowing blood to bypass the most clogged arteries.

The costs are enormous. More than one of every fifty elective patients will die because of complications[31] during the $46,000 procedure.[32] Other side effects include heart attack, respiratory complications, bleeding complications, infection, high blood pressure and stroke. When the vessels around the heart are clamped shut during the operation, plaque breaks off of the inner walls. Blood then carries this debris to the brain, where it causes numerous "mini" strokes. Researchers have compared the intellectual capabilities of patients before and after the operation, and found that a stunning 79% of patients "showed impairment in some aspect of cognitive function" seven days after the operation.[33]

Why do we put ourselves through this? The most pronounced benefit of this procedure is relief of angina, or chest pain. About 70–80% of patients who undergo bypass surgery remain free of this crippling chest pain for one year.[34] *But this benefit doesn't last.* Within three years of the operation, up to one-third of patients will suffer from chest pain again.[35] Within ten years half of the bypass patients will have died, had a heart attack or had their chest pain return.[36] Long-term studies indicate that only certain subsets of heart disease patients live longer because of their bypass operation.[12] Furthermore, these studies demonstrate that *those patients who undergo bypass operation do not have fewer heart attacks than those who do not have surgery.*[12]

Remember which plaque buildups cause heart attacks? The deadly buildups are the smaller, less stable plaques that tend to rupture. The bypass operation, however, is targeted to the largest, most visible plaques, which may be responsible for chest pain, but not for heart attacks.

Angioplasty is a similar story. The procedure is expensive and carries significant risks. After identifying blockages in a coronary artery, a balloon is inserted into the artery and inflated. It pushes the plaque back against the vessel, thereby allowing more blood to flow. Roughly one out of sixteen patients will experience an "abrupt vessel closure" during the procedure, which can lead to death, heart attack or an emergency bypass operation.[37] Assuming that doesn't happen, there is still a good chance that the procedure will fail. Within four months after the procedure, 40% of the arteries that were "squished" open will close up again, effectively nullifying the procedure.[38] Nonetheless, barring these unfavorable outcomes, angioplasty does a good job of providing temporary relief of chest pain. Of course, angioplasty does little to treat the small blockages that are most likely to lead to heart attacks.

So, upon closer examination, our seemingly beneficent mechanical advances in the field of heart disease are severely disappointing. *Bypass surgery and angioplasty do not address the cause of heart disease, prevent heart attacks or extend the lives of any but the sickest heart disease patients.*

What's going on here? Despite the positive public relations surrounding the past fifty years of heart disease research, we must ask ourselves: are we winning this war? Maybe we should ask ourselves what we might do differently. For example, whatever happened to the dietary lessons learned fifty years ago? Whatever happened to the dietary treatments discovered by Dr. Lester Morrison, as discussed earlier?

Those discoveries largely faded away. I only learned about this 1940s and 1950s research in recent years. I am bewildered because the professionals I heard during my graduate student days in the late 1950s and early 1960s vigorously denied that any such work was being done or even being contemplated. In the meanwhile, America's eating habits have only gotten worse. According to the U.S. Department of Agriculture, we consume significantly more meat and added fat than we did thirty years ago.[39] Clearly we are not moving in the right direction.

As this information has resurfaced in the past two decades, the fight against the status quo has been heating up again. A few rare doctors are proving that there is a better way to defeat heart disease. They are demonstrating revolutionary success, using the most simple of all treatments: food.

DR. CALDWELL B. ESSELSTYN, JR.

If you were to guess the location of the best cardiac care center in the country, maybe the world, what city would you name? New York? Los Angeles? Chicago? A city in Florida, perhaps, near elderly people? As it turns out, the best medical center for cardiac care is located in Cleveland, Ohio, according to *US News and World Report*. Patients fly in to the Cleveland Clinic from all over the world for the most advanced heart treatment available, administered by prestigious doctors.

One of the doctors at the Clinic, Dr. Caldwell B. Esselstyn, Jr. has quite a resume. As a student at Yale University, Dr. Esselstyn rowed in the 1956 Olympics, winning a gold medal. After being trained at the Cleveland Clinic, he went on to earn the Bronze Star as an army surgeon in the Vietnam War. He then became a highly successful doctor at one of the top medical institutions in the world, the Cleveland Clinic, where he was president of the staff, member of the Board of Governors, chairman of the Breast Cancer Task Force and head of the Section of Thyroid and Parathyroid Surgery. Having published over 100 scientific papers, Dr. Esselstyn was named one of the best doctors in America in 1994–1995.[40] From knowing this man personally, I get the feeling that he has excelled at virtually everything he has done in his life. He reached the pinnacle of success in his professional and personal life, and did it with grace and humility.

The quality I find most appealing about Dr. Esselstyn, however, is not his resume or awards; it is his principled search for the truth. Dr. Esselstyn has had the courage to take on the establishment. For the Second National Conference on Lipids in the Elimination and Prevention of Coronary Artery Disease (which he organized and in which he kindly asked me to participate) Dr. Esselstyn wrote:

> Eleven years into my career as a surgeon, I became disillusioned with the treatment paradigm of U.S. medicine in cancer and heart disease. Little had changed in 100 years in the management of cancer, and in neither heart disease nor cancer was there a serious

effort at prevention. I found the epidemiology of these diseases provocative, however: Three-quarters of the humans on this planet had no heart disease, a fact strongly associated with diet.[41]

Dr. Esselstyn started to reexamine the standard medical practice. "Aware that medical, angiographic and surgical interventions were treating only the symptoms of heart disease and believing that a fundamentally different approach to treatment was necessary," Dr. Esselstyn decided to test the effects of a whole foods, plant-based diet on people with established coronary disease.[42] By using a minimal amount of cholesterol-lowering medication and a very low-fat, plant-based diet, he has gotten the most spectacular results ever recorded in the treatment of heart disease.[42, 43]

In 1985, Dr. Esselstyn began his study with the primary goal of reducing his patients' blood cholesterol to below 150 mg/dL. He asked each patient to record everything he or she ate in a food diary. Every two weeks, for the next five years, Dr. Esselstyn met with his patients to discuss the process, administer blood tests and record blood pressure and weight. He followed up this daytime meeting with an evening telephone call to report the results of the blood tests and further discuss how the diet was working. In addition, all of his patients met together a few times a year to talk about the program, socialize and exchange helpful information. In other words, Dr. Esselstyn was diligent, involved, supportive and compassionately stern on a personal level with his patients.

The diet they, including Dr. Esselstyn and his wife Ann, followed was free of all added fat and almost all animal products. Dr. Esselstyn and his colleagues report, "[Participants] were to avoid oils, meat, fish, fowl and dairy products, except for skim milk and nonfat yogurt."[42] About five years into the program, Dr. Esselstyn recommended to his patients that they stop consuming any skim milk and yogurt, as well.

Five of his patients dropped out of the study within the first two years; that left eighteen. These eighteen patients originally had come to Dr. Esselstyn with severe disease. *Within the eight years leading up to the study, these eighteen people had suffered through forty-nine coronary events,* including angina, bypass surgery, heart attacks, strokes and angioplasty. These were not healthy hearts. One might imagine that they were motivated to join the study by the panic created when premature death is near.[42, 43]

These eighteen patients achieved remarkable success. At the start of the study, the patients' average cholesterol level was 246 mg/dL. *During the course of the study, the average cholesterol was 132 mg/dL, well below the 150 mg/dL target!*[43] Their levels of "bad" LDL cholesterol dropped just as dramatically.[42] In the end, though, the most impressive result was not the blood cholesterol levels, but how many coronary events occurred since the start of the study.

In the following eleven years, there was exactly ONE coronary event among the eighteen patients who followed the diet. That one event was from a patient who strayed from the diet for two years. After straying, the patient consequently experienced clinical chest pain (angina) and then resumed a healthy plant-based diet. The patient eliminated his angina, and has not experienced any further events.[43]

Not only has the disease in these patients been stopped, it has even been reversed. *Seventy percent of his patients have seen an opening of their clogged arteries.*[43] Eleven of his patients had agreed to angiography, a procedure in which specific arteries in the heart can be "x-rayed." Of these eleven, the blockages in the arteries were, on average, reduced in size by 7% over the first five years of his study. This may sound like a small change but it should be noted that the volume of blood delivered is at least 30% greater when the diameter is increased by 7%.[44] More importantly, this is the difference between the presence of pain (from angina) and absence of pain, indeed between life and death. Authors of the five-year report note, "This is the longest study of minimal fat nutrition used in combination with cholesterol-lowering drugs conducted to date, and our finding of a mean decrease of arterial stenosis [blockage] of 7.0% is greater than any reports in previous research."[42]

One physician took special note of Dr. Esselstyn's study. He was only forty-four years of age and seemingly healthy when he found himself with a heart problem, culminating in a heart attack. Because of the nature of his heart disease, there was nothing that conventional medicine could safely offer him. He visited Dr. Esselstyn, decided to commit to the dietary program, and *after thirty-two months, without any cholesterol-lowering medication, he reversed his heart disease and lowered his blood cholesterol to 89 mg/dL.* What follows is the dramatic image of this patient's diseased artery before and after Dr. Esselstyn's dietary advice (Chart 5.4).[8] The light part of the picture is blood flowing through an artery. The picture on the left (A) has a section marked by a parenthesis where severe coronary disease reduced the amount of blood flow. After

**CHART 5.4: CORONARY ARTERY BEFORE AND AFTER
CONSUMING PLANT-BASED DIET**

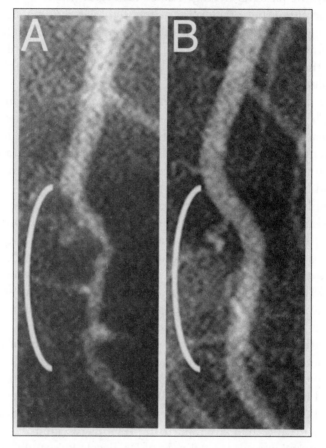

adopting a whole foods, plant-based diet, that same artery opened up, reversing the ravages of heart disease and allowing a much more normal blood flow, as shown in the picture on the right (B).

Is it possible that Dr. Esselstyn just got a lucky group of patients? The answer is no. Patients this sick with heart disease don't spontaneously heal themselves. Another way to check the likelihood of this degree of success is to look at the five patients that dropped out of the dietary program and resumed their standard care. *As of 1995, these five people had fallen prey to ten new coronary events.*[42] Meanwhile, as of 2003, seventeen years into the study, all but one patient following the diet are still alive, headed into their seventies and eighties.[45]

Can any sane person dispute these findings? It seems impossible. If you remember nothing else about this chapter, remember the forty-nine to zero score; forty-nine coronary events prior to a whole foods, plant-based diet, and zero events for those patients who adhered to a whole foods, plant-based diet. Dr. Esselstyn has done what "Big Science" has been trying to do, without success, for over fifty-five years: *he defeated heart disease.*

DR. DEAN ORNISH

In the past fifteen years another giant in this field, Dr. Dean Ornish, has been instrumental in bringing diet to the forefront of medical thought. A graduate of Harvard Medical School, he has been featured prominently in popular media, succeeded in having his heart disease treatment plan covered by a number of insurance carriers and written several best-selling books. If you have heard of the diet/heart disease connection, chances are that it may well be because of Dr. Ornish's work.

His best-known research is the Lifestyle Heart Trial, in which he treated twenty-eight heart disease patients with lifestyle changes alone.[46] He put these patients on an experimental treatment plan and twenty additional patients on the standard treatment plan. He followed both groups carefully and measured several health indicators, including artery blockages, cholesterol levels and weight.

Dr. Ornish's treatment plan was very different from the standards of high-tech modern medicine. He put the twenty-eight patients in a hotel for the first week of treatment and told them what they had to do to take control of their health. He asked them to eat a low-fat, plant-based diet for at least a year. Only about 10% of their calories were to come from fat. They could eat as much food as they wanted, as long as it was on the acceptable food list, which included fruits, vegetables and grains. As researchers noted, "No animal products were allowed except egg white and one cup per day of non-fat milk or yogurt."[46] In addition to diet, the group was to practice various forms of stress management, including meditation, breathing exercises and relaxation exercises for at least one hour per day. The patients were also asked to exercise three hours per week at levels customized to the severity of their disease. To help the patients make these lifestyle changes, the group met twice a week for four hours at a time for mutual support. Dr. Ornish and his research group did not use any drugs, surgery or technology to treat these patients.[46]

The experimental patients adhered to pretty much everything that the researchers asked of them and were rewarded with improved health and vitality. On average, their total cholesterol dropped from 227 mg/dL to 172 mg/dL, and their "bad" LDL cholesterol dropped from 152 mg/dL to 95 mg/dL. And after one year, the frequency, duration and severity of their chest pains plummeted. Further, it was clear that the closer the patients adhered to the lifestyle recommendations, the more their hearts healed. The patients who had the best adherence over the course of the year saw the blockages in their arteries diminish by over 4%. Four percent may seem like a small number, but remember that heart disease builds up over a lifetime, so a 4% change in only a year is a fantastic result. *In all, 82% of the patients in the experimental group had regression in their heart disease over the course of a year.*

The control group did not fare so well, despite the fact that they received the usual care. Their chest pain became worse in terms of frequency, duration and severity. For example, although the experimental group experienced a 91% reduction in the frequency of chest pain, the control group experienced a 165% rise in the frequency of chest pain. Their cholesterol levels were significantly worse than those of the experimental patients, and the blockages in their arteries also became worse. The patients in the group who were the least attentive to diet and lifestyle changes had blockages that increased in size by 8% over the course of the year.[46]

Between Dr. Ornish, Dr. Esselstyn and others before them, like Dr. Morrison, I believe that we have found the strategic link in our heart disease battle plan. Their dietary treatments not only relieve the symptoms of chest pain, but they also treat the cause of heart disease and can eliminate future coronary events. There are no surgical or chemical heart disease treatments, at the Cleveland Clinic or anywhere else, that can compare to these impressive results.

THE FUTURE

The future is filled with hope. We now know enough to nearly eliminate heart disease. We know not only how to prevent the disease, but how to successfully treat it. We do not need to crack open our breast plates to reroute our arteries, and we do not need a lifetime of powerful drugs in our blood. By eating the right food, we can keep our hearts healthy.

The next step is to implement this dietary approach on a large scale, which is exactly what Dr. Dean Ornish is currently working on. His research group has begun the Multicenter Lifestyle Demonstration Project, which represents the future of heart disease health care. Teams of health professionals at eight diverse sites have been trained to treat heart disease patients with Dr. Ornish's lifestyle intervention program. Patients eligible to participate are those who have documented heart disease severe enough to warrant surgery. Instead of surgery, they may enroll in a one-year lifestyle program. This program was started in 1993, and by 1998 there were forty insurance programs that covered the costs for selected patients.[32]

As of 1998, almost 200 people had taken part in the Lifestyle Project, and the results are phenomenal. After one year of treatment, 65% of patients had eliminated their chest pain. The effect was long lasting, as well. After three years, over 60% of the patients continued reporting no chest pain.[32]

The health benefits are equaled by the economic benefits. Over one million heart disease surgeries are undertaken every year.[32] In 2002, physician services and hospital care for heart disease patients cost $78.1 billion (that does not include drug costs, home health care or nursing home care).[2] The angioplasty procedure alone costs $31,000, and by-pass surgery costs $46,000.[32] In marked contrast, the year-long lifestyle intervention program only costs $7,000. By comparing the patients who underwent the lifestyle program with those patients who underwent the traditional route of surgery, Dr. Ornish and his colleagues demonstrated that the lifestyle intervention program cut costs by an average of $30,000 per patient.[32]

Much work remains to be done. The health care establishment is structured to profit from chemical and surgical intervention. Diet still takes the back seat to drugs and surgery. One criticism that is constantly leveled at the dietary argument is that patients will not make such fundamental changes. One doctor charges that Dr. Esselstyn's patients change their eating habits simply because of Esselstyn's "zealous belief."[47] This criticism is not only wrong and insulting to patients; it is also self-fulfilling. If doctors do not believe that patients will change their diets, they will neglect to talk about diet, or will do it in an off-handed, disparaging way. There is no greater disrespect a doctor can show patients than that of withholding potentially lifesaving information based on the assumption that patients do not want to change their lifestyle.

Well-meaning institutions are not exempt from such closed-mindedness. The American Heart Association recommends a diet for heart disease that favors moderation, rather than scientific truth. The National Cholesterol Education Program does the same thing. These organizations pitch moderate diets with trivial changes as being healthy lifestyle "goals." If you are at high risk for heart disease, or if you already have the disease, they recommend that you adopt a diet containing 30% of total calories as fat (7% of total calories as saturated fat) and less than 200 mg/day of dietary cholesterol.[48, 49] According to them, we should also keep our total blood cholesterol level under the "desirable" level of 200 mg/dL.[49]

These venerable organizations are not giving the American public the most up-to-date scientific information. While we are told that a total blood cholesterol level of 200 mg/dL is "desirable," *we know that 35% of heart attacks strike Americans who have cholesterol levels between 150 and 200 mg/dL*[50] (a truly safe cholesterol level is under 150 mg/dL). We also know that the most aggressive reversal of heart disease ever demonstrated occurred when fat was about 10% of total calorie intake. Studies have clearly demonstrated that many patients who follow the more moderate government recommended diets see a *progression of heart disease.*[51] The innocent victims are health-conscious Americans who follow these recommendations, keeping their total cholesterol around 180 or 190 mg/dL, only to be rewarded with a heart attack leading to a premature death.

To top it off, the National Cholesterol Education Program dangerously writes, "Lifestyle changes are the most cost-effective means to reduce risk for CHD[coronary heart disease]. Even so, to achieve maximal benefit, many persons will require LDL [cholesterol]-lowering drugs."[49] No wonder America's health is failing. The dietary recommendations for the most diseased hearts among us, given by supposedly reputable institutions, are severely watered down and followed by the caveat that we'll probably need a lifetime of drugs anyway.

Our leading organizations fear that if they advocate more than modest changes, no one will listen to them. But the establishment-recommended diets are not nearly as healthy as the diets espoused by Drs. Esselstyn and Ornish. The fact is that a blood cholesterol level of 200 mg/dL is not safe, a 30% fat diet is not "low-fat," and eating foods containing any cholesterol above 0 mg is unhealthy. Our health institutions are intentionally misleading the public about heart disease, all in the name of "moderation."

Whether scientists, doctors and policy makers think the public will change or not, the layperson must be aware that a whole foods, plant-based diet is far and away the healthiest diet. In the seminal paper regarding the landmark Lifestyle Heart Trial, the authors, Dr. Ornish and his scientific colleagues, write, "*The point of our study was to determine what is true, not what is practicable* [my emphasis]."[46]

We now know what is true: a whole foods, plant-based diet can prevent and treat heart disease, saving hundreds of thousands of Americans every year.

Dr. William Castelli, the long-time director of the Framingham Heart Study, a cornerstone of heart disease research, espouses a whole foods, plant-based diet.

Dr. Esselstyn, who has demonstrated the most significant reversal of heart disease in all of medical history, espouses a whole foods, plant-based diet.

Dr. Ornish, who has pioneered reversal of heart disease without drugs or surgery and proved widespread economic benefit for patients and insurance providers, espouses a whole foods, plant-based diet.

Now is a time of great hope and challenge, a time when people can control their health. One of the best and most caring doctors I have ever met puts it best:

> *The collective conscience and will of our profession*
> *is being tested as never before. Now is the time*
> *for us to have the courage for legendary work.*

> — Dr. Caldwell B. Esselstyn, Jr.[8]

6

Obesity

PERHAPS YOU'VE HEARD THE NEWS.

Perhaps you've caught a glimpse of the staggering statistics on obesity among Americans.

Perhaps you've simply noticed that, compared to a few years ago, more people at the grocery store are overweight.

Perhaps you've been in classrooms, on playgrounds or at day care centers and noticed how many kids are already crippled with a weight problem and can't run twenty feet without getting winded.

Our struggle with weight is hard to miss these days. Open a newspaper or a magazine, or turn on the radio or TV—you know that America has a weight problem. In fact, two out of three adult Americans are overweight, and one-third of the adult population is obese. Not only are these numbers high, but the rate at which they have been rising is ominous (Chart 1.2, page 13).[1]

But what do the terms "overweight" and "obese" mean? The standard expression of body size is the body mass index (BMI). It represents body weight (in kilograms, kg) relative to body height (in meters squared, m^2). By most official standards, being overweight is having a BMI above twenty-five, and being obese is having a BMI over thirty. The same scale is used for both men and women. You can determine your own BMI using Chart 6.1, which lists the necessary information in pounds and inches for your convenience.

CHART 6.1: BODY MASS INDEX TABLE

	Normal						Overweight					Obese		
BMI (kg/m)	19	20	21	22	23	24	25	26	27	28	29	30	35	40
Height (in.)	Weight (lb.)													
58	91	96	100	105	110	115	119	124	129	134	138	143	167	191
59	94	99	104	109	114	119	124	128	133	138	143	148	173	198
60	97	102	107	112	118	123	128	133	138	143	148	153	179	204
61	100	106	111	116	122	127	132	137	143	148	153	158	185	211
62	104	109	115	120	126	131	136	142	147	153	158	164	191	218
63	107	113	118	124	130	135	141	146	152	158	163	169	197	225
64	110	116	122	128	134	140	145	151	157	163	169	174	204	232
65	114	120	126	132	138	144	150	156	162	168	174	180	210	240
66	118	124	130	136	142	148	155	161	167	173	179	186	216	247
67	121	127	134	140	146	153	159	166	172	178	185	191	223	255
68	125	131	138	144	151	158	164	171	177	184	190	197	230	262
69	128	135	142	149	155	162	169	176	182	189	196	203	236	270
70	132	139	146	153	160	167	174	181	188	195	202	209	243	278
71	136	143	150	157	165	172	179	186	193	200	208	215	250	286
72	140	147	154	162	169	177	184	191	199	206	213	221	258	294
73	144	151	159	166	174	182	189	197	204	212	219	227	265	302
74	148	155	163	171	179	186	194	202	210	218	225	233	272	311
75	152	160	168	176	184	192	200	208	216	224	232	240	279	319
76	156	164	172	180	189	197	205	213	221	230	238	246	287	328

THE CHILDREN

Perhaps the most depressing element of our supersize mess is the growing number of overweight and obese children. About 15% of America's youth (ages six to nineteen) are overweight. Another 15% are at risk of becoming overweight.[2]

Overweight children face a wide range of psychological and social challenges. As you know, children have a knack for being open and blunt; sometimes the playground can be a merciless place. Overweight children find it more difficult to make friends and are often thought of as lazy and sloppy. They are more likely to have behavioral and learning difficulties, and the low self-esteem likely to be formed during adolescence can last forever.[3]

Young people who are overweight also are highly likely to face a host of medical problems. They often have elevated cholesterol levels, which can be a predictor for any number of deadly diseases. They are more likely to have problems with glucose intolerance, and, consequently, diabetes. Type 2 diabetes, formerly seen only in adults, is skyrocketing among adolescents. (See chapters seven and nine for a more thorough discussion of childhood diabetes.) Elevated blood pressure is nine times more likely to occur among obese kids. Sleep apnea, which can cause neuro-cognitive problems, is found in one in ten obese children. A wide variety of bone problems is more common in obese kids. Most importantly, an obese young person is much more likely to be an obese adult,[3] greatly increasing the likelihood of lifelong health problems.

CONSEQUENCES FOR THE ADULT

If you are obese, you may not be able to do many things that could make your life more enjoyable. You may find that you cannot play vigorously with your grandchildren (or your children), walk long distances, participate in sports, find a comfortable seat in a movie theatre or airplane or have an active sex life. In fact, even sitting still in a chair may be impossible without experiencing back or joint pain. For many, standing is hard on the knees. Carrying around too much weight can dramatically affect physical mobility, work, mental health, self-perception and social life. So you see, this isn't about death; it really is about missing many of the more enjoyable things in life.[4]

Clearly no one *desires* to be overweight. So why is it that two out of three adult Americans are overweight? Why is one-third of the population obese?

The problem is not a lack of money. In 1999, medical care costs relating to obesity alone were estimated to be $70 billion.[5] In 2002, a mere three years later, the American Obesity Association listed these costs at $100 billion.[6] This is not all. Add another $30–40 billion out-of-pocket money that we spend trying to keep off the weight in the first place.[5] Going on special weight-loss diet plans and popping pills to cut our appetites or rearrange our metabolism have become a national pastime.

This is an economic black hole that sucks our money away without offering anything in return. Imagine paying $40 to a service man to fix your leaky kitchen sink, and then two weeks later, the sink pipes explode and flood the kitchen and it costs $500 to repair. I bet you wouldn't ask that guy to fix your sink again! So then why do we endlessly try those weight-loss plans, books, drinks, energy bars and assorted gimmicks when they don't deliver as promised?

I applaud people for trying to achieve a healthy weight. I don't question the worthiness or dignity of overweight people any more than I question cancer victims. My criticism is of a societal system that allows and even encourages this problem. I believe, for example, that we are drowning in an ocean of very bad information, too much of it intended to put money into someone else's pockets. What we really need, then, is a new solution comprised of good information for individual people to use at a price that they can afford.

THE SOLUTION

The solution to losing weight is a whole foods, plant-based diet, coupled with a reasonable amount of exercise. It is a long-term lifestyle change, rather than a quick-fix fad, and it can provide sustained weight loss while minimizing risk of chronic disease.

Have you ever known anyone who regularly consumes fresh fruits, vegetables and whole grain foods—and rarely, if ever, consumes meats or junk foods like chips, French fries and candy bars? What is his or her weight like? If you know many people like this, you have probably noticed that they tend to have a healthy weight. Now think of traditional cultures around the world. Think of traditional Asian cultures (Chinese, Japanese, Indian), where a couple of billion people have been eating a mostly plant-based diet for thousands of years. It's hard to imagine these people—at least until recently—as anything other than slender.

Now imagine a guy buying two hot dogs and ordering his second beer at a baseball game, or a woman ordering a cheeseburger and fries at your local fast food joint. The people in these images look different, don't they? Unfortunately, the guy munching his hot dogs and sipping his beer is rapidly becoming the "all-American" image. I have had visitors from other countries tell me that one of the first things they notice when they arrive in our good land is the exceptional number of fat people.

Solving this problem does not require magic tricks or complex equations involving blood types or carbohydrate counting or soul searching. Simply trust your observations on who is slim, vigorous and healthy, and who is not. Or trust the findings of some impressive research studies, large and small, showing time and time again that vegetarians and vegans are slimmer than their meat-eating counterparts. People in these studies who are vegetarian or vegan are anywhere from five to thirty pounds slimmer than their fellow citizens.[7–13]

In a separate intervention study, overweight subjects were told to eat as much as they wanted of foods that were mostly low-fat, whole-food and plant-based. In three weeks these people lost an average of seventeen pounds.[14] At the Pritikin Center, 4,500 patients who had gone through their three-week program got similar results. By feeding a mostly plant-based diet and promoting exercise, the Center found that its clients lost 5.5% of their body weight over three weeks.[15]

Published results for still more intervention studies using a low-fat, whole foods, mostly plant-based diet:

- About two to five pounds lost after twelve days[16]
- About ten pounds lost in three weeks[17, 18]
- Sixteen pounds lost over twelve weeks[19]
- Twenty-four pounds lost after one year[20]

All of these results show that consuming a whole foods, plant-based diet will help you to lose weight and, furthermore, it can happen quickly. The only question is how much weight you can lose. In most of these studies, the people who shed the most pounds were those who started with the most excess weight.[21] After the initial weight loss, the weight can be kept off for the long term by staying on the diet. Most importantly, losing weight this way is consistent with long-term health.

Some people, of course, can be on a plant-based diet and still not lose weight. There are a few very good reasons for this. First and foremost, losing body weight on a plant-based diet is much less likely to occur if the diet includes too many refined carbohydrates. *Sweets, pastries and pastas won't do it.* These foods are high in readily digested sugars and starches and, for the pastries, oftentimes very high in fat as well. As mentioned in chapter four, these highly processed, unnatural foods are not part of a plant-based diet that works to reduce body weight and promote health. This is one of the main reasons that I usually refer to the optimal diet as a *whole foods*, plant-based diet.

Notice that a strict vegetarian diet is not necessarily the same thing as a whole foods, plant-based diet. Some people become vegetarian only to replace meat with dairy foods, added oils and refined carbohydrates, including pasta made with refined grains, sweets and pastries. I refer to these people as "junk-food vegetarians" because they are not consuming a nutritious diet.

The second reason weight loss may be elusive is if a person never engages in any physical activity. A reasonable amount of physical activity, sustained on a regular basis, can pay important dividends.

Thirdly, certain people have a family predisposition for overweight bodies that may make their challenge more difficult. If you are one of these people, I can only say that you probably need to be especially rigorous in your diet and exercise. In rural China, we noticed that obese people simply did not exist, even though Chinese immigrants in Western countries do succumb to obesity. Now, as the dietary and lifestyle practices of people in China are becoming more like ours, so too have their bodies become more like ours. For some of these people with genetic predispositions, it doesn't take much bad food before their change in diet starts to cause problems.

Keeping body weight off is a long-term lifestyle choice. Gimmicks that produce impressively large, quick weight losses don't work in the long term. Short-term gains should not come along with long-term pain, like kidney problems, heart disease, cancer, bone and joint ailments and other problems that may be brought on with popular diet fads. If the weight was gained slowly, over a period of months and years, why would you expect to take it off healthily in a matter of weeks? Treating weight loss as a race doesn't work; it only makes the dieter more eager to quit the diet and go back to the eating habits that put them in need of losing weight in the first place. One very large study of 21,105 vegetarians and vegans[13] found that body mass index was "...lower among those who had adhered to their diet for five or more years" compared to people who had been on the diet for less than five years.

WHY THIS WILL WORK FOR YOU

So there is a solution to the weight-gain problem. But how can you apply it to your own life?

First of all, throw away ideas about counting calories. Generally speaking, you can eat as much as you want and still lose weight—*as long you eat the right type of food.* (See chapter twelve for details.) Secondly, stop expecting sacrifice, deprivation or blandness; there's no need. Feeling hungry is a sign that something is wrong, and prolonged hunger causes your body to slow the overall rate of metabolism in defense. Moreover, there are mechanisms in our bodies that naturally allow the right kind of plant-based foods to nourish us, without our having to think about every morsel of food we put in our mouths. It is a worry-free way to eat. Give your body the right food and it will do the right thing.

In some studies, those who follow a whole foods, low-fat, plant-based diet consume fewer calories. It's not because they're starving themselves. In fact, they will likely spend more time eating and eat a larger volume of food than their meat-eating counterparts.[22] That's because fruits, vegetables and grains—as whole foods—are much less energy-dense than animal foods and added fats. There are fewer calories in each spoonful or cupful of these foods. Remember that fat has nine calories per gram while carbohydrates and protein have only four calories per gram. In addition, whole fruits, vegetables and grains have a lot of fiber, which makes you feel full[22, 23] and yet contributes almost no calories to your meal. So by eating a healthy meal, you may reduce the calories that you consume, digest and absorb, even if you eat significantly more food.

This idea on its own, however, is not yet a sufficient explanation for the benefits of a whole foods, plant-based diet. The same criticisms I made against the Atkins diet and the other popular "low-carb" diets (chapter four) can also be applied to short-term studies in which subjects consume fewer calories while eating a plant-based diet. Over the long term, these subjects will find it very difficult to continue consuming an abnormally low level of calories; weight loss due to calorie restriction rarely leads to long-term weight loss. This is why other studies play such a crucial part in explaining the health benefits of a whole foods, plant-based diet, studies that show that the weight-loss effect is due to more than simple calorie restriction.

These studies document the fact that *vegetarians consume the same amount or even significantly more calories than their meat-eating counterparts, and yet are still slimmer.*[11, 24, 25] The China Study demonstrated that rural Chinese consuming a plant-based diet actually consume significantly more calories per pound of body weight than Americans. Most people would automatically assume that these rural Chinese would therefore be heavier than their meat-eating counterparts. But here's the kicker: the rural *Chinese are still slimmer while consuming a greater volume of food and more calories.* Much of this effect is undoubtedly due to greater physical activity...but this comparison is between average

Americans and the least active Chinese, those who do office work. Furthermore, studies done in Israel[24] and the United Kingdom,[11] neither of which represent primarily agrarian cultures, also show that vegetarians may consume the same or significantly more calories and still weigh less.

What's the secret? One factor that I've mentioned previously is the process of thermogenesis, which refers to our production of body heat during metabolism. Vegetarians have been observed to have a slightly higher rate of metabolism during rest,[26] meaning they burn up slightly more of their ingested calories as body heat rather than depositing them as body fat.[27] A relatively small increase in metabolic rate translates to a large number of calories burned over the course of twenty-four hours. Most of the scientific basis for the importance of this phenomenon was presented in chapter four.

EXERCISE

The slimming effect of physical activity is obvious. Scientific evidence concurs. A recent review of all the credible studies compared the relationship between body weight and exercise[28] and showed that people who were more physically active had less body weight. Another set of studies showed that exercising on a regular basis helped to keep off weight originally lost through exercise programs. No surprise here, either. Starting and stopping an exercise program is not a good idea. It is better to build it into your lifestyle so that you will become and continue to be more fit over all, not just burn off calories.

How much exercise is needed to keep the pounds off? A rough estimate derived from a good review[28] suggested that exercising a mere fifteen to forty-five minutes per day, every day, will maintain a body weight that is eleven to eighteen pounds lighter than it would otherwise be. Interestingly, we should not forget our "spontaneous" physical activity, the kind that is associated with chores of daily life. This can account for 100–800 calories per day (kcal/day).[29, 30] People who are regularly "up and about" doing physical things are going to be well ahead of those who get trapped in a sedentary lifestyle.

The advantages of combining diet and exercise to control body weight were brought home to me by a very simple study involving our experimental animals. Recall that our experimental animals were fed diets containing either the traditional 20% casein (cow's milk protein) or the much lower 5% casein. The rats consuming the 5% casein diets had strikingly less cancer, lower blood cholesterol levels and longer lives. They also consumed slightly more calories but burned them off as body heat.

Some of us had noticed over the course of these experiments that the 5% casein animals seemed to be more active than the 20% casein animals. To test this idea, we housed rats fed either 5% or 20% casein diets in cages equipped with exercise wheels outfitted with meters to record the number of turns of the wheel. *Within the very first day, the 5% casein-fed animals voluntarily "exercised" in the wheel about twice as much as the 20% casein-fed animals.*[31] Exercise remained considerably higher for the 5% casein animals throughout the two weeks of the study.

Now we can combine some really interesting observations on body weight. A plant-based diet operates on calorie balance to keep body weight under control in two ways. First, it discharges calories as body heat instead of storing them as body fat, and it doesn't take many calories to make a big difference over the course of a year. Second, a plant-based diet encourages more physical activity. And, as body weight goes down, it becomes easier to be physically active. Diet and exercise work together to decrease body weight and improve overall health.

GOING IN THE RIGHT DIRECTION

Obesity is the most ominous harbinger of poor health that Western nations currently face. Tens of millions of people will fall prey to disability, putting our health care systems under greater strain than has previously been seen.

There are many people and institutions working to reduce this problem, but their point of attack is often illogical and misinformed. First, there are the many quick-fix promises and gimmicks. Obesity is not a condition that can be fixed in a few weeks or even a few months, and you should beware of diets, potions and pills that create rapid weight loss with no promise of good health in the future. *The diet that helps to reduce weight in the short run needs to be the same diet that creates and maintains health in the long run.*

Second, the tendency to focus on obesity as an independent, isolated disease[32, 33] is misplaced. Considering obesity in this manner directs our attention to a search for specific cures while ignoring control of the other diseases to which obesity is strongly linked. That is, we sacrifice context.

Also, I would urge that we ignore the suggestion that knowing its genetic basis might control obesity. A few years ago,[34-36] there was great publicity given to the discovery of "the obesity gene." Then there was the discovery of a second gene related to obesity, and a third gene, and a fourth and on and on. The purpose behind the obesity gene search is to allow researchers to develop a drug capable of knocking out or inactivating the underlying cause of obesity. This is extremely shortsighted, as well as unproductive. Believing that specific identifiable genes are the basis of obesity (i.e., it's all in the family) also allows us to fatalistically blame a cause that we cannot control.

We *can* control the cause. It is right at the end of our fork.

7
Diabetes

TYPE 2 DIABETES, the most common form, often accompanies obesity. As we, as a nation, continue to gain weight, our rate of diabetes spirals out of control. In the eight years from 1990 to 1998, the incidence of diabetes increased 33%.[1] Over 8% of American adults are diabetic, and over 150,000 young people have the disease. That translates to 16 million Americans. The scariest figure? One-third of those people with diabetes don't yet know that they have it.[2]

You know the situation is serious when our children, at the age of puberty, start falling prey to the form of diabetes usually reserved for adults over forty. One newspaper recently illustrated the epidemic with the story of a girl who weighed 350 pounds at the age of fifteen, had the "adult-onset" form of diabetes and was injecting insulin into her body three times a day.[3]

What is diabetes, why should we care about it and how do we stop it from happening to us?

TWO FACES OF THE SAME DEVIL

Almost all cases of diabetes are either Type 1 or Type 2. Type 1 develops in children and adolescents, and thus is sometimes referred to as juvenile-onset diabetes. This form accounts for 5% to 10% of all diabetes cases. Type 2, which accounts for 90% to 95% of all cases, used to occur primarily in adults age forty and up, and thus was called adult-onset diabetes.[2] But because up to 45% of new diabetes cases in children are Type 2 diabetes,[4] the age-specific names are being dropped, and the two forms of diabetes are simply referred to as Type 1 and Type 2.[4]

145

In both types, the disease begins with dysfunctional glucose metabolism. Normal metabolism goes like this:

- We eat food.
- The food is digested and the carbohydrate part is broken down into simple sugars, much of which is glucose.
- Glucose (blood sugar) enters the blood, and insulin is produced by the pancreas to manage its transport and distribution around the body.
- Insulin, acting like an usher, opens doors for glucose into different cells for a variety of purposes. Some of the glucose is converted to short-term energy for immediate cell use, and some is stored as long-term energy (fat) for later use.

As a person develops diabetes, this metabolic process collapses. Type 1 diabetics cannot produce adequate insulin because the insulin-producing cells of their pancreas have been destroyed. This is the result of the body attacking itself, making Type 1 diabetes an autoimmune disease. (Type 1 diabetes and other autoimmune diseases are discussed in chapter nine.) Type 2 diabetics can produce insulin, but the insulin doesn't do its job. This is called insulin resistance, which means that once the insulin starts "giving orders" to dispatch the blood sugar, the body doesn't pay attention. The insulin is rendered ineffective, and the blood sugar is not metabolized properly.

Imagine your body as an airport, complete with vast parking areas. Each unit of your blood sugar is an individual traveler. After you eat, your blood sugar rises. In our analogy, then, that means lots of travelers would start to arrive at the airport. The people would drive in, park in a lot and walk to the stop where the shuttle bus is supposed to pick them up. As your blood sugar continues to rise, all the airport parking lots would fill to capacity, and all the people would congregate at the shuttle bus stops. The shuttle buses, of course, represent insulin. In the diabetic airport, unfortunately, there are all sorts of problems with the buses. In the Type 1 diabetic airport, the shuttle buses simply don't exist. The only shuttle bus manufacturer in the known universe, Pancreas Company, was shut down. In the Type 2 diabetic airport, there are some shuttle buses, but they don't work very well.

In both cases, travelers never get to where they want to go. The airport system breaks down, and chaos ensues. In real life, this corresponds with a rise in blood sugar to dangerous levels. In fact, diabetes is diagnosed by the observation of elevated blood sugar levels, or its "spillage" into urine.

What are the long-term health risks of glucose metabolism being disrupted? Here's a summary, taken from a report from the Centers for Disease Control[2]:

Diabetes Complications

Heart Disease
- 2–4 times the risk of death from heart disease.

Stroke
- 2–4 times the risk of stroke.

High Blood Pressure
- Over 70% of people with diabetes have high blood pressure.

Blindness
- Diabetes is the leading cause of blindness in adults.

Kidney Disease
- Diabetes is the leading cause of end-stage kidney disease.
- Over 100,000 diabetics underwent dialysis or kidney transplantation in 1999.

Nervous System Disease
- 60% to 70% of diabetics suffer mild to severe nervous system damage.

Amputation
- Over 60% of all lower limb amputations occur with diabetics.

Dental Disease
- Increased frequency and severity of gum disease that can lead to tooth loss.

Pregnancy Complications

Increased Susceptibility to Other Illnesses

Death

Modern drugs and surgery offer no cure for diabetics. At best, current drugs allow diabetics to maintain a reasonably functional lifestyle, but these drugs will never treat the cause of the disease. As a consequence, diabetics face a lifetime of drugs and medications, making diabetes an enormously costly disease. The economic toll of diabetes in the U.S.: over $130 billion a year.[2]

But there is hope. In fact, there is much more than hope. The food we eat has enormous influence over this disease. The right diet not only prevents but also treats diabetes. What, then, is the "right" diet? You can probably guess what I'm going to say, but let the research speak for itself.

NOW YOU SEE IT, NOW YOU DON'T

Like most chronic diseases, diabetes shows up more often in some parts of the world than in others. This has been known for a hundred years. It has also been well documented that those populations with low rates of diabetes eat different diets than those populations with high rates of diabetes. But is that just a coincidence, or is there something else at work?

CHART 7.1: DIETS AND DIABETES RATES, CIRCA 1925[4, 5]

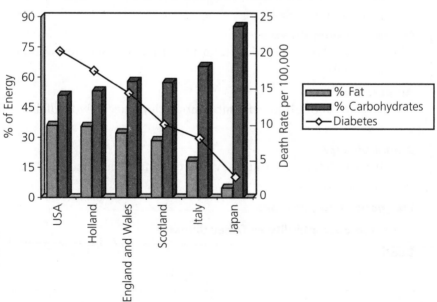

Almost seventy years ago, H.P. Himsworth compiled all the existing research in a report comparing diets and diabetes rates in six countries. What he found was that some cultures were consuming high-fat diets, while others had diets high in carbohydrates. These fat vs. carbohydrate consumption patterns were the result of animal vs. plant food consumption. Chart 7.1 documents the diet and disease conditions for these countries in the early part of the twentieth century.[5]

As carbohydrate intake goes up and fat intake goes down, the number of deaths from diabetes plummets from 20.4 to 2.9 per 100,000 people. The verdict? A high-carbohydrate, low-fat diet—a plant-based diet—may help to prevent diabetes.

Thirty years later, the question was reexamined. After examining four countries from Southeast Asia and South America, researchers again found that high-carbohydrate diets were linked to low rates of diabetes. Researchers noted that the country with the highest rate of diabetes, Uruguay, had a diet that was "typically 'Western' in character, being high in calories, animal protein, [total] fat and animal fat." Countries with low rates of diabetes used a diet that was "relatively lower in protein (particularly animal protein), fat and animal fat. A high proportion of calories is derived from carbohydrates, particularly from rice."[6]

These same researchers enlarged their study to eleven countries through Central and South America and Asia. The strongest association they found with diabetes was excess weight.[7] Populations eating the most "Western" type of diet also had the highest cholesterol levels, which in turn was strongly associated with the rate of diabetes.[7] Is this starting to sound familiar?

WITHIN ONE POPULATION

These old, cross-cultural studies can be crude, resulting in conclusions that are not entirely reliable. Perhaps the difference in diabetes rates in the above studies were not due to diet, but to genetics. Perhaps other unmeasured cultural factors, like physical activity, were more relevant. A better test would be a study of diabetes rates in a single population.

The Seventh-day Adventists population is a good example. They are an interesting group of people to study because of their dietary habits: their religion encourages them to stay away from meat, fish, eggs, coffee, alcohol and tobacco. As a result, half of them are vegetarian. But 90% of these vegetarians still consume dairy and/or egg products, thus deriving a significant amount of their calories from animal sources. It should also be noted that the meat-eating Adventists are not the meatiest of eaters. They consume about three servings of beef a week, and less than one serving a week of fish and poultry.[8] I know plenty of people who consume this amount of meat (including fish and poultry) every two days.

In dietary studies involving the Adventists, scientists compare "moderate" vegetarians to "moderate" meat eaters. This is not a big difference. *Even so, the Adventist vegetarians are much healthier than their meat eating counterparts.*[8] *Those Adventists that "deprived" themselves of meat also "deprived" themselves of the ravages of diabetes. Compared to the meat eaters, the vegetarians had about one-half the rate of diabetes.*[8, 9] They also had almost half the rate of obesity.[8]

In another study, scientists measured diets and diabetes in a population of Japanese American men in Washington State.[10] These men were the sons of Japanese immigrants to the U.S. Remarkably, they had more than four times the prevalence of diabetes than the average rate found in similar-aged men who stayed in Japan. So what happened?

For Japanese Americans, the ones who developed diabetes also ate the most animal protein, animal fat and dietary cholesterol, each of which is only found in animal-based foods.[10] Total fat intake also was higher among the diabetics. These same dietary characteristics also resulted in excess weight. These second-generation Japanese Americans ate a meatier diet with less plant-based food than men born in Japan. The researchers wrote, "Apparently, the eating habits of Japanese men living in the United States resemble more the American eating style than the Japanese." The consequence: four times as much incidence of diabetes.[10]

Some other studies:

- Researchers found that increased fat intake was associated with an increased rate of Type 2 diabetes among 1,300 people in the San Luis valley in Colorado. They said, "The findings support the hypothesis that high-fat, low-carbohydrate diets are associated with the onset of non-insulin-dependent [Type 2] diabetes mellitus in humans."[11]
- In the past twenty-five years, the rate at which children in Japan contract Type 2 diabetes has more than tripled. Researchers note that consumption of animal protein and animal fat has drastically increased in the past fifty years. Researchers say that this dietary

shift, along with low exercise levels, might be to blame for this explosion of diabetes.[12]

- In England and Wales the rate of diabetes markedly dropped from 1940 to 1950, largely during World War II when food consumption patterns changed markedly. During the war and its aftermath, fiber and grain intake went up and fat intake went down. People ate "lower" on the food chain because of national necessity. Around 1950, though, people gave up the grain-based diets and returned to eating more fat, more sugar and less fiber. Sure enough, diabetes rates started going up.[13]
- Researchers studied 36,000 women in Iowa for six years. All were free of diabetes at the start of the study, but more than 1,100 cases of diabetes developed after six years. The women who were least likely to get diabetes were those that ate the most whole grains and fiber[14]—those whose diets contained the most carbohydrates (the complex kind found in whole foods).

All of these findings support the idea that both across and within populations, high-fiber, whole, plant-based foods protect against diabetes, and high-fat, high-protein, animal-based foods promote diabetes.

CURING THE INCURABLE

All of the research cited above was *observational* and an observed association, even if frequently seen, may only be an incidental association that masks the real cause-effect relationship of environment (including diet) and disease. There is, however, also research of the "controlled" or intervention variety. This involves changing the diets of people who already have either full-blown Type 1 or Type 2 diabetes or mild diabetic symptoms (impaired glucose tolerance).

James Anderson, M.D., is one of the most prominent scientists studying diet and diabetes today, garnering dramatic results using dietary means alone. One of his studies examined the effects of a high-fiber, high-carbohydrate, low-fat diet on twenty-five Type 1 diabetics and twenty-five Type 2 diabetics in a hospital setting.[15] None of his fifty patients were overweight and all of them were taking insulin shots to control their blood sugar levels.

His experimental diet consisted mostly of whole plant foods and the equivalent of only a cold cut or two of meat a day. He put his patients on the conservative, American-style diet recommended by the American

Diabetes Association for one week and then switched them over to the experimental "veggie" diet for three weeks. He measured their blood sugar levels, cholesterol levels, weight and medication requirements. The results were impressive.

Type 1 diabetics cannot produce insulin. It is difficult to imagine any dietary change that might aid their predicament. *But after just three weeks, the Type 1 diabetic patients were able to lower their insulin medication by an average of 40%!* Their blood sugar profiles improved dramatically. *Just as importantly, their cholesterol levels dropped by 30%!*[15] Remember, one of the dangers of being diabetic is the secondary outcomes, heart disease and stroke. Lowering risk factors for those secondary outcomes by improving the cholesterol profile is almost as important as treating high blood sugar.

Type 2 diabetics, unlike Type 1, are more "treatable" because they haven't incurred such extensive damage to their pancreas. So when Anderson's Type 2 patients ate the high-fiber, low-fat diet, the results were even more impressive. Of the twenty-five Type 2 patients, twenty-four were able to discontinue their insulin medication! Let me say that again. *All but one person were able to discontinue their insulin medication in a matter of weeks!*[15]

One man had a twenty-one-year history of diabetes and was taking thirty-five units of insulin a day. After three weeks of intensive dietary treatment, his insulin dosage dropped to eight units a day. After eight weeks at home, his need for insulin shots vanished.[15] Chart 7.2 shows a sample of patients and how eating a plant-based diet lowered their insulin medications. This is a huge effect.

In another study of fourteen lean diabetic patients, Anderson found that diet alone could lower total cholesterol levels by 32% *in just over two weeks.*[16] Some of the results are shown in Chart 7.3.

These benefits, representing a decrease in blood cholesterol from 206 mg/dL to 141 mg/dL, are astounding—especially considering the speed with which they appear. Dr. Anderson also found no evidence that this cholesterol decrease was temporary as long as people continued on the diet; it remained low for four years.[17]

Another group of scientists at the Pritikin Center achieved equally spectacular results by prescribing a low-fat, plant-based diet and exercise to a group of diabetic patients. *Of forty patients on medication at the start of the program, thirty-four were able to discontinue all medication after only twenty-six days.*[18] This research group also demonstrated that

CHART 7.2: INSULIN DOSAGE RESPONSE TO DIET

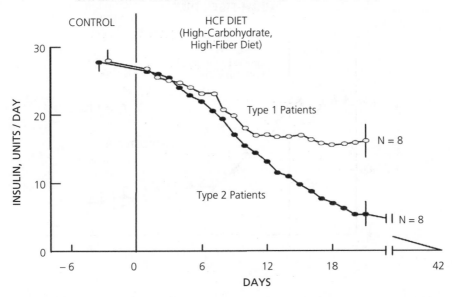

the benefits of a plant-based diet will last for years if the same diet is continued.[19]

These are examples of some very dramatic research, but they only scratch the surface of all the supporting research that has been done. One scientific paper reviewed nine publications citing the use of high-carbohydrate, high-fiber diets and two more standard-carbohydrate, high-fiber diets to treat diabetic patients.[20] All eleven studies resulted in improved blood sugar and cholesterol levels. (Dietary fiber supplements, by the way, although beneficial, did not have same consistent effects as a change to a plant-based, whole foods diet.)[21]

THE PERSISTENCE OF HABIT

As you can see by these findings, we can beat diabetes. Two recent studies considered a combination of diet and exercise effects on this disease.[22, 23] One study placed 3,234 non-diabetic people at risk for diabetes (elevated blood sugar) into three different groups.[22] One group, the control, received standard dietary information and a drug placebo (no effect), one received the standard dietary information and the drug metformin, and a third group received "intensive" lifestyle intervention, which included a moderately low-fat diet and exercise plan to lose at least 7% of their weight. After almost three years, the lifestyle group had

CHART 7.3: BLOOD CHOLESTEROL ON HIGH-CARBOHYDRATE, HIGH-FIBER DIET

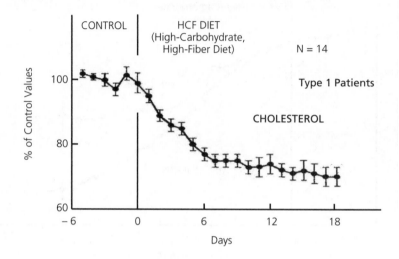

58% fewer cases of diabetes than the control group. The drug group reduced the number of cases only by 31%. Compared to the control, both treatments worked, but clearly a lifestyle change is much more powerful and safer than simply taking a drug. Moreover, the lifestyle change would be effective in solving other health problems, whereas the drug would not.

The second study also found that the rate of diabetes could be reduced by 58% just by modest lifestyle changes, including exercise, weight loss and a moderately low-fat diet.[23] Imagine what would happen if people fully adopted the healthiest diet: a whole foods, plant-based diet. I strongly suspect that virtually all Type 2 diabetes cases could be prevented.

Unfortunately, misinformation and ingrained habits are wreaking havoc on our health. Our habit of eating hot dogs, hamburgers and French fries is killing us. Even Dr. James Anderson, who achieved profound results with many patients by prescribing a near-vegetarian diet, is not immune to habitual health advice. He writes, "Ideally, diets providing 70% of calories as carbohydrate and up to 70 gm fiber daily offer the greatest health benefits for individuals with diabetes. However, these diets allow only one to two ounces of meat daily and are impractical for home use for many individuals."[20] Why does Professor Anderson, a very

fine researcher, say that such a diet is "impractical" and thereby prejudice his listeners before they even consider the evidence?

Yes, changing your lifestyle may seem impractical. It may seem impractical to give up meat and high-fat foods, but I wonder how practical
it is to be 350 pounds and have Type 2 diabetes at the age of fifteen, like
the girl mentioned at the start of this chapter. I wonder how practical it
is to have a lifelong condition that can't be cured by drugs or surgery; a
condition that often leads to heart disease, stroke, blindness or amputation; a condition that might require you to inject insulin into your body
every day for the rest of your life.

Radically changing our diets may be "impractical," but it might also
be worth it.

8

Common Cancers:
Breast, Prostate, Large Bowel
(Colon and Rectal)

MUCH OF MY CAREER has been concentrated on the study of cancer. My laboratory work was focused on several cancers, including those of the liver, breast and pancreas, and some of the most impressive data from China were related to cancer. For this lifetime work, the American Institute for Cancer Research kindly presented me with their Research Achievement award in 1998.

An exceptional number of books have summarized the evidence on the effects of nutrition on a variety of cancers, each with their own particularities. But what I've found is that the nutritional effects on the cancers I've chosen to discuss here are virtually the same for all cancers, regardless of whether they are initiated by different factors or are located in different parts of the body. Using this principle, I can limit my discussion to three cancers, which will allow me space in the rest of the book to address diseases other than cancer, demonstrating the breadth of evidence linking food to many health concerns.

I have chosen to comment on three cancers that affect hundreds of thousands of Americans and that generally represent other cancers as well: two reproductive cancers that get plenty of attention, breast and prostate, and one digestive cancer, large bowel—the second leading cause of cancer death, behind lung cancer.

BREAST CANCER

It was spring almost ten years ago. I was in my office at Cornell when I was told that a woman with a question regarding breast cancer was on the phone.

"I have a strong history of breast cancer in my family," the woman, Betty, said. "My mother and grandmother both died from the disease, and my forty-five-year-old sister was recently diagnosed with it. Given this family problem, I can't help but be afraid for my nine-year-old daughter. She's going to start menstruating soon and I worry about her risks of getting breast cancer." Her fear was evident in her voice. "I've seen a lot of research showing that family history is important, and I'm afraid that it's inevitable that my daughter will get breast cancer. One of the options I've been thinking about is a mastectomy for my daughter, to remove both breasts. Do you have any advice?"

This woman was in an exceptionally difficult position. Does she let her daughter grow up into a deathtrap, or grow up without breasts? Although extreme, this question represents a variety of similar questions faced every day by thousands of women around the world.

These questions were especially encouraged by the early reports on the discovery of the breast cancer gene, BRCA-1. Headline articles in the *New York Times* and other newspapers and magazines trumpeted this discovery as an enormous advance. The hoopla surrounding BRCA-1, which now also includes BRCA-2, reinforced the idea that breast cancer was due to genetic misfortune. This caused great fear among people with a family history of breast cancer. It also generated excitement among scientists and pharmaceutical companies. The possibility was high that new technologies would be able to assess overall breast cancer risk in women by doing genetic testing; they hoped they might be able to manipulate this new gene in a way that would prevent or treat breast cancer. Journalists busily started translating selective bits of this information for the public, relying heavily on the genetic fatalistic attitude. No doubt this contributed to the concern of mothers like Betty.

"Well, let me first tell you that I am not a physician," I said. "I can't help you with diagnosis or treatment advice. That's for your physician to do. I can speak about the current research in a more general way, however, if that is of any help to you."

"Yes," she said, "that's what I wanted."

I told her a little bit about the China Study and about the important role of nutrition. I told her that just because a person has the gene for a disease does not mean that they are destined to get the cancer: prominent studies reported that only a tiny minority of cancers can be solely blamed on genes.

I was surprised at how little she knew about nutrition. She thought genetics was the only factor that determined risk. She didn't realize that food was an important factor in breast cancer as well.

We talked for twenty or thirty minutes, a brief time for such an important matter. By the end of the conversation I had the feeling that she was not satisfied with what I told her. Perhaps it was my conservative, scientific way of talking, or my reluctance to give her a recommendation. Maybe, I thought, she had already made up her mind to do the procedure.

She thanked me for my time and I wished her well. I remember thinking about how often I receive questions from people about specific health situations, and that this was one of the most unusual.

But Betty wasn't alone. One other woman also talked to me regarding the possibility of her young daughter undergoing surgery to remove both breasts. Other women who already had one breast removed wondered whether to have the second breast removed as a preventative measure.

It's clear that breast cancer is an important concern in our society. One out of eight American women will be diagnosed with this disease during their lifetimes—one of the highest rates in the world. Breast cancer grassroots organizations are widespread, strong, relatively well funded and exceptionally active compared to other health activist organizations. This disease, perhaps more than any other, incites panic and fear in many women.

When I think back to that conversation I had with Betty, I now feel that I could have made a stronger statement about the role nutrition plays in breast cancer. I still would not have been able to give her clinical advice, but the information I now know might have been of more use to her. So what would I tell her now?

RISK FACTORS

There are at least four important breast cancer risk factors that are affected by nutrition, as shown in Chart 8.1. Many of these relationships were confirmed in the China Study after being well established in other research.

**CHART 8.1: BREAST CANCER RISK FACTORS
AND NUTRITIONAL INFLUENCE**

Risk of breast cancer increases when a woman has...	A diet high in animal foods and refined carbohydrates...
...early age of menarche (first menstruation)	...lowers the age of menarche
...late age of menopause	...raises the age of menopause
...high levels of female hormones in the blood	...increases female hormone levels
...high blood cholesterol	...increases blood cholesterol levels

With the exception of blood cholesterol, these risk factors are variations on the same theme: exposure to excess amounts of female hormones, including estrogen and progesterone, leads to an increased risk of breast cancer. Women who consume a diet rich in animal-based foods, with a reduced amount of whole, plant-based foods, reach puberty earlier and menopause later, thus extending their reproductive lives. They also have higher levels of female hormones throughout their lifespan, as shown in Chart 8.2.

According to our China Study data, lifetime exposure to estrogen[1] is at least 2.5–3.0 times higher among Western women when compared

**CHART 8.2: DIETARY INFLUENCE ON FEMALE HORMONE EXPOSURE
OVER A WOMAN'S LIFETIME (SCHEMATIC)**

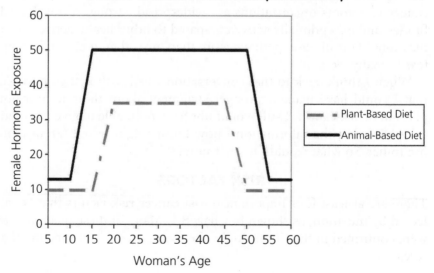

with rural Chinese women. This is a huge difference for such a critically important hormone.[2] To use the words of one of the leading breast cancer research groups in the world,[3] "there is overwhelming evidence that estrogen levels are a critical determinant of breast cancer risk."[4, 5] Estrogen directly participates in the cancer process.[6, 7] It also tends to indicate the presence of other female hormones[8-12] that play a role in breast cancer risk.[6, 7] Increased levels of estrogen and related hormones are a result of the consumption of typical Western diets, high in fat and animal protein and low in dietary fiber.[3, 13-18]

The difference in estrogen levels between rural Chinese women and Western women[19] is all the more remarkable because a previous report[20] found that a mere 17% decrease in estrogen levels could account for a huge difference in breast cancer rates when comparing different countries. Imagine, then, what 26–63% lower blood estrogen levels and eight to nine fewer reproductive years of blood estrogen exposure could mean, as we found in the China Study.

This idea that breast cancer is centered on estrogen exposure[3, 21, 22] is profound because diet plays a major role in establishing estrogen exposure. This suggests that the risk of breast cancer is preventable if we eat foods that will keep estrogen levels under control. The sad truth is that most women simply are not aware of this evidence. If this information were properly reported by responsible and credible public health agencies, I suspect that many more young women might be taking very real, very effective steps to avoid this awful disease.

THE COMMON ISSUES

Genes

Understandably, women who are most afraid of this disease have a family history of breast cancer. Family history implies that genes do play a role in the development of breast cancer. But I hear too many people say, in effect, that "it's all in the family" and deny that they can do anything to help themselves. This fatalistic attitude removes a sense of personal responsibility for one's own health and profoundly limits available options.

It is true that if you have a family history of breast cancer, you are at an increased risk of getting the disease.[23, 24] However, one research group found that less than 3% of all breast cancer cases can be attributed to family history.[24] Even though other groups have estimated that a higher percentage of cases are due to family history,[25] the vast majority of breast cancer in American women is not due to family history or genes. But genetic fatalism continues to define the nation's mindset.

Among the genes that influence breast cancer risk, BRCA-1 and BRCA-2 have received the most attention since their discovery in 1994.[26-29] These genes, when mutated, confer a higher risk both for breast and ovarian cancers.[30, 31] These mutated genes may be passed on from generation to generation; that is, they are inherited genes.

In the excitement over these discoveries, however, other information has been ignored. First, only 0.2% of individuals in the general population (1 in 500) carry the mutated forms of these genes.[25] Because of the rarity of these genetic aberrations, only a few percent of the breast cancer cases in the general population can be attributed to mutated BRCA-1 or BRCA-2 genes.[32, 33] Second, these genes are not the only genes that participate in the development of this disease[32]; many more will surely be discovered. Third, the mere presence of BRCA-1, BRCA-2 or any other breast cancer gene does not guarantee disease occurrence. Environmental and dietary factors play a central role in determining whether these genes are expressed.

A recent paper[31] reviewed twenty-two studies that assessed the risk of breast (and ovarian) cancer among women who carried mutated BRCA-1 and BRCA-2 genes. Overall, disease risk was 65% for breast cancer and 39% for ovarian cancer by age seventy for BRCA-1 women, and 45% and 11%, respectively, for BRCA-2 women. Women with these genes certainly face high risks for breast cancer. But even among these high-risk women, there is still good reason to believe that more attention to diet is likely to pay handsome rewards. *About half of the women who carry these rare, potent genes do not get breast cancer.*

In short, although the discovery of BRCA-1 and BRCA-2 added an important dimension to the breast cancer story, the excessive emphasis given to these particular genes and genetic causation in general is not warranted.

I do not mean to diminish the importance of knowing all there is to know about these genes for the small minority of women who carry them. But we need to remind ourselves that these genes need to be "expressed" in order for them to participate in disease formation, and nutrition can affect this. We've already seen in chapter three how a diet high in animal-based protein has the potential to control genetic expression.

Screening and Non-Nutritional Prevention

With all of this new information regarding genetic risk and family history, women are often encouraged to get screened for breast cancer. Screening is a reasonable step, especially for women who may have tested positive for the BRCA genes. But it's important to remember that doing a mammography or getting a genetic test to see if you harbor BRCA genes does not constitute prevention of breast cancer.

Screening is merely an observation to see whether the disease has progressed to an observable state. Some studies[34-36] have found that groups of women who undergo frequent mammography have slightly lower mortality rates than groups of women who do not undergo frequent mammography. This implies that our cancer treatments are more likely to be successful if the cancer is found at an earlier stage. This is likely to be true, but there is some concern over the way statistics are used in this debate.

One of the statistics used to support early detection and the ensuing treatments is that once diagnosed with breast cancer, the likelihood of surviving for at least five years is higher than ever before.[37] What this really means is that with the aggressive campaign for regular screening, many women are discovering their breast cancer at an earlier stage of disease. When disease is discovered at an earlier stage it is less likely to lead to death within five years, *regardless of treatment. As a consequence, we may have an improved five-year survival rate simply because women find out that they have breast cancer earlier in the disease progression, not because our treatments have improved over time.*[38]

Beyond the current screening methods, there are other non-nutritional options for prevention that have been promoted. They are especially of interest to women who have a high risk of breast cancer due to family history and/or to the presence of the BRCA genes. These options include taking a drug such as tamoxifen and/or mastectomy.

Tamoxifen is one of the most popular drugs taken to prevent breast cancer,[39, 40] but the long-term benefits of this option are not clear. One major U.S. study showed that tamoxifen administered over a period of four years to women at increased risk of breast cancer reduced the number of cases by an impressive 49%.[41] This benefit, however, may be limited to women whose estrogen levels are very high. It was this result that led the U.S. Food and Drug Administration to approve use of tamoxifen by women who met certain criteria.[42] Other studies suggest that the enthusiasm for this drug is not warranted. Two less substantial European trials[43, 44] have failed to show any statistically significant tamoxifen benefit, raising some doubt about how dramatic the benefit really is. Moreover, there is the additional concern that tamoxifen raises the risks for stroke, uterine cancer, cataracts, deep vein thrombosis and pulmonary embolism, although the overall benefits of breast cancer prevention are still believed to outweigh the risks.[42] Other chemicals have also been investigated as alternatives to tamoxifen, but these drugs are encumbered by limited effectiveness and/or some of the same troublesome side effects.[45, 46]

Drugs such as tamoxifen and its newer analogues are considered *anti-estrogen* drugs. In effect, they work by reducing the activity of estrogen, which is known to be associated with elevated breast cancer risk.[4, 5] My question is quite simple: why don't we ask why estrogen is so high in the first place, and once we recognize its nutritional origin, why don't we then correct that cause? We now have enough information to show that a diet low in animal-based protein, low in fat and high in whole plant foods will reduce estrogen levels. Instead of suggesting dietary change as a solution, we spend hundreds of millions of dollars developing and publicizing a drug that may or may not work and that almost certainly will have unintended side effects.

The ability of dietary factors to control female hormone levels has long been known in the research community, but a recent study was particularly impressive.[47] Several female hormones, which increase with the onset of puberty, were lowered by 20–30% (even 50% lower levels for progesterone!) simply by having girls eight to ten years of age consume a modestly low-fat, low animal-based food diet for seven years.[47] These results are extraordinary because they were obtained with a modest dietary change and were produced during a critical time of a young girl's life, when the first seeds of breast cancer were being sowed. These girls consumed a diet of no more than 28% fat and less than 150 mg cholesterol/day: a moderate plant-based diet. I believe that had they consumed a diet devoid of animal-based foods and had they started this diet earlier in life, they would have seen even greater benefits, including a delay in puberty and an even lower risk of breast cancer later in life.

Women at high risk for breast cancer are given three options: watch and wait, take tamoxifen medication for the remainder of their lives or undergo mastectomy. There should be a fourth option: consuming a diet free of animal-based foods and low in refined carbohydrates, aided by regular monitoring for those at high risk. I stand by the usefulness of this fourth option even for women who have already had a first mastectomy. Using diet as an effective treatment of already-diagnosed disease has been well documented in human studies with advanced heart disease,[48, 49] clinically documented Type 2 diabetes (see chapter seven), advanced melanoma[50] (a deadly skin cancer) and, in experimental animal studies,[51] liver cancer.

Environmental Chemicals

There is another breast cancer conversation that has been taking place for some years now. It concerns environmental chemicals. These widely distributed chemicals have been shown to disrupt hormones, although it is not clear which hormones in humans are being disrupted. These chemicals may also cause reproductive abnormalities, birth defects and Type 2 diabetes.

There are many different types of offending chemicals, most of which are commonly associated with industrial pollution. One group, including dioxins and PCBs, persist in the environment because they are not metabolized when consumed. Thus they are not excreted from the body. Because of this lack of metabolism, these chemicals accumulate in body fat and breast milk of lactating mothers. Some of these chemicals are known to promote the growth of cancer cells, although humans may not be at significant risk unless one consumes excessive quantities of meat, milk and fish. Indeed, 90–95% of our exposure to these chemicals comes from consuming animal products—yet another reason why consuming animal-based foods can be risky.

There is a second group of these environmental chemicals that are also commonly perceived to be significant causes of breast[52] and other cancers. They are called PAHs (Polycyclic Aromatic Hydrocarbons) and are found in auto exhaust, factory smoke stacks, petroleum tar products and tobacco smoke, among other processes common to an industrial society. Unlike the PCBs and dioxins, when we consume PAHs (in food and water), we can metabolize and excrete them. But there is a snag: when the PAHs are metabolized within the body, they produce intermediate products that react with DNA to form tightly bound complexes, or adducts (see chapter three). This is the first step in causing cancer. In fact, these chemicals have recently been shown to adversely affect the BRCA-1 and BRCA-2 genes of breast cancer cells grown in the laboratory.[53]

In chapter three, I described studies in my laboratory showing that when a very potent carcinogen is put into the body, the rate at which it causes problems is mostly controlled by nutrition. Thus the rate at which PAHs are metabolized into products that bind to DNA is very much controlled by what we eat. Very simply, consuming a Western-type diet will increase the rate at which chemical carcinogens like PAHs bind to DNA to form products that cause cancer.

So when a recent study found slightly increased levels of PAH-DNA adducts in women with breast cancer in Long Island, New York,[54] it may well have been that these women were consuming a more meaty diet, which increased the binding of the PAHs to DNA. It is entirely possible that the quantity of PAHs being consumed had nothing to do with increasing breast cancer risk. In fact, in this study, the number of PAH-DNA adducts in these women seem to be *unrelated* to PAH exposure.[54] How is this possible? Perhaps all of the women in this Long Island study consumed a relatively uniform, low level of PAHs, and the only ones who subsequently got breast cancer were the ones who ate a diet high in fat and animal protein, thus causing more of the ingested PAHs to bind to their DNA.

In this same Long Island study, breast cancer was not associated with PCBs and dioxins, the chemicals that can't be metabolized.[55] As a result of the Long Island study, the hype associating environmental chemicals with breast cancer has been somewhat muted. This and other findings suggest that environmental chemicals seem to play a far less significant role for breast cancer than the kind of foods we choose to eat.

Hormone Replacement Therapy

I must briefly mention one final breast cancer issue: whether to use hormone replacement therapy (HRT), which increases breast cancer risk. HRT is taken by many women in order to alleviate unpleasant effects of menopause, protect bone health and prevent coronary heart disease.[56] However, it is now becoming widely acknowledged that HRT is not as beneficial as once thought, and it may have certain severe side effects. So what are the facts?

I am writing this commentary at an opportune time because the results of some large trials of HRT use have been released in the last year.[56] Of special interest are two large randomized intervention trials: the Women's Health Initiative (WHI)[57] and the Heart and Estrogen/ Progestin Replacement Study (HERS).[58] Among women who take HRT, after 5.2 years the WHI trial is showing a 26% *increase* in breast cancer cases while the HERS study is seeing an even greater 30% increase.[59] These studies are consistent. It appears that increased exposure to female hormones, via HRT, does indeed lead to more breast cancer.

It has been thought that HRT is associated with lower rates of coronary heart disease.[56] However, this is not necessarily true. In the large WHI trial, for every 10,000 healthy postmenopausal women who took HRT, there were seven more women with heart disease, eight more with strokes and eight more with pulmonary embolism[57]—the opposite of what had been expected. HRT may *increase* cardiovascular disease risk after all. On the other hand, HRT did have a beneficial effect on colorectal cancer and bone fracture rate. Among every 10,000 women, there were six fewer colorectal cancers and five fewer bone fractures.[57]

So how do you make a decision with such information? Just by adding and subtracting the numbers we can see that HRT may well be the cause of more harm than good. We can tell each individual woman to make her own decision depending on which disease and which unpleasantry she fears the most, as many physicians are likely to do. But this can be a tough decision for women who are having a difficult time with menopause. These women must choose between living unaided through the emotional and physical symptoms of menopause in order to preserve a low risk of breast cancer, or taking HRT to manage their menopause discomforts while increasing their risk of breast cancer and, possibly, cardiovascular disease. To say that this scenario troubles me would be an understatement. We have spent well over a billion dollars on the research and development of these HRT medical preparations, and all we get is some apparent pluses and probably even more minuses. Calling this troubling doesn't begin to describe it.

Instead of relying on HRT, I suggest that there is a better way, using food. The argument goes like this:

- During the reproductive years, hormone levels are elevated, although the levels among women who eat plant-based diets are not as elevated.
- When women reach the end of their reproductive years, it is entirely natural for reproductive hormones of all women to drop to a low "base" level.
- As reproductive years come to an end, the lower hormone levels among plant eaters don't crash as hard as they do among animal eaters. Using hypothetical numbers to illustrate the concept, the

levels of plant eaters may crash from forty to fifteen, rather than
sixty to fifteen for animal eaters.

- These abrupt hormone changes in the body are what cause menopausal symptoms.
- Therefore, a plant-based diet leads to less severe hormone crash
and a gentler menopause.

This argument is eminently reasonable based on what we know, although more studies would be helpful. But even if future studies fail to
confirm these details, a plant-based diet still offers the lowest risk for
both breast cancer and heart disease for other reasons. It might just be
the best of all worlds, something that no drug can offer.

In each of the various issues involving breast cancer risk (tamoxifen
use, HRT use, environmental chemical exposure, preventive mastectomy), I am convinced that these practices are distractions that prevent
us from considering a safer and far more useful nutritional strategy. It is
critical that we change the way we think about this disease, and that we
provide this information to the women who need it.

LARGE BOWEL CANCER
(INCLUDING COLON AND RECTUM)

At the end of June 2002, George W. Bush handed the presidency over to
Dick Cheney for a period of roughly two hours while he underwent a
colonoscopy. Because of the implications President Bush's colonoscopy
had for world politics, the story made national news, and colon and rectal screening were briefly thrust into the spotlight. Across the country,
whether the comedians were making jokes or the news anchors were
describing the drama, everybody was suddenly, briefly, talking about
this thing called a colonoscopy and what it was for. It was a rare moment in which the country turned its focus to some of the most prolific
killer diseases, colon and rectal cancers.

Because colon and rectal cancers are both cancers of the large bowel,
and because of their other similarities, they often are grouped together
under the term colorectal cancer. Colorectal cancer is the fourth most
common cancer worldwide, in terms of overall mortality.[60] It is the second most common in the United States, with 6% of Americans getting the
cancer during their lifetime.[37] Some even claim that, by age seventy, one-
half of the population of "Westernized" countries will develop a tumor in
the large bowel and 10% of these cases will progress to a malignancy.[61]

GEOGRAPHIC DISPARITY

North America, Europe, Australia and wealthier Asian countries (Japan, Singapore) have very high rates of colorectal cancer, while Africa, Asia and most of Central and South America have very low rates of this cancer. For example, the Czech Republic has a death rate of 34.19 per 100,000 males, while Bangladesh has a death rate of 0.63 per 100,000 males![62, 63] Chart 8.3 shows a comparison of average death rates between more developed countries and less developed countries; all these rates are age-adjusted.

The fact that rates of colorectal cancer vary hugely between countries has been known for decades. The question has always been why. Are the differences due to genetics, or to environment?

It seems that environmental factors, including diet, play the most important roles in colorectal cancer. Migrant studies have shown that as people move from a low-cancer risk area to a high-cancer risk area, they assume an increased risk within two generations.[64] This suggests that diet and lifestyle are important causes of this cancer. Other studies have also found that rates of colorectal cancer change rapidly as a population's diet or lifestyle changes.[64] These rapid changes in cancer rates within one population cannot possibly be explained by changes in inherited genes. In the context of human society, it takes thousands of

CHART 8.3: COLORECTAL CANCER DEATH RATE IN "MORE DEVELOPED" COUNTRIES AND "LESS DEVELOPED" COUNTRIES

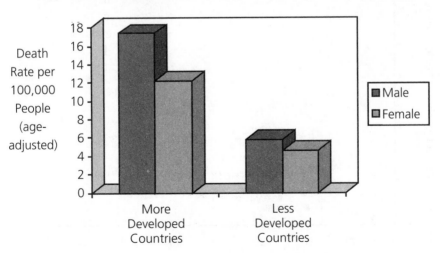

years to get widespread, permanent changes in the inherited genes that are passed from one generation to the next. Clearly, something about environment or lifestyle is either preventing or enhancing the risk of getting colorectal cancer.

In a landmark paper published almost thirty years ago, researchers compared environmental factors and cancer rates in thirty-two countries around the world.[65] One of the strongest links between any cancer and any dietary factor was between colon cancer and meat intake. Chart 8.4 shows this link for women in twenty-three different countries.

In this report, countries where more meat, more animal protein, more sugar and fewer cereal grains were consumed had far higher rates of colon cancer.[65] Another researcher whom I mentioned in chapter four, Denis Burkitt, hypothesized that intake of dietary fiber was essential for digestive health in general. He compared stool samples and fiber intakes in Africa and Europe and proposed that colorectal cancers were largely the result of low fiber intake.[66] Fiber, remember, is only found in plant foods. It is the part of the plant that our body cannot digest. Using data from another famous study that compared diets in seven different countries, researchers found that eating an additional ten grams of dietary fiber a day lowered the long-term risk of colon cancer by 33%.[67] There are ten grams of fiber in one cup of red raspberries, one Asian pear or

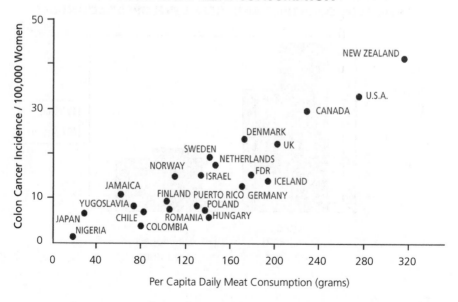

**CHART 8.4: FEMALE COLON CANCER INCIDENCE
AND DAILY MEAT CONSUMPTION**

one cup of peas. A cup of just about any variety of bean would provide significantly more than ten grams of fiber.

From all this research, it seems clear that something can be said for the importance of diet in colorectal cancer. But what exactly stops colon and rectal cancer? Is it fiber? Is it fruits and vegetables? Is it carbohydrates? Is it milk? Each of these foods or nutrients has been suggested to play a role. The debate has raged, and solid answers are seldom agreed upon.

THE SPECIFIC CURE

Most of the debate over the past twenty-five years on dietary fiber and its link to large bowel cancer began with Burkitt's work in Africa. Because of Burkitt's prominence, many people have believed that fiber is the source of colorectal health. Perhaps you have already heard that fiber is good for preventing colon cancer. At least you probably have heard that fiber "keeps things running well." Isn't that what prunes are known for?

Yet nobody has ever been able to prove that fiber is the magic bullet for preventing colorectal cancer. There are important technical reasons why a definitive conclusion regarding fiber is difficult to make.[68] Each of these reasons is related either directly or indirectly to the fact that dietary fiber is not a single, simple substance producing a single, simple benefit. Fiber represents hundreds of substances, and "its" benefits operate through an exceptionally complex series of biochemical and physiological events. Each time researchers assess the consumption of dietary fiber, they must decide which of the hundreds of fiber sub-fractions to measure and which methods to use. It is nearly impossible to establish a standard procedure because it is virtually impossible to know what each fiber sub-fraction does in the body.

The uncertainty of having a standard procedure prompted us to measure fiber in more than a dozen ways in our China Study. As summarized in chapter four, as consumption of almost all of these fiber types went up, colon and rectal cancer rates went down.[69] But we could make no clear interpretations[70] as to which type of fiber was especially important.

Despite the uncertainties, I continue to believe that Burkitt's[66] initial hypothesis that *fiber-containing diets* prevent colorectal cancers is correct and that some of this effect is due to the aggregate effect of all the fiber types. In fact, the hypothesis that dietary fiber prevents large bowel cancers has become even more convincing. In 1990, a group of researchers reviewed sixty different studies that had been done on fiber and colon cancer.[71] They found that most of the studies supported the idea that fiber protects against colon cancer. They noted that the combined results showed that the people who consumed the most fiber had a 43% lower risk of colon cancer than the people who consumed the least fiber.[71] Those who consume the most vegetables had a 52% lower risk than those who consume the least vegetables.[71] But even in this large review of the evidence, researchers noted, "the data do not permit discrimination between effects due to fiber and non-fiber effects due to vegetables."[71] So is fiber, all by itself, the magic bullet we've been looking for? We still, in 1990, didn't know.

Two years later, in 1992, a different group of researchers reviewed thirteen studies that had compared people with and without colorectal cancer (case-control design).[72] They found that those who had consumed the most fiber had a 47% lower risk of colorectal cancer than those who consumed the least.[72] In fact, they found that if Americans ate an additional thirteen grams of fiber a day *from food sources* (not as supplements), about a third of all colorectal cancer cases in the U.S. could be avoided.[72] If you'll remember, thirteen grams, in real world terms, is the amount found in about a cup of any variety of beans.

More recently, a mammoth study called the EPIC study collected data on fiber intake and colorectal cancer in 519,000 people across Europe.[73] They found that the 20% of people who consumed the most fiber in their diet, about thirty-four grams per day, had a 42% lower risk of colorectal cancer than the 20% who consumed the least fiber in their diet, about thirteen grams per day.[73] It's important to note once again that, as with all of these studies, dietary fiber was obtained in food, not as supplements. So all we can say is "fiber-containing diets" seem to significantly reduce the risk of colorectal cancer. We still can't say anything definitive about isolated fiber itself. This means that attempts to add isolated fiber to foods may not produce benefits. But consuming plant foods naturally high in fiber is clearly beneficial. These foods include vegetables (the non-root parts), fruits and whole grains.

In reality, we can't even be sure how much of the prevention of colorectal cancer is due to fiber-containing foods, because as people eat more of these foods they usually consume less animal-based foods. In other words, are fruits, vegetables and whole grains protective, or is meat dangerous? Or is it both? A recent study in South Africa helped to answer these questions. White South Africans have seventeen times more large bowel cancer than black South Africans, and this was first thought to be due to the much higher consumption of dietary fiber among black South Africans provided by unrefined maize.[74] However, in more recent years, black South Africans have been increasingly consuming commercially *refined* maize-meal—maize minus its fiber. They now eat even less fiber than the white South Africans. Yet, colon cancer rates among blacks remain at a low level,[75] which calls into question how much of the cancer-protective effect is due to dietary fiber alone. A more recent study[76] showed that the higher colon cancer rates among white South Africans could well be due to their elevated consumption of animal protein (77 vs. 25 g/day), total fat (115 vs. 71 g/day) and cholesterol (408 vs. 211 mg/day), as seen in Chart 8.5. The researchers suggested that the much higher colon cancer rates among white South

CHART 8.5: INTAKE OF ANIMAL PROTEIN, TOTAL FAT AND CHOLESTEROL AMONG BLACK AND WHITE SOUTH AFRICANS

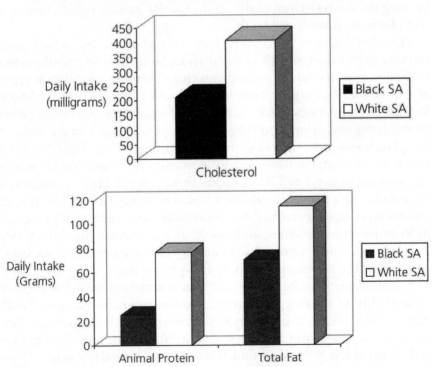

Africans may be more related to the quantity of animal protein and fat in their diets than their lacking the protective factor of dietary fiber.[76]

What is clear is that diets naturally high in fiber and low in animal-based foods can prevent colorectal cancer. Even in the absence of more specific details, we can still make important public health recommendations. *The data clearly show that a whole foods, plant-based diet can dramatically lower colorectal cancer rates. We don't need to know which fiber is responsible, what mechanism is involved or even how much of the effect is independently due to fiber.*

OTHER FACTORS

It has been recently noted that the same risk factors that promote colorectal cancer, a diet low in fruits and vegetables and high in animal foods and refined carbohydrates, can also promote insulin resistance syndrome.[77–79] From there, scientists have hypothesized that insulin resistance may be responsible for colon cancer.[77–82] Insulin resistance was described in chapter six as a diabetic condition. And what's good for keeping insulin resistance under control is also good for colon cancer: a diet of whole, plant-based foods.

This diet happens to be very high in carbohydrates, which have recently been under assault in the marketplace. Because carbohydrate-confusion persists, let me remind you that there are two different types of carbohydrates: refined carbohydrates and complex carbohydrates. Refined carbohydrates are the starches and sugars obtained from plants by mechanically stripping off their outer layers, which contain most of the plant's vitamins, minerals, protein and fiber. This "food" (regular sugar, white flour, etc.) has very little nutritional value. Foods such as pastas made from refined flour, sugary cereals, white bread, candies and sugar-laden soft drinks should be avoided as much as possible. But do eat whole, complex carbohydrate-containing foods such as unprocessed fresh fruits and vegetables, and whole grain products like brown rice and oatmeal. These unprocessed carbohydrates, especially from fruits and vegetables, are exceptionally health-promoting.

You also may have heard that calcium is beneficial in fighting colon cancer. This, of course, gets extended to the argument that cow's milk fights colon cancer. It has been hypothesized that high-calcium diets prevent colon cancer in two ways: first, it inhibits the growth of critical cells in the colon,[83, 84] and second, it binds up intestinal bile acids. These bile acids arise in the liver, move to the intestine and are thought to get into the large bowel and promote colon cancer development. By binding these bile acids, calcium is said to prevent colon cancer.

One research group demonstrated that high-calcium diets—generally meaning diets high in dairy foods—inhibit the growth of certain cells in the colon,[84] *but this effect was not entirely consistent for the various indicators of cell growth. Furthermore, it is not clear whether these presumably favorable biochemical effects really lead to less cancer growth.*[83, 85]Another research group demonstrated that calcium does reduce the presumably dangerous bile acids, but also observed that *a high-wheat diet did an even better job of reducing the bile acids.*[86] But—and this is the really odd part—when a combination high-calcium and high-wheat diet was consumed, the binding effect on bile acids was weaker than for each individual supplement taken alone.[86] It just goes to show that when individually-observed nutrient effects are combined, as in a dietary situation, the expected may become the unexpected.

I doubt that a high-calcium diet, obtained through calcium supplements or through calcium-rich cow's milk, has a beneficial effect on colon cancer. In rural China where calcium consumption is modest and almost no dairy food is consumed,[87] colon cancer rates are not higher; instead they are much lower than in the U.S. The parts of the world that consume the most calcium, Europe and North America, have the highest rates of colorectal cancer.

Another lifestyle choice that is clearly important for this disease is exercise. Increased exercise is convincingly associated with less colorectal cancer. In one summary from the World Cancer Research Fund and the American Institute for Cancer Research, seventeen out of twenty studies found that exercise protected against colon cancer.[64] Unfortunately, there seems to be no convincing evidence as to why or how this occurs.

SCREENING FOR TROUBLE

The benefits of exercise bring me back to President George W. Bush. He is known to enjoy staying physically fit with a regular running routine, and that is undoubtedly one of the reasons why he received a clean bill of health when he had a colonoscopy. But what is a colonoscopy anyway, and is it really worth the effort to get checked? When people go to the doctor to get a colonoscopy, the doctor inspects the large bowel using a rectal probe and looks for abnormal tissue growth. The most commonly found abnormality is a polyp. Although it is not yet clear exactly how tumors are related to polyps, most scientists would agree[88, 89] that they share similar dietary associations and genetic characteristics. Those people who have noncancerous problems in the large bowel, such as polyps, often are the same people who later develop cancerous tumors.

So getting screened for polyps or other problems is a reasonable way to establish risk for large bowel cancer in the future. But what if you have a polyp? What is the best thing to do? Will surgical removal of the polyp lessen colon cancer risk? A nationwide study has shown that, when polyps were removed, there was a 76–90% decrease in the expected cases of colon cancer.[89, 90] This certainly supports the idea of routine screening.[89, 91] It is commonly recommended that people get a colonoscopy once every ten years starting at the age of fifty. If you have a higher risk of colorectal cancer, it is recommended that you start at the age of forty and screen more frequently.

How do you know if you are at a higher risk for colorectal cancer? We can very roughly assess our personal genetic risk in several ways. We can consider the probability of our getting colon cancer based on the number of immediate family members who already have the disease, we can screen for the presence of polyps, and we now can clinically test for the presence of suspect genes.[92]

This is an excellent example of how genetic research can lead to a better understanding of complex diseases. However, in the enthusiasm for studying the genetic basis for this cancer, two things often get overlooked. First, the proportion of colon cancer cases attributed to known inherited genes is only about 1–3%.[89] Another 10–30%[89] tend to occur in some families more than others (called familial clustering), an effect possibly reflective of a significant genetic contribution. These numbers, however, exaggerate the number of cancers that are solely "due to genes."

Except for the very few people whose colon cancer risk is largely determined by known inherited genes (1–3%), most of the family-con-nected colon cancer cases (i.e, the additional 10–30%) are still largely determined by environmental and dietary factors. After all, place of resi-dence and diet are often shared experiences within families.

Even if you have a high genetic risk, a healthy plant-based diet is capable of negating most, if not all, of that risk by controlling the ex-pression of these genes. Because a high-fiber diet can only prevent colon cancer—extra fiber won't ever *promote* colon cancer—dietary recom-mendations should be the same regardless of one's genetic risk.

PROSTATE CANCER

I suspect that most people do not know exactly what a prostate is, even though prostate cancer is commonly discussed. The prostate is a male reproductive organ about the size of a walnut, located between the bladder and the colon. It is responsible for producing some of the fluid that helps sperm on its quest to fertilize the female's egg.

For such a little thing, it sure can cause a lot of problems. Several of my friends now have prostate cancer or closely related conditions, and they aren't alone. As one recent report pointed out, "Prostate cancer is one of the most commonly diagnosed cancers among men in the United States, representing about 25% of all tumors...."[93] As many as half of all men seventy years and older have latent prostate cancer,[94] a silent form of the cancer which is not yet causing discomfort. Prostate cancer is not only extremely prevalent, but also slow-growing. Only 7% of diagnosed prostate cancer victims die within five years.[95] This makes it difficult to know how and if the cancer should be treated. The main question for the patient and doctor is: will this cancer become life threatening before death comes from other causes?

One of the markers used to determine the likelihood of prostate cancer becoming life threatening is the blood level of prostate specific antigen (PSA). Men are diagnosed as having prostate problems when their PSA levels are above four. But this test alone is hardly a firm diagnosis of cancer, especially if the PSA level is barely above four. The ambiguity of this test leads to some very difficult decision-making. Occasionally my friends ask for my opinion. Should they have a little surgery or a lot? Is a PSA value of 6.0 a serious problem or just a wake-up call? If it's a wake-up call, then what must they do to reduce such a number? While I cannot speak to the clinical condition of an individual, I can speak to the research, and of the research I have seen, there is no doubt that diet plays a key role in this disease.

Although there is debate regarding the specifics of diet and this cancer, let's start with some very safe assumptions that have long been accepted in the research community:

- Prostate cancer rates vary widely between different countries, even more than breast cancer.
- High prostate cancer rates primarily exist in societies with "Western" diets and lifestyles.

- In developing countries, men who adopt Western eating practices or move to Western countries suffer more prostate cancer.

These disease patterns are similar to those of other diseases of affluence. Mostly this tells us that although prostate cancer certainly has a genetic component, environmental factors play the dominant role. So what environmental factors are important? You can guess that I'm going to say plant-based foods are good and animal-based foods are bad, but do we know anything more specific? Surprisingly, one of the most consistent, specific links between diet and prostate cancer has been dairy consumption.

A 2001 Harvard review of the research could hardly be more convincing[96]:

> ...twelve of...fourteen case-control studies and seven of...nine cohort studies [have] observed a positive association for some measure of dairy products and prostate cancer; *this is one of the most consistent dietary predictors for prostate cancer in the published literature* [my emphasis]. In these studies, men with the highest dairy intakes had approximately double the risk of total prostate cancer, and up to a fourfold increase in risk of metastatic or fatal prostate cancer relative to low consumers.[96]

Let's consider that again: dairy intake is "one of the most consistent dietary predictors for prostate cancer in the published literature," and those who consume the most dairy have double to quadruple the risk.

Another review of published literature done in 1998 reached a similar conclusion:

> In ecologic data, correlations exist between per capita meat and dairy consumption and prostate cancer mortality rate [one study cited]. In case control and prospective studies, the major contributors of animal protein, meats, dairy products and eggs have frequently been associated with a higher risk of prostate cancer... [twenty-three studies cited]. Of note, numerous studies have found an association primarily in older men [six studies cited] though not all [one study cited].... The consistent associations with dairy products could result from, at least in part, their calcium and phosphorous content.[97]

In other words, an enormous body of evidence shows that animal-based foods are associated with prostate cancer. In the case of dairy, the high intake of calcium and phosphorus also could be partly responsible for this effect.

This research leaves little room for dissent; each of the above studies represents analyses of over a dozen individual studies, providing an impressive bulk of convincing literature.

THE MECHANISMS

As we have seen with other forms of cancer, large-scale observational studies show a link between prostate cancer and an animal-based diet, particularly one based heavily on dairy. Understanding the mechanisms behind the observed link between prostate cancer and dairy clinches the argument.

The first mechanism concerns a hormone that increases cancer cell growth, a hormone that our bodies make, as needed. This growth hormone, Insulin-like Growth Factor 1 (IGF-1), is turning out to be a predictor of cancer just as cholesterol is a predictor for heart disease. Under normal conditions, this hormone efficiently manages the rates at which cells "grow"—that is, how they reproduce themselves and how they discard old cells, all in the name of good health.

Under unhealthy conditions, however, IGF-1 becomes more active, increasing the birth and growth of new cells while simultaneously inhibiting the removal of old cells, both of which favor the development of cancer [seven studies cited[98]]. So what does this have to do with the food we eat? It turns out that consuming animal-based foods increases the blood levels of this growth hormone, IGF-1.[99–101]

With regard to prostate cancer, people with higher than normal blood levels of IGF-I have been shown to have 5.1 times the risk of advanced-stage prostate cancer.[98] There's more: when men also have low blood levels of a protein that binds and inactivates IGF-I,[102] they will have *9.5 times the risk of advanced-stage prostate cancer*,[98] Let's put a few stars by these numbers. They are big and impressive—and fundamental to this finding is the fact that we make more IGF-I when we consume animal-based foods like meat and dairy.[99–101]

The second mechanism relates to vitamin D metabolism. This "vitamin" is not a nutrient that we need to consume. Our body can make all that we need simply by being in sunlight fifteen to thirty minutes every couple of days. In addition to the production of vitamin D being affected by sunlight, it is also affected by the food that we eat. The formation of the most active form of vitamin D is a process that is closely monitored and controlled by our bodies. This process is a great example of our bodies' natural balancing act, affecting not only prostate cancer, but breast cancer, colon cancer, osteoporosis and autoimmune diseases like Type 1 diabetes. Because of its importance for multiple diseases, and because of the complexity involved in explaining how it all works, I have provided in Appendix C an abbreviated scheme, just enough to illustrate my point. This web of reactions illustrates many similar and highly integrated reaction networks showing how food controls health.

The main component of this process is an active form of vitamin D produced in the body from the vitamin D that we get from food or sunshine. This active or "supercharged" D produces many benefits throughout the body, including the prevention of cancer, autoimmune diseases and diseases like osteoporosis. This all-important supercharged D is not something that you get from food or from a drug. A drug composed of isolated supercharged D would be far too powerful and far too dangerous for medical use. Your body uses a carefully composed series of controls and sensors to produce just the right amount of supercharged D for each task at exactly the right time.

As it turns out, our diet can determine how much of this supercharged D is produced and how it works once it is produced. Animal protein that we consume has the tendency to block the production of supercharged D, leaving the body with low levels of this vitamin D in the blood. If these low levels persist, prostate cancer can result. Also, persistently high intakes of calcium create an environment where supercharged D declines, thus adding to the problem.

So what food substance has both animal protein and large amounts of calcium? *Milk and other dairy foods.* This fits in perfectly with the evidence that links dairy consumption with prostate cancer. This information provides what we call biological plausibility and shows how the observational data fit together. To review the mechanisms:

- Animal protein causes the body to produce more IGF-1, which in turn throws cell growth and removal out of whack, stimulating cancer development.
- Animal protein suppresses the production of "supercharged" D.
- Excessive calcium, as found in milk, also suppresses the production of "supercharged" D.

- "Supercharged" D is responsible for creating a wide variety of health benefits in the body. Persistently low levels of supercharged D create an inviting environment for different cancers, autoimmune diseases, osteoporosis and other diseases.

The important story here is how the effects of food—both good and bad—operate through a symphony of coordinated reactions to prevent diseases like prostate cancer. In discovering the existence of these networks, we sometimes wonder which specific function comes first and which comes next. We tend to think of these reactions within the network as independent. But this surely misses the point. What impresses me is the multitude of reactions working together in so many ways to produce the same effect: in this case, to prevent disease.

There is no single "mechanism" that fully explains what causes diseases such as cancer. Indeed, it would be foolish to even think along these lines. But what I do know is this: the totality and breadth of the evidence, operating through highly coordinated networks, supports the conclusions that consuming dairy and meat are serious risk factors for prostate cancer.

BRINGING IT TOGETHER

Roughly half a million Americans this year will go to the doctor's office and be told that they have cancer of the breast, prostate or large bowel. People who get one of these cancers represent 40% of all new cancer patients. These three cancers devastate the lives of not only the victims themselves, but also their family and friends.

When my mother-in-law died of colon cancer at the age of fifty-one, none of us knew that much about nutrition or what it meant for health. It wasn't that we didn't care about the health of our loved ones—of course we did. We just didn't have the information. Yet, over thirty years later, not much has changed. Of the people you know who have cancer, or are at risk of having cancer, how many of them have considered the possibility of adopting a whole foods, plant-based diet to improve their chances? I'm guessing very few of them have done so. Probably they, too, don't have the information.

Our institutions and information providers are failing us. Even cancer organizations, at both the national and local level, are reluctant to discuss or even believe this evidence. Food as a key to health represents a powerful challenge to conventional medicine, which is fundamentally built on drugs and surgery (see Part IV). The widespread communities of nutrition professionals, researchers and doctors are, as a whole, either unaware of this evidence or reluctant to share it. Because of these failings, Americans are being cheated out of information that could save their lives.

There is enough evidence now that doctors should be discussing the option of pursuing dietary change as a potential path to cancer prevention and treatment. There is enough evidence now that the U.S. government should be discussing the idea that the toxicity of our diet is the single biggest cause of cancer. There is enough evidence now that local breast cancer alliances, and prostate and colon cancer institutions, should be discussing the possibility of providing information to Americans everywhere on how a whole foods, plant-based diet may be an incredibly effective anti-cancer medicine.

If these discussions were to happen, it is possible that, next year, fewer than 500,000 people would go to the doctor's office and be told they have cancer of the breast, prostate or large bowel. The year after that, even fewer friends, coworkers and family members would be given the most dreaded of all diagnoses. And the following year, even fewer.

The possibility that this future could be our reality is real, and as long as this future holds such promise for the health of people everywhere, it is a future worth working for.

9
Autoimmune Diseases

No GROUP OF DISEASES is more insidious than autoimmune diseases. They are difficult to treat, and progressive loss of physical and mental function is a common outcome. Unlike heart disease, cancer, obesity and Type 2 diabetes, with autoimmune diseases the body systematically attacks itself. The afflicted patient is almost guaranteed to lose.

A quarter million people in the U.S. are diagnosed with one of the forty separate autoimmune diseases each year.[1, 2] Women are 2.7 times more likely to be afflicted than are men. About 3% of Americans (one in every thirty-one people) have an autoimmune disease, a staggering total of 8.5 million people; some people put the total at as many as 12–13 million people.[3]

The more common of these diseases are listed in Chart 9.1.[2] The first nine comprise 97% of all autoimmune disease cases.[2] The most studied are multiple sclerosis (MS), rheumatoid arthritis, lupus, Type 1 diabetes and rheumatic heart disease.[2] These are also the primary autoimmune diseases that have been studied in reference to diet.

Others not listed in Chart 9.1 include inflammatory bowel disease,[4] Crohn's disease,[4] rheumatic heart disease[3] and (possibly) Parkinson's disease.[5]

Each disease name may sound very different, but as one recent review points out,[2] "...it is important to consider...these disorders as a group." They show similar clinical backgrounds,[3, 6, 7] they sometimes occur in the same person and they are often found in the same populations.[2] MS and Type 1 diabetes, for example, have "near(ly) identical

> ### CHART 9.1: COMMON AUTOIMMUNE DISEASES
> ### (FROM MOST COMMON TO LEAST COMMON)
>
> | | |
> |---|---|
> | 1. Graves' disease (Hyperthyroidism) | 10. Sjogren's disease |
> | 2. Rheumatoid arthritis | 11. Myasthenia gravis |
> | 3. Thyroiditis (Hypothyroidism) | 12. Polymyositis/dermatomyositis |
> | 4. Vitiligo | 13. Addison's disease |
> | 5. Pernicious anemia | 14. Scleroderma |
> | 6. Glomerulonephritis | 15. Primary biliary cirrhosis |
> | 7. Multiple sclerosis | 16. Uveitis |
> | 8. Type 1 diabetes | 17. Chronic active hepatitis |
> | 9. Systemic lupus erythematosus | |

ethnic and geographic distribution."[8] Autoimmune diseases in general become more common the greater the distance from the equator. This phenomenon has been known since 1922.[9] MS, for example, is over a hundred times more prevalent in the far north than at the equator.[10]

Because of some of these common features, it is not too far-fetched to think of the autoimmune diseases as one grand disease living in different places in the body and taking on different names. We refer in this way to cancer, which is specifically named depending on what part of the body it resides in.

All autoimmune diseases are the result of one group of mechanisms gone awry, much like cancer. In this case, the mechanism is the immune system mistakenly attacking cells in its own body. Whether it is the pancreas as in Type 1 diabetes, the myelin sheath as in MS or joint tissues as in arthritis, all autoimmune diseases involve an immune system that has revolted. It is an internal mutiny of the worst kind, one in which our body becomes its own worst enemy.

IMMUNITY FROM INVADERS

The immune system is astonishingly complex. I often hear people speaking about this system as if it were an identifiable organ like a lung. Nothing could be further from the truth. It is a system, not an organ.

In essence, our immune system is like a military network designed to defend against foreign invaders. The "soldiers" of this network are the white blood cells, which are comprised of many different sub-groups, each having its own mission. These sub-groups are analogous to a navy, army, air force and marines, with each group of specialists doing highly specialized work.

The "recruitment center" for the system is in the marrow of our bones. The marrow is responsible for generating specialized cells called stem cells. Some of these cells are released into circulation for use elsewhere in the body; these are called B-cells (for bone). Other cells formed in the bone marrow remain immature, or unspecialized, until they travel to the thymus (an organ in the chest cavity just above the heart) where they become specialized; these are called T-cells (for thymus). These "soldier" cells, along with other specialized cells, team up to create intricate defense plans. They meet at major intersections around the body, including the spleen (just inside the left lower rib cage) and the lymph nodes. These meeting points are like command and control centers, where the "soldier cells" rearrange themselves into teams to attack foreign invaders.

These cells are remarkably adaptable when they form their teams. They are able to respond to different circumstances and different foreign substances, even those they have never before seen. The immune response to these strangers is an incredibly creative process. It is one of the true wonders of nature.

The foreign invaders are protein molecules called antigens. These foreign cells can be a bacterium or a virus looking to corrupt the body's integrity. So when our immune system notices these foreign cells, or antigens, it destroys them. Each of these foreign antigens has a separate identity, which is determined by the sequence of amino acids that comprises its proteins. It is analogous to each and every person having a different face. Because numerous amino acids are available for creating proteins, there are infinite varieties of distinctive "faces."

To counter these antigens, our immune system must customize its defense to each attack. It does this by creating a "mirror image" protein for each attacker. The mirror image is able to fit perfectly onto the antigen and destroy it. Essentially, the immune system creates a mold for each face it encounters. Every time it sees that face after the initial encounter, it uses the custom-made mold to "capture" the invader and destroy it. The mold may be a B-cell antibody or a T-cell-based receptor protein.

Remembering each defense against each invader is what immunization is all about. An initial exposure to chicken pox, for example, is a difficult battle, but the second time you encounter that virus you will know exactly how to deal with it, and the war will be shorter, less painful and much more successful. You may not even get sick.

IMMUNITY FROM OURSELVES

Even though this system is a wonder of nature when it is defending the body against foreign proteins, it is also capable of attacking the same tissues that it is designed to protect. This self-destructive process is common to all autoimmune diseases. It is as if the body were to commit suicide.

One of the fundamental mechanisms for this self-destructive behavior is called molecular mimicry. It so happens that some of the foreign invaders that our soldier cells seek out to destroy look the same as our own cells. The immune system "molds" that fit these invaders also fit our own cells. The immune system then destroys, under some circumstances, everything that fits the mold, including our own cells. This is an extremely complex self-destructive process involving many different strategies on the part of the immune system, all of which share the same fatal flaw of not being able to distinguish "foreign" invader proteins from the proteins of our own body.

What does all of this have to do with what we eat? It so happens that the antigens that trick our bodies into attacking our own cells may be in food. During the process of digestion, for example, some proteins slip into our bloodstream from the intestine without being fully broken down into their amino acid parts. The remnants of undigested proteins are treated as foreign invaders by our immune system, which sets about making molds to destroy them and sets into motion the self-destructive autoimmune process.

One of the foods that supply many of the foreign proteins that mimic our own body proteins is cow's milk. Most of the time, our immune system is quite smart. Just like an army arranges for safeguards against friendly fire, the immune system has safeguards to stop itself from attacking the body it's supposed to protect. Even though an invading antigen looks just like one of the cells in our own body, the system can still distinguish our own cells from the invading antigen. In fact, the immune system may use our own cells to practice making molds against the invader antigen *without actually destroying the friendly cell.*

This is analogous to training camps in preparations for war. When our immune system is working properly, we can use the cells in our body that look like the antigens as a training exercise, without destroying them, to prepare our soldier cells to repulse the invading antigens. It is one more example[1] of the exceptional elegance of nature's ability to regulate itself.

The immune system uses a very delicate process to decide which proteins should be attacked and which should be left alone.[11] The way this process, which is incredibly complex, breaks down with autoimmune diseases is not yet understood. We just know that the immune system loses its ability to differentiate between the body's cells and the invading antigen, and instead of using the body's cells for "training," it destroys them along with the invaders.

TYPE 1 DIABETES

In the case of Type 1 diabetes, the immune system attacks the pancreas cells responsible for producing insulin. This devastating, incurable disease strikes children, creating a painful and difficult experience for young families. What most people don't know, though, is that there is strong evidence that this disease is linked to diet and, more specifically, to dairy products. The ability of cow's milk protein to initiate Type 1 diabetes[12–14] is well documented. The possible initiation of this disease goes like this:

- A baby is not nursed long enough and is fed cow's milk protein, perhaps in an infant formula.
- The milk reaches the small intestine, where it is digested down to its amino acid parts.
- For some infants, cow's milk is not fully digested, and small amino acid chains or fragments of the original protein remain in the intestine.
- These incompletely digested protein fragments may be absorbed into the blood.
- The immune system recognizes these fragments as foreign invaders and goes about destroying them.
- Unfortunately, some of the fragments look exactly the same as the cells of the pancreas that are responsible for making insulin.
- The immune system loses its ability to distinguish between the cow's milk protein fragments and the pancreatic cells, and destroys them both, thereby eliminating the child's ability to produce insulin.
- The infant becomes a Type 1 diabetic, and remains so for the rest of his or her life.

This process boils down to a truly remarkable statement: *cow's milk may cause one of the most devastating diseases that can befall a child.* For obvious reasons, this is one of the most contentious issues in nutrition today.

One of the more remarkable reports on this cow's milk effect was published over a decade ago, in 1992, in the *New England Journal of Medicine*.[12] The researchers, from Finland, obtained blood from Type 1 diabetic children, aged four to twelve years. Then they measured the levels of antibodies that had formed in the blood against an incompletely digested protein of cow's milk called bovine serum albumin (BSA). They did the same process with non-diabetic children and compared the two groups (remember, an antibody is the mirror image, or "mold," of a foreign antigen). Children who had antibodies to cow's milk protein must have previously consumed cow's milk. It also means that undigested protein fragments of the cow's milk proteins had to have entered the infant's circulation in order to cause the formation of antibodies in the first place.

The researchers discovered something truly remarkable. Of the 142 diabetic children measured, *every single one had antibody levels higher than 3.55.* Of the seventy-nine normal children measured, *every single one had antibody levels less than 3.55.*

There is absolutely no overlap between antibodies of healthy and diabetic children. All of the diabetic children had levels of cow's milk antibodies that were higher than those of all of the non-diabetic children. This implies two things: children with more antibodies consumed more cow's milk, and second, increased antibodies may cause Type 1 diabetes.

These results sent shock waves through the research community. It was the complete separation of antibody responses that made this study so remarkable. This study,[12] and others even earlier,[15–17] initiated an avalanche of additional studies over the next several years that continue to this day.[13, 18, 19]

Several studies have since investigated this effect of cow's milk on BSA antibody levels. All but one showed that cow's milk increases BSA antibodies in Type 1 diabetic children,[18] although the responses were quite variable in their magnitude.

Over the past decade, scientists have investigated far more than just the BSA antibodies, and a more complete picture is coming into view. Very briefly, it goes something like this[13, 19]: infants or very young children of a certain genetic background,[20, 21] who are weaned from the breast too early[22] onto cow's milk and who, perhaps, become infected with a virus that may corrupt the gut immune system,[19] are likely to have a high risk for Type 1 diabetes. A study in Chile[23] considered the first two factors, cow's milk and genes. Genetically susceptible children weaned too early onto cow's milk-based formula had a risk of Type 1 diabetes that was 13.1 times greater than children who did not have these genes and who were breast-fed for at least three months (thus minimizing their exposure to cow's milk). Another study in the U.S. showed that genetically susceptible children fed cow's milk as infants had a risk of disease that was 11.3 times greater than children who did not have these genes and who were breast-fed for at least three months.[24] This eleven to thirteen times greater risk is incredibly large (1,000–1,200%!); anything over three to four times is usually considered very important. To put this in perspective, smokers have approximately ten times greater risk of getting lung cancer (still less than the eleven to thirteen times risk here) and people with high blood pressure and cholesterol have a 2.5–3.0 times greater risk of heart disease (Chart 9.2).[18]

So how much of the eleven to thirteen times increased risk of Type 1 diabetes is due to early exposure to cow's milk, and how much is due

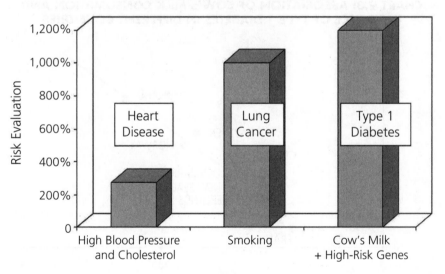

CHART 9.2: RELATIVE RISKS OF VARIOUS FACTORS ON VARIOUS DISEASE OUTCOMES

to genes? These days, there is a popular opinion that Type 1 diabetes is due to genetics, an opinion often shared by doctors as well. But genetics alone cannot account for more than a very small fraction of cases of this disease. Genes do not act in isolation; they need a trigger for their effects to be produced. It has also been observed that after one member of identical twin pairs gets Type 1 diabetes, there is only a 13–33% chance of the second twin getting the disease, even though both twins have the same genes.[13, 20, 21, 25, 26] If it were all due to genes, closer to 100% of the identical twins would get the disease. In addition, it is possible that the 13–33% risk for the second twin is due to the sharing of a common environment and diet, factors affecting both twins.

Consider, for example, the observation shown in Chart 9.3, which highlights the link between one aspect of environment, cow's milk consumption, and this disease. Cow's milk consumption by children zero to fourteen years of age in twelve countries[27] shows an almost perfect correlation with Type 1 diabetes.[28] The greater the consumption of cow's milk, the greater the prevalence of Type 1 diabetes. In Finland, Type 1 diabetes is thirty-six times more common than in Japan.[29] Large amounts of cow's milk products are consumed in Finland but very little is consumed in Japan.[27]

CHART 9.3: ASSOCIATION OF COW'S MILK CONSUMPTION AND INCIDENCE OF TYPE 1 DIABETES IN DIFFERENT COUNTRIES

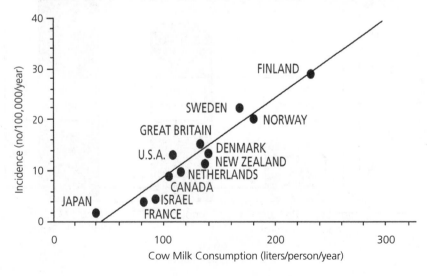

As we have seen with other diseases of affluence, when people migrate from areas of the world where disease incidence is low to areas of the world where disease incidence is high, they quickly adopt the high incidence rates as they change their diet and lifestyle.[30-32] This shows that even though individuals may have the necessary gene(s), the disease will occur only in response to certain dietary and/or environmental circumstances.

Disease trends over time show the same thing. The worldwide prevalence of Type 1 diabetes is increasing at an alarming rate of 3% per year.[33] This increase is occurring for different populations even though there may be substantial differences in disease rates. This relatively rapid increase cannot be due to genetic susceptibility. The frequency of any one gene in a large population is relatively stable over time, unless there are changing environmental pressures that allow one group to reproduce more successfully than another group. For example, if all families with Type 1 diabetic relatives had a dozen babies and all the families without Type 1 diabetic relatives died off, then the gene or genes that may be responsible for Type 1 diabetes would become much more common in the population. This, of course, is not what is happening, and the fact that Type 1 diabetes is increasing 3% every year is very strong evidence that genes are not solely responsible for this disease.

It seems to me that we now have impressive evidence showing that cow's milk is likely to be an important cause of Type 1 diabetes. When the results of all these studies are combined (both genetically susceptible and not susceptible), we find that children weaned too early and fed cow's milk have, on average, a 50–60% higher risk of Type 1 diabetes (1.5–1.6 times increased risk).[34]

The earlier information on diet and Type 1 diabetes was impressive enough to cause two significant developments. The American Academy of Pediatrics in 1994 "strongly encouraged" that infants in families where diabetes is more common not be fed cow's milk supplements for their first two years of life. Second, many researchers[19] have developed prospective studies—the kind that follow individuals into the future—to see if a careful monitoring of diet and lifestyle could explain the onset of Type 1 diabetes.

Two of the better known of these studies have been underway in Finland, one starting in the late 1980s[15] and the other in the mid-1990s.[35] One has shown that cow's milk consumption increases the risk of Type 1 diabetes five- to sixfold,[36] while the second[35] tells us that cow's milk increases the development of at least another three to four antibodies in addition to those presented previously (p. 190). In a separate study, antibodies to beta-casein, another cow's milk protein, were significantly elevated in bottle-fed infants compared to breast-fed infants; children with Type 1 diabetes also had higher levels of these antibodies.[37] In short, of the studies that have reported results, *the findings strongly confirm the danger of cow's milk, especially for genetically susceptible children.*

THE CONTROVERSY OF CONTROVERSY

Imagine looking at the front page of the newspaper and finding the following headline: "Cow's Milk the Likely Cause of Lethal Type 1 Diabetes." Because the reaction would be so strong, and the economic impact monumental, this headline won't be written anytime soon, regardless of the scientific evidence. Stifling this headline is accomplished under the powerful label of "controversy." With so much at stake, and so much information understood by so few people, it is easy to generate and sustain controversy. Controversies are a natural part of science. Too often, however, controversy is not the result of legitimate scientific debate, but instead reflects the perceived need to delay and distort research results. For example, if I say cigarettes are bad for you and provide a mountain of evidence to support my contention, the tobacco companies might come along and pick out one unsolved detail and then claim that the whole idea of cigarettes being unhealthy is mired in controversy, thereby nullifying all my conclusions. This is easy to do, because there will always be unsolved details; this is the nature of science. Some groups use controversy to stifle certain ideas, impede constructive research, confuse the public and turn public policy into babble rather than substance. Sustaining controversy as a means of discrediting findings that cause economic or social discomfort is one of the greatest sins in science.

It can be difficult for the layperson to assess the legitimacy of a highly technical controversy such as that regarding cow's milk and Type 1 diabetes. This is true even if the layperson is interested in reading scientific articles.

Take a recent scientific review[38] of the cow's milk-Type 1 diabetes association. In ten human studies (all case-control) summarized in a paper published as part of a "controversial topics series,"[38] the authors concluded that five of the ten studies showed a statistically significant positive association between cow's milk and Type 1 diabetes and five did not. Obviously, this at first seems to demonstrate considerable uncertainty, going a long way to discredit the hypothesis.

However, the five studies that were counted as "negative" did not show that cow's milk *decreased* Type 1 diabetes. These five studies showed *no statistically significant effect either way.* In contrast, there are a total of five statistically significant studies and all five showed the same result: early cow's milk consumption is associated with *increased* risk of Type 1 diabetes. There is only one chance in sixty-four that this was a random or chance result.

There are many, many reasons, some seen and some unseen, why an experiment would find no statistically significant relationship between two factors, even when a relationship really exists. Perhaps the study didn't include enough people, and statistical certainty was unattainable. Perhaps most of the subjects had very similar feeding practices, limiting detection of the relationship you might otherwise see. Maybe trying to measure infant feeding practices from years ago was inaccurate enough that it obscured the relationship that does exist. Perhaps the researchers were studying the wrong period of time in an infant's life.

The point is, if five of the ten studies did find a statistically significant relationship, and *all five* showed that cow's milk consumption is linked to increasing Type 1 diabetes, and *none* show that cow's milk consumption is linked to decreasing Type 1 diabetes, I could hardly justify saying, as the authors of this review did, that the hypothesis "has become quite murky with inconsistencies in the literature."[38]

In this same review,[38] the authors summarized additional studies that indirectly compared breast-feeding practices associated with cow's milk consumption and Type 1 diabetes. This compilation involved fifty-two possible comparisons, twenty of which were statistically significant. Of these twenty significant findings, *nineteen favored an association of cow's milk with disease, and only one did not.* Again the odds heavily favored the hypothesized association, something that the authors failed to note.

I cite this example not only to support the evidence showing a cow's milk effect on Type 1 diabetes, but also to illustrate one tactic that is often used to make something controversial when it is not. This practice is more common than it should be and is a source of unnecessary confusion. When researchers do this—even if they do it unintentionally—they often have a serious prejudice against the hypothesis in the first place. Indeed, shortly after I wrote this, I heard a brief National Public Radio interview on the Type 1 diabetes problem with the senior author of this review paper.[38] Suffice it to say, the author did not acknowledge the evidence for the cow's milk hypothesis.

Because this issue has mammoth financial implications for American agriculture, and because so many people have such intense personal biases against it, it is unlikely that this diabetes research will reach the American media anytime soon. However, the depth and breadth of evidence now implicating cow's milk as a cause of Type 1 diabetes is overwhelming, even though the very complex mechanistic details are not yet fully understood. We not only have evidence of the danger of cow's milk, we also have considerable evidence showing that the association between diabetes and cow's milk is biologically plausible. Human breast milk is the perfect food for an infant, and one of the most damaging things a mother can do is to substitute the milk of a cow for her own.

MULTIPLE SCLEROSIS
AND OTHER AUTOIMMUNE DISEASES

Multiple sclerosis (MS) is a particularly difficult autoimmune disease, both for those who have it and for those who care for its victims. It is a lifelong battle involving a variety of unpredictable and serious disabilities. MS patients often pass through episodes of acute attacks while gradually losing their ability to walk or to see. After ten to fifteen years, they often are confined to a wheelchair, and then to a bed for the rest of their lives.

About 400,000 people in the U.S. alone have the disease, according to the National Multiple Sclerosis Society.[39] It is a disease that is initially diagnosed between twenty and forty years of age and strikes women about three times more often than men.

Even though there is widespread medical and scientific interest in this disease, most authorities claim to know very little about causes or cures. Major multiple sclerosis Internet Web sites all claim that the disease is an enigma. They generally list genetics, viruses and environmental factors as possibly playing roles in the development of this disease but pay almost no heed to a possible role for diet. This is peculiar considering the wealth of intriguing information on the effects of food that is available from reputable research reports.[40-42] Once again cow's milk appears to play an important role.

The "multiple" symptoms of this disease represent a nervous system gone awry. The electrical signals carrying messages to and from the central nervous system (brain and spinal cord) and out through the peripheral nervous system to the rest of the body are not well coordinated and controlled. This is because the insulating cover or sheath of the nerve fibers, the myelin, is being destroyed by an autoimmune reaction. Think of what would happen to your household wiring if the electrical insulation became thin or was stripped away, leaving bare wires. The electrical signals would be short-circuited. That is what happens with MS; the wayward electrical signals may destroy cells and "burn" patches of neighboring tissue, leaving little scars or bits of sclerotic tissue. These "burns" can become serious and ultimately destroy the body.

The initial research showing an effect of diet on MS goes back more than half a century to the research of Dr. Roy Swank, who began his work in Norway and at the Montreal Neurological Institute during the 1940s. Later, Dr. Swank headed the Division of Neurology at the University of Oregon Medical School.[43]

Dr. Swank became interested in the dietary connection when he learned that MS appeared to be more common in the northern climates.[43] There is a huge difference in MS prevalence as one moves away from the equator: MS is over 100 times more prevalent in the far north than at the equator,[10] and seven times more prevalent in south Australia (closer to the South Pole) than in north Australia.[44] This distribution is very similar to the distribution of other autoimmune diseases, including Type 1 diabetes and rheumatoid arthritis.[45, 46]

Although some scientists speculated that magnetic fields might be responsible for the disease, Dr. Swank thought it was diet, especially animal-based foods high in saturated fats.[43] He found that inland dairy-consuming areas of Norway had higher rates of MS than coastal fish-consuming areas.

Dr. Swank conducted his best-known trial on 144 MS patients recruited from the Montreal Neurological Institute. He kept records on these patients for the next thirty-four years.[47] He advised his patients to consume a diet low in saturated fat, most of whom did, but many of whom did not. He then classified them as good dieters or poor dieters, based on whether they consumed less than 20 g/day or more than 20 g/day of saturated fat. (For comparison, a bacon cheeseburger with condiments has about sixteen grams of saturated fat. One small frozen chicken pot pie has almost ten grams of saturated fat.)

As the study continued, Dr. Swank found that progression of disease was greatly reduced by the low-saturated fat diet, which worked even for people with initially advanced conditions. He summarized his work in 1990,[47] concluding that for the sub-group of patients who began the

**CHART 9.4: MS DEATH RATE AFTER 144 PATIENTS DIETED
FOR THIRTY-FOUR YEARS**

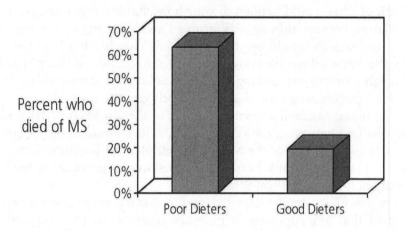

low-saturated fat diet during the earlier stages of their disease, "about
95%...remained only mildly disabled for approximately thirty years."
Only 5% of these patients died. *In contrast, 80% of the patients with early-
stage MS who consumed the "poor" diet (higher saturated fat) died of MS.*
The results from all 144 patients, including those who started the diet
at a later stage of disease, are shown in Chart 9.4.

This work is remarkable. To follow people for thirty-four years is an
exceptional demonstration of perseverance and dedication. Moreover,
if this were a study testing a potential drug, these findings would make
any pharmaceutical manufacturer jingle the coins in his or her pocket.
Swank's first results were published more than a half century ago,[48] then
again[49] and again[50] and again[47] for the next forty years.

More recently, additional studies[42, 51, 52] have confirmed and extended
Swank's observations and gradually have begun to place more emphasis on cow's milk. These new studies show that consuming cow's milk
is strongly linked to MS both when comparing different countries[52]
and when comparing states within the U.S.[51] Chart 9.5, published by
French researchers, compares the consumption of cow's milk with MS
for twenty-six populations in twenty-four countries.[52]

This relationship, which is virtually identical to that for Type 1
diabetes, is remarkable, and it is not due to variables such as the availability of medical services or geographic latitude.[51] In some studies[52, 53]
researchers suggest this strong correlation with fresh cow's milk might

CHART 9.5: ASSOCIATION OF COW'S MILK CONSUMPTION
AND MULTIPLE SCLEROSIS

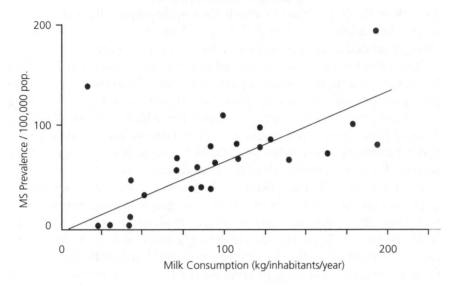

be due to the presence of a virus in the milk. These more recent studies also suggest that saturated fat alone probably was not fully responsible for Swank's results. The consumption of meat high in saturated fat, like milk, was also associated with MS in these multi-country studies,[54] while the consumption of fish, containing more omega-3 fat, was associated with low rates of disease.[55]

The association of cow's milk with MS, shown in Chart 9.5, may be impressive, but it does not constitute proof. For example, where do genes and viruses come into play? Each of these, in theory, might account for the unusual geographic distribution of this disease.

In the case of viruses, no definite conclusions are yet possible. A variety of different virus types have been suggested and a variety of effects on the immune system may be involved. However, nothing very convincing has been proven. Some of the evidence is based on finding more viral antibodies in MS patients than in controls, some is based on sporadic outbreaks of MS among isolated communities, and some is based on finding virus-like genes among MS cases.[13, 19, 56]

With regard to genes, we can begin to puzzle out their association with MS by asking the usual question: what happens to people who migrate from one population to another, keeping their genes the same but changing their diets and their environment? The answer is the same as it was for cancer, heart disease and Type 2 diabetes. People acquire the risk of the population to which they move, especially if they move before their adolescent years.[57, 58] This tells us that this disease is more strongly related to environmental factors than it is to genes.[59]

Specific genes have been identified as possible candidates for causing MS but, according to a recent report,[3] there may be as many as twenty-five genes playing such a role. Therefore, it will undoubtedly be a long time before we determine with any precision which genes or combinations of genes predispose someone to MS. Genetic predisposition may make a difference as to who gets MS, but even at best, genes can only account for about one-fourth of the total disease risk.[60]

Although MS and Type 1 diabetes share some of the same unanswered questions on the exact roles of viruses and genes and the immune system, they also share the same alarming evidence regarding diet. For both diseases, a "Western" diet is strongly associated with disease incidence. Despite the efforts of those who would rather dismiss or mire these observational studies in controversy, they paint a consistent picture. Intervention studies conducted on people already suffering from these diseases only reinforce the findings of the observational studies. Dr. Swank did brilliant work on MS, and you may recall from chapter seven that Dr. James Anderson successfully reduced the medication requirements for Type 1 diabetics using diet alone. It's important to note that both of these doctors used a diet that was significantly more moderate than a total whole foods, plant-based diet. I wonder what would happen to these autoimmune patients if the ideal diet were followed. I would bet on even greater success.

THE COMMONALITY OF AUTOIMMUNE DISEASES

What about other autoimmune diseases? There are dozens of autoimmune diseases and I have mentioned only two of the more prominent ones. Can we say anything about autoimmune diseases as a whole?

To answer this question, we need to identify how much these diseases have in common. The more they have in common, the greater the probability that they also will share a common cause (or causes). This is like seeing two people you don't know, both of whom have a similar body type, hair color, eye color, facial features, physical and vocal mannerisms and age, and concluding that they come from the same parents. Just as we hypothesized that diseases of affluence such as cancer and heart disease have common causes because they share similar geography and similar biochemical biomarkers (chapter four), we can also hypothesize that MS, Type 1 diabetes, rheumatoid arthritis, lupus and other autoimmune diseases may share a similar cause if they exhibit similar characteristics.

First, by definition, each of these diseases involves an immune system that has gone awry in such a way that it attacks "self" proteins that look the same as foreign proteins.

Second, all the autoimmune diseases that have been studied have been found to be more common at the higher geographic latitudes where there is less constant sunshine.[9, 10, 61]

Third, some of these diseases have a tendency to afflict the same people. MS and Type 1 diabetes, for example, have been shown to coexist in the same individuals.[62–65] Parkinson's disease, a non-autoimmune disease with autoimmune characteristics, is often found with MS, both within the same geographic regions[66] and within the same individuals.[5] MS also has been associated—either geographically or within the same individuals—with other autoimmune diseases like lupus, myasthenia gravis, Graves' disease and eosinophilic vasculitis.[63] Juvenile rheumatoid arthritis, another autoimmune disease, has been shown to have an unusually strong association with Hashimoto thyroiditis.[67]

Fourth, of those diseases studied in relation to nutrition, the consumption of animal-based foods—especially cow's milk—is associated with greater disease risk.

Fifth, there is evidence that a virus (or viruses) may trigger the onset of several of these diseases.

A sixth and most important characteristic binding together these diseases is the evidence that their "mechanisms of action" have much in common—jargon used to describe the "how to" of disease formation. As we consider common mechanisms of action, we might start with sunlight exposure, because this somehow seems linked to the autoimmune diseases. Sunlight exposure, which decreases with increasing latitude, could be important—but clearly there are other factors. The consumption of animal-based foods, especially cow's milk, also increases with distance from the equator. In fact, in one of the more extensive studies, cow's milk was found to be as good of a predictor of MS as latitude (i.e., sunshine).[51] In Dr. Swank's studies in Norway, MS was less common near the coastal areas of the country where fish intake was more common. This gave rise to the idea that the omega-3 fats common to fish might have a protective effect. What is almost never mentioned, however, is that dairy consumption (and saturated fat) was much lower in the fish-eating areas. Is it possible that cow's milk and lack of sunshine are having a similar effect on MS and other autoimmune diseases because they operate through a similar mechanism? This could be very interesting, if true.

As it turns out, the idea is not so crazy. This mechanism involves, once again, vitamin D. There are experimental animal models of lupus, MS, rheumatoid arthritis and inflammatory bowel disease (e.g., Crohn's disease, ulcerative colitis), each of which is an autoimmune disease.[6, 7, 68] Vitamin D, operating through a similar mechanism in each case, prevents the experimental development of each of these diseases. This becomes an even more intriguing story when we think about the effect of food on vitamin D.

The first step in the vitamin D process occurs when you go outside on a sunny day. When the sunshine hits your exposed skin, the skin produces vitamin D. The vitamin D then must be activated in the kidney in order to produce a form that helps repress the development of autoimmune diseases. As we've seen before, this critically important activation step can be inhibited by foods that are high in calcium and by acid-producing animal proteins like cow's milk (some grains also produce excess acid). Under experimental conditions, the activated vitamin D operates in two ways: it inhibits the development of certain T-cells and their production of active agents (called cytokines) that initiate the autoimmune response, and/or it encourages the production of other T-cells that oppose this effect.[69, 70] (An abbreviated schematic of this vitamin D network is shown in Appendix C.) This mechanism of action appears to be a strong commonality between all autoimmune diseases so far studied.

Knowing the strength of the evidence against animal foods, cow's milk in particular, for both MS and Type 1 diabetes, and knowing how much in common all of the autoimmune diseases have, it is reasonable to begin thinking about food and its relationship to a much broader group of autoimmune diseases. Obviously caution is called for; more research is needed to make conclusive statements about cross-autoimmune disease similarities. But the evidence we have now is already striking.

Today almost no indication of the dietary connection to these diseases has reached public awareness. The Web site of the Multiple Sclerosis International Federation, for example, reads, "There is no credible evidence that MS is due to poor diet or dietary deficiencies." They warn that dietary regimens can be "expensive" and "can alter the normal nutritional balance."[71] If changing your diet is expensive, I don't know what they would say about being bedridden and incapacitated. As far as altering the "normal nutritional balance" is concerned, what is normal? Does this mean the diet that we now eat is "normal"—the diet that is largely responsible for diseases that cripple, kill and make profoundly miserable millions of Americans every year? Are massive rates of heart disease, cancer, autoimmune diseases, obesity and diabetes "normal"? If this is normal, I propose we start seriously considering the abnormal.

There are 400,000 Americans who are victims of multiple sclerosis, and millions more with other autoimmune diseases. While statistics, research results and clinical descriptions form the basis for much of my discussion of diet and disease, the importance of the information comes down to the *intimate experience of individual people*. Any one of these serious diseases I've talked about in this chapter can forever alter the life of any person—a family member, a friend, a neighbor, a coworker or you yourself.

It is time to sacrifice our sacred cows. Reason must prevail. Professional societies, doctors and government agencies need to stand up and do their duty, so that children being born today do not face tragedies that otherwise could be prevented.

10

Wide-Ranging Effects: Bone, Kidney, Eye and Brain Diseases

ONE OF THE MOST CONVINCING ARGUMENTS for a plant-based diet is the fact that it prevents a broad range of diseases. If I have a conversation with someone about a single study showing the protective effect of fruits and vegetables on heart disease, they may agree that it's all very nice for fruits and vegetables, but they will probably still go home to meatloaf and gravy. It doesn't matter how big the study, how persuasive the results or how respectable the scientists who conducted the investigation. The fact is that most people have a healthy skepticism about one study standing alone—as well they should.

But if I tell them about dozens and dozens of studies showing that the countries with low rates of heart disease consume low amounts of animal-based foods, and dozens and dozens of studies showing that individuals who eat more whole, plant-based foods get less heart disease, and I go on to document still more studies showing that a diet low in animal-based foods and high in unprocessed plant-based foods can slow or reverse heart disease, then people are more inclined to pay some attention.

If I keep talking and go through this process not only for heart disease, but obesity, Type 2 diabetes, breast cancer, colon cancer, prostate cancer, multiple sclerosis and other autoimmune diseases, it's quite possible that people may never eat meatloaf and gravy again.

What has become so convincing about the effect of diet on health is the breadth of the evidence. While a single study might be found to support almost any idea under the sun, what are the chances that hundreds, even thousands, of different studies show a protective benefit of plant-based foods and/or harmful effects of animal-based foods for so many different diseases? We can't say it's due to coincidence, bad data, biased research, misinterpreted statistics or "playing with numbers." This has got to be the real deal.

I have so far presented only a small sample of the breadth of evidence that supports plant-based diets. To show you just how broad this evidence is, I will cover five more seemingly unrelated diseases common in America: osteoporosis, kidney stones, blindness, cognitive dysfunction and Alzheimer's disease. These disorders are not often fatal and are often regarded as the inevitable consequences of aging. Therefore, we don't think it's unnatural when grandpa gets blurry spots in his vision, can't remember the names of his friends or needs a hip replacement operation. But, as we shall see, even these diseases have a dietary link.

OSTEOPOROSIS

Did you ever have an elementary school teacher tell you that if you didn't have bones, you would just be a shapeless blob on the floor? Or maybe you learned about the human skeleton from that popular song, "...the ankle bone is connected to the shin bone, the shin bone is connected to the knee bone," etc. At that same time in your life, you probably were told to drink milk to build strong bones and teeth. Because none of us want to be shapeless blobs, and because our celebrities have been paid to advertise milk's presumed benefits, we drank it. Milk is to bone health as bees are to honey.

Americans consume more cow's milk and its products per person than most populations in the world. So Americans should have wonderfully strong bones, right? Unfortunately not. A recent study showed that American women aged fifty and older have one of the highest rates of hip fractures in the world.[1] The only countries with higher rates are in Europe and in the south Pacific (Australia and New Zealand)[1] where they consume even more milk than the United States. What's going on?

An excess rate of hip fractures is often used as a reliable indicator of osteoporosis, a bone disease that especially affects women after menopause. It is often claimed to be due to an inadequate intake of calcium. Therefore, health policy people often recommend higher calcium consumption. Dairy products are particularly rich in calcium, so the dairy industry eagerly supports efforts to boost calcium consumption. These efforts have something to do with why you were told to drink your milk for strong bones—the politics of which are discussed in Part IV.

Something is amiss, though, because those countries that use the most cow's milk and its products also have the highest fracture rates and the worst bone health. One possible explanation is found in a report showing an impressively strong association between animal protein intake and bone fracture rate for women in different countries.[2] Authored in 1992 by researchers at Yale University School of Medicine, the report summarized data on protein intake and fracture rates taken from thirty-four separate surveys in sixteen countries that were published in twenty-nine peer-reviewed research publications. All the subjects in these surveys were women fifty years and older. It found that a very impressive 70% of the fracture rate was attributable to the consumption of animal protein.

These researchers explained that animal protein, unlike plant protein, increases the acid load in the body.[3] An increased acid load means that our blood and tissues become more acidic. The body does not like this acidic environment and begins to fight it. In order to neutralize the acid, the body uses calcium, which acts as a very effective base. This calcium, however, must come from somewhere. It ends up being pulled from the bones, and the calcium loss weakens them, putting them at greater risk for fracture.

We have had evidence for well over a hundred years that animal protein decreases bone health. The explanation of animal protein causing excess metabolic acid, for example, was first suggested in the 1880s[4] and was documented as long ago as 1920.[5] We also have known that animal protein is more effective than plant protein at increasing the metabolic acid load in the body.[6, 7, 8]

When animal protein increases metabolic acid and draws calcium from the bones, the amount of calcium in the urine is increased. This effect has been established for over eighty years[5] and has been studied in some detail since the 1970s. Summaries of these studies were published in 1974,[9] 1981[10] and 1990.[11] Each of these summaries clearly shows that the amount of animal protein consumed by many of us on a daily basis is capable of causing substantial increases in urinary cal-

CHART 10.1: ASSOCIATION OF URINARY CALCIUM EXCRETION WITH DIETARY PROTEIN INTAKE

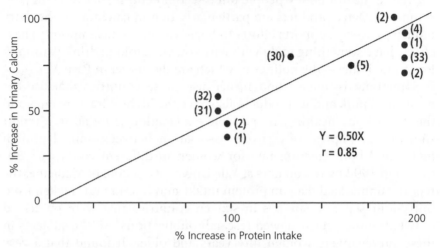

% Increase in Protein Intake

cium. Chart 10.1 is taken from the 1981 publication.[10] Doubling protein intake (mostly animal-based) from 35–78 g/day causes an alarming 50% increase in urinary calcium. This effect occurs well within the range of protein intake that most of us consume; average American intake is around 70–100 g/day. Incidentally, as mentioned in chapter four, a six-month study funded by the Atkins Center found that those people who adopted the Atkins Diet excreted 50% more calcium in their urine after six months on the diet.[12]

The initial observations on the association between animal protein consumption and bone fracture rates are very impressive, and now we have a plausible explanation as to how the association might work, a mechanism of action.

Disease processes are rarely as simple as "one mechanism does it all," but the work being done in this field makes a strong argument. A more recent study, published in 2000, comes from the Department of Medicine at the University of California at San Francisco. Using eighty-seven surveys in thirty-three countries, it compared the ratio of vegetable to animal protein consumption to the rate of bone fractures (Chart 10.2).[1] A high ratio of vegetable to animal protein consumption was found to be impressively associated with a virtual disappearance of bone fractures.

These studies are compelling for several reasons. They were published in leading research journals, the authors were careful in their analyses and

CHART 10.2: ASSOCIATION OF ANIMAL VERSUS PLANT PROTEIN INTAKE AND BONE FRACTURE RATES FOR DIFFERENT COUNTRIES

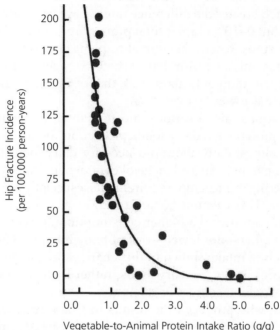

interpretation of data, they included a large number of individual research reports, and the statistical significance of the association of animal protein with bone fracture rates is truly exceptional. They cannot be dismissed as just another couple of studies; the most recent study represents a summary of eighty-seven separate surveys!

The Study of Osteoporotic Fractures Research Group at the University of California at San Francisco published yet another study[13] of over 1,000 women aged sixty-five and up. Like the multi-country study, researchers characterized women's diets by the proportions of animal and plant protein. After seven years of observations, the women with the highest ratio of animal protein to plant protein had 3.7 times more bone fractures than the women with the lowest ratio. Also during this time the women with the high ratio lost bone almost four times as fast as the women with the lowest ratio.

Experimentally, this study is high quality because it compared protein consumption, bone loss and broken bones for the same subjects. This 3.7-fold effect is substantial, and is very important because the women with the lowest bone fracture rates still consumed, on average, about half of their total protein from animal sources. I can't help but wonder how much greater the difference might have been had they consumed not 50% but 0–10% of their total protein from animal sources. In our rural China study, where the animal to plant ratio was about 10%, the fracture rate is only one-fifth that of the U.S. Nigeria shows an animal-to-plant protein ratio only about 10% that of Germany, and the hip fracture incidence is lower by over 99%.[1]

These observations raise a serious question about the widely advertised claim that protein-rich dairy foods protect our bones. And yet we still are warned almost daily about our need for dairy foods to provide calcium for strong bones. An avalanche of commentary warns that most of us are not meeting our calcium requirements, especially pregnant and lactating women. This calcium bonanza, however, is not justified. In one study of ten countries,[14] a higher consumption of calcium was associated with a higher—not lower—risk of bone fracture (Chart 10.3). Much of the calcium intake shown in this chart, especially in high consumption countries, is due to dairy foods, rather than calcium supplements or non-dairy food sources of calcium.

Mark Hegsted, who produced the results in Chart 10.3, was a long-time Harvard professor. He worked on the calcium issue beginning in the early 1950s, was a principal architect of the nation's first dietary guidelines in 1980 and in 1986 published this graph. Professor Hegsted believes that excessively high intakes of calcium consumed over a long time impair the body's ability to control how much calcium it uses and when. Under healthy conditions, the body uses an activated form of vitamin D, calcitriol, to adjust how much calcium it absorbs from food and how much it excretes and distributes in the bone. Calcitriol is considered a hormone; when more calcium is needed, it enhances calcium absorption and restricts calcium excretion. If too much calcium is consumed over a long period of time, the body may lose its ability to regulate calcitriol, permanently or temporarily disrupting the regulation of calcium absorption and excretion. Ruining the regulatory mechanism in this way is a recipe for osteoporosis in menopausal and post-menopausal women. Women at this stage of life must be able to enhance their utilization of calcium in a timely manner, especially if they continue to consume a diet high in animal protein. The fact that the body loses its ability to control finely tuned mechanisms when they are subjected to continuous abuse is a well-established phenomenon in biology.

CHART 10.3: ASSOCIATION OF RATES OF HIP FRACTURES WITH CALCIUM INTAKE FOR DIFFERENT COUNTRIES

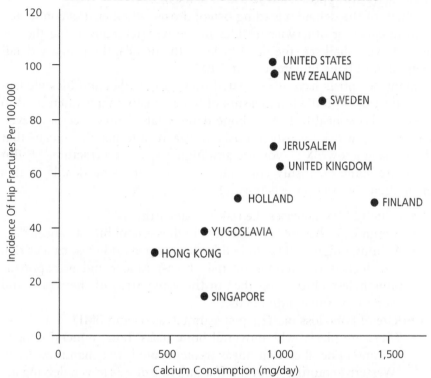

Given these findings, it seems perfectly plausible that animal protein and even calcium—when consumed at excessive levels—are capable of increasing the risk of osteoporosis. Dairy, unfortunately, is the only food that is rich in both of these nutrients. Hegsted, backed by his exceptional experience in calcium research, said in his 1986 paper, "...hip fractures are more frequent in populations where dairy products are commonly consumed and calcium intakes are relatively high."

Years later, the dairy industry still suggests that we should be consuming more of its products to build strong bones and teeth. The confusion, conflict and controversy rampant in this area of research allow anybody to say just about anything. And of course, huge amounts of money are at stake as well. One of the most cited osteoporosis experts—one funded by the dairy industry—angrily wrote in a prominent editorial[15] that the findings favoring a diet with a higher ratio of plant-to-animal protein cited above could have been "influenced to some extent by currents in the larger society." The "currents" he was referring to were the animal rights activists opposed to the use of dairy foods.

Much of the debate regarding osteoporosis, whether it is conducted with integrity or otherwise, resides in the research concerning the details. As you shall see, the devil lurks in the details, the primary detail being that of bone mineral density (BMD).

Many scientists have investigated how various diet and lifestyle factors affect BMD. BMD is a measure of bone density that is often used to diagnose bone health. If your bone density falls below a certain level, you may be at risk for osteoporosis. In practical terms, this means that if you have a low BMD, you are at a higher risk for a fracture.[16–18] But there are some devilishly contradictory and confusing details in this great circus of osteoporosis research. To name a few:

- A high BMD increases the risk of osteoarthritis.[19]
- A high BMD has been linked to a higher risk of breast cancer.[20, 21]
- Although high BMD is linked both to increased breast cancer risk and decreased osteoporotic risk, breast cancer and osteoporosis nonetheless cluster together in the same areas of the world and even in the same individuals.[22]
- Rate of bone loss matters just as much as overall BMD.[23]
- There are places where overall bone mass, bone mineral density or bone mineral content measurements are lower than they are in "Western" countries, but the fracture rate also is lower, defying accepted logic of how we define "big, strong bones."[24–26]
- Being fat is linked to greater BMD,[24, 27] even though areas of the world that have higher rates of obesity also have higher rates of osteoporosis.

Something is wrong with the idea that BMD reliably represents osteoporosis and, by inference, indicates the kind of diet that would lower fracture rates. In contrast, an alternative, but much better, predictor of osteoporosis is the dietary ratio of animal-to-plant protein.[1, 13] The higher the ratio, the higher the risk of disease. And guess what? BMD is not significantly associated with this ratio.[13]

Clearly the conventional recommendations regarding animal foods, dairy and bone mineral density, which are influenced and advertised by the dairy industry, are besieged by serious doubts in the literature. Here is what I would recommend you do, based on the research, to minimize your risk of osteoporosis:

- Stay physically active. Take the stairs instead of the elevator, go for walks, jogs, bicycle rides. Swim, do yoga or aerobics every couple of days and don't be afraid to buy barbells to use once in a while. Play a sport or join a social group that incorporates exercise. The possibilities are endless, and they can be fun. You'll feel better, and your bones will be much healthier for the effort.
- Eat a variety of whole plant foods, and avoid animal foods, including dairy. Plenty of calcium is available in a wide range of plant foods, including beans and leafy vegetables. As long as you stay away from refined carbohydrates, like sugary cereals, candies, plain pastas and white breads, you should have no problem with calcium deficiency.
- Keep your salt intake to a minimum. Avoid highly processed and packaged foods, which contain excess salt. There is some evidence that excessive salt intake can be a problem.

KIDNEYS

At the Web site for the UCLA Kidney Stone Treatment Center,[28] you will discover that kidney stones may cause the following symptoms:

- Nausea, vomiting
- Restlessness (trying to find comfortable position to ease the pain)
- Dull pain (ill-defined, lumbar, abdominal, intermittent pain)
- Urgency (urge to empty the bladder)
- Frequency (frequent urination)
- Bloody urine with pain (gross hematuria)
- Fever (when complicated by infection)
- Acute renal colic (severe colicky flank pain radiating to groin, scrotum, labia)

Acute renal colic deserves some explanation. This agonizing symptom is the result of a crystallized stone trying to pass through the thin tube in your body (ureter) that transports urine from the kidney to the bladder. In describing the pain involved, the Web site states, "This is probably one of the worst pains humans experience. Those who have had it will never forget it....The severe pain of renal colic needs to be controlled by potent pain killers. Don't expect an aspirin to do the trick. Get yourself to a doctor or an emergency room."[28]

I don't know about you, but just thinking about these things gives me a shiver. Unfortunately, up to 15% of Americans, more men than women, will be diagnosed with having a kidney stone in their lifetime.[29]

There are several kinds of kidney stones. Although one is a genetically rare type[30] and another is related to urinary infection, the majority involve stones made of calcium and oxalate. These calcium oxalate stones are relatively common in developed countries and relatively rare in developing countries.[31] Again, this illness falls into the same global patterns as all the other Western diseases.

I first was made aware of the dietary connection with this disease at the Faculty of Medicine of the University of Toronto. I was invited to give a seminar on our China Study findings and while there I met Professor W. G. Robertson from the Medical Research Council in Leeds, England. This chance encounter was extremely rewarding. Dr. Robertson, as I have come to learn, is one of the world's foremost experts on diet and kidney stones. Dr. Robertson's research group has investigated the relationship between food and kidney stones with great depth and breadth, both in theory and in practice. Their work began more than thirty years ago and continues to the present day. A search of the scientific publications authored or co-authored by Robertson shows at least 100 papers published since the mid-1960s.

One of Robertson's charts depicts a stunning relationship between animal protein consumption and the formation of kidney stones (Chart 10.4).[32] It shows that consuming animal protein at levels above twenty-one grams per person per day (slightly less than one ounce) for the United Kingdom for the years of 1958 to 1973 is closely correlated with a high number of kidney stones formed per 10,000 individuals per year. This is an impressive relationship.

Few researchers have worked out the details of a research question more thoroughly than Robertson and his colleagues. They have developed a model for estimating the risk of stone formation with remarkable accuracy.[33] Although they have identified six risk factors for kidney stones,[34, 35] animal protein consumption was the major culprit. Consumption of animal protein at levels commonly seen in affluent countries leads to the development of four of the six risk factors.[34, 35]

Not only is animal protein linked to risk factors for future formation of stones, but it affects recurring stones as well. Robertson published findings showing that, among the patients who had recurrent kidney stones, he was able to resolve their problem simply by shifting their diet away from animal protein foods.[36]

CHART 10.4: ASSOCIATION BETWEEN ANIMAL PROTEIN INTAKE AND FORMATION OF URINARY CALCULI

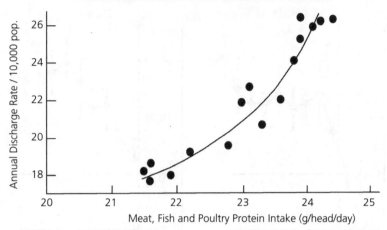

How does this work? When enough animal protein-containing foods are consumed, the concentrations of calcium and oxalate in the urine increase sharply, usually within hours. Chart 10.5 shows these impressive changes, published by Robertson's group.[35]

The individuals in this study consumed only fifty-five grams per day of animal protein, to which was added another thirty-four grams per day of animal protein in the form of tuna fish. This amount of animal protein consumption is well within the levels most Americans regularly eat. Men consume around 90–100 grams of total protein per day, the majority of which comes from animal foods; women consume about 70–90 grams per day.

When the kidney is under a persistent, long-term assault from increased calcium and oxalate, kidney stones may result.[35] The following, excerpted from a 1987 review by Robertson,[37] emphasizes the role of diet, especially foods containing animal proteins:

> Urolithiasis [kidney stone formation] is a worldwide problem which appears to be aggravated by the high dairy-produce, highly energy-rich and low-fibre diets consumed in most industrialized countries.... Evidence points, in particular, to a high-meat protein intake as being the dominant factor.... On the basis of epidemiological and biochemical studies a move toward a more vegetarian, less energy-rich diet would be predicted to reduce the risk of stone in the population.

CHART 10.5: EFFECT OF ANIMAL PROTEIN INTAKE
ON CALCIUM AND OXALATE IN THE URINE

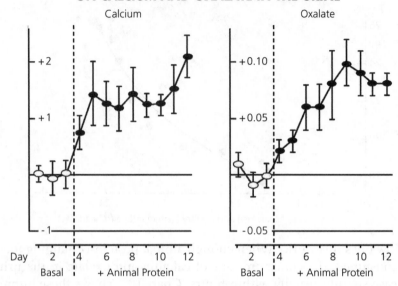

A substantial and convincing effect on stone formation has been demonstrated for animal-based foods. Recent research also shows that kidney stone formation can be initiated by the activity of free radicals,[38] and may thus be prevented by consumption of antioxidant-containing plant-based foods (see chapter four). For yet another organ and another disease, we see opposing effects (in this case on stone formation) by animal- and plant-based foods.

EYE PROBLEMS

People who can see well often take vision for granted. We treat our eyes more as little bits of technology than as living parts of the body, and are all too willing to believe that lasers are the best course of action for maintaining healthy eyes. But during the past couple of decades, research has shown that these bits of "technology" are actually greatly affected by the foods we eat. Our breakfasts, lunches and dinners have a particular effect on two common eye diseases, cataracts and macular degeneration—diseases which afflict millions of older Americans.

Yes, that's right. I'm about to tell you that if you eat animal foods instead of plant foods, you just might go blind.

Macular degeneration is the leading cause of irreversible blindness among people over age sixty-five. Over 1.6 million Americans suffer from this disease, many of whom become blind.[39] As the name implies, this condition involves destruction of the macula, which is the biochemical intersection in the eye—where the energy of the light coming in is transformed into a nerve signal. The macula occupies center stage, so to speak, and it must be functional for sight to occur.

Around the macula there are fatty acids that can react with incoming light to produce a low level of highly reactive free radicals.[40] These free radicals (see chapter four) can destroy, or degenerate, neighboring tissue, including the macula. But fortunately for us, free radical damage can be repressed thanks to the antioxidants in vegetables and fruits.

Two studies, each involving a team of experienced researchers at prestigious institutions, provide compelling evidence that food can protect against macular degeneration. Both studies were published a decade ago. One evaluated diet[41] and the other assessed nutrients in blood.[42] The findings of these two studies suggested that as much as 70–88% of blindness caused by macular degeneration could be prevented if the right foods are eaten.

The study on dietary intakes[41] compared 356 individuals fifty-five to eighty years of age who were diagnosed with advanced macular degeneration (cases) with 520 individuals with other eye diseases (controls). Five ophthalmology medical centers collaborated on the study.

Researchers found that a higher intake of total carotenoids was associated with a lower frequency of macular degeneration. Carotenoids are a group of antioxidants found in the colored parts of fruits and vegetables. When carotenoid intakes were ranked, those individuals who consumed the most had 43% less disease than those who consumed the least. Not surprisingly, five out of six plant-based foods measured also were associated with lower rates of macular degeneration (broccoli, carrots, spinach or collard greens, winter squash and sweet potato). Spinach or collard greens conferred the most protection. There was 88% less disease for people who ate these greens five or more times per week when compared with people who consumed these greens less than once per month. The only food group not showing a preventive effect was the cabbage/cauliflower/brussels sprout group, which sports the least color of the six food groups.[43]

These researchers also looked at the potential protection from disease as a result of the consumption of five of the individual carotenoids consumed in these foods. All but one of these five showed a highly significant protective effect, especially the carotenoids found in the dark green leafy vegetables. In contrast, supplements of a few vitamins, including retinol (preformed "vitamin" A), vitamin C and vitamin E showed little or no beneficial effects. Yet again, we see that while supplements may give great wealth to supplement manufacturers, they will not give great health to you and me.

When all was said and done, this study found that *macular degeneration risk could be reduced by as much as 88%, simply by eating the right foods.*[41]

At this point you may be wondering, "Where can I get some of those carotenoids?" Green leafy vegetables, carrots and citrus fruits are all good sources. Herein lies a problem, however. Among the hundreds (maybe thousands) of antioxidant carotenoids in these foods, only a dozen or so have been studied in relation to their biological effects. The abilities of these chemicals to scavenge and reduce free radical damage are well established, but the activities of the individual carotenoids vary enormously depending on dietary and lifestyle conditions. Such variations make it virtually impossible to predict their individual activities, either good or bad. The logic of using them as supplements is much too particular and superficial. It ignores the dynamic of nature. It's much safer to consume these carotenoids in their natural context, in highly colored fruits and vegetables.

The second study[42] compared a total of 421 macular degeneration patients (cases) with 615 controls. Five of the leading clinical centers specializing in eye diseases and their researchers participated in this study. The researchers measured the levels of antioxidants in the blood, rather than the antioxidants consumed. Four kinds of antioxidants were measured: carotenoids, vitamin C, selenium and vitamin E. Except for selenium, each of these nutrient groups was associated with fewer cases of macular degeneration, although only the carotenoids showed statistically significant results. Risk of macular degeneration was reduced by two-thirds for those people with the highest levels of carotenoids in their blood, when compared with the low-carotenoid group.

This reduction of about 65–70% in this study is similar to the reduction of upwards of 88% in the first study. These two studies consistently demonstrated the benefits of antioxidant carotenoids consumed as food. Given experimental limitations, we can only approximate the proportion of macular degeneration caused by poor dietary habits, and we cannot know which antioxidants are involved. What we can say, however, is that eating antioxidant-containing foods, especially those containing the carotenoids, will prevent most blindness cases resulting from macular degeneration. This in itself is a remarkable recommendation.

Cataracts are slightly less serious than macular degeneration because there are effective surgical options available to restore vision loss caused by this disease. But when you look at the numbers, cataracts are a much larger burden on our society. By the age of eighty, half of all Americans will have cataracts.[39] Currently there are 20 million Americans age forty and older with the disease.

Cataract formation involves the clouding of the eye lens. Corrective surgery involves removing the cloudy lens and replacing it with an artificial lens. The development of the opaque condition, like the degeneration of the macula and so many other disease conditions in our body, is closely associated with the damage created by an excess of reactive free radicals.[44] Once again, it is reasonable to assume that eating antioxidant-containing foods should be helpful.

Starting in 1988, researchers in Wisconsin began to study eye health and dietary intakes in over 1,300 people. Ten years later, they published a report[45] on their findings. The people who consumed the most lutein, a specific type of antioxidant, had one-half the rate of cataracts as the people who consumed the least lutein. Lutein is an interesting chemical because, in addition to being readily available in spinach, along with other dark leafy green vegetables, it also is an integral part of the lens tissue itself.[46, 47] Similarly, those who consumed the most spinach had 40% less cataracts.

These two eye conditions, macular degeneration and cataracts, both occur when we fail to consume enough of the highly colored green and leafy vegetables. In both cases, excess free radicals, increased by animal-based foods and decreased by plant-based foods, are likely to be responsible for these conditions.

MIND-ALTERING DIETS

By the time this book hits the shelves, I will be seventy years old. I recently went to my high school's fiftieth reunion, where I learned that many of my classmates had died. I receive the AARP magazine, get discounts on various products for being advanced in age and receive social security checks every month. Some euphemists might call me a "mature adult." I just say old. What does it mean to be old? I still run every morning, sometimes six or more miles a day. I still have an active work life, perhaps more active than ever. I still enjoy all the same leisure activities, whether visiting grandchildren, dining with friends, gardening, traveling, golfing, lecturing or making outdoor improvements like building fences or tinkering with this or that as I used to do on the farm. Some things have changed, though. Clearly there is a difference between the seventy-year-old me and the twenty-year-old me. I am slower, not as strong, work fewer hours every day and am prone to taking naps more frequently than I used to.

We all know that getting old brings with it diminished capacities compared with our younger days. But there is good science to show that thinking clearly well into our later years is not something we need to give up. Memory loss, disorientation and confusion are not inevitable parts of aging, but problems linked to that all-important lifestyle factor: diet.

There is now good dietary information for the two chief conditions referring to mental decline. On the modest side, there is a condition called "cognitive impairment" or "cognitive dysfunction." This condition describes the declining ability to remember and think as well as one once did. It represents a continuum of disease ranging from cases that only hint at declining abilities to those that are much more obvious and easily diagnosed.

Then there are mental dysfunctions that become serious, even life threatening. These are called dementia, of which there are two main types: vascular dementia and Alzheimer's disease. Vascular dementia is primarily caused by multiple little strokes resulting from broken blood vessels in the brain. It is common for elderly people to have "silent" strokes in their later years. A stroke is considered silent if it goes undetected and undiagnosed. Each little stroke incapacitates part of the brain. The other type of dementia, Alzheimer's, occurs when a protein substance called beta-amyloid accumulates in critical areas of the brain as a plaque, rather like the cholesterol-laden plaque that builds up in cardiovascular diseases.

Alzheimer's is surprisingly common. It is said that 1% of people at age sixty-five have evidence of Alzheimer's, a figure that doubles every five years thereafter.[48] I suppose this is why we blandly accept "senility" as part of the aging process.

It has been estimated that 10–12% of individuals with mild cognitive impairment progress to the more serious types of dementia, whereas only 1–2% of individuals without cognitive impairment acquire these diseases.[49, 50] This means that people with cognitive impairment have about a tenfold risk of Alzheimer's.

Not only does cognitive impairment often lead to more serious dementia, it is also associated with cardiovascular disease,[51–53] stroke[54] and adult-onset Type 2 diabetes.[55, 56] All of these diseases cluster in the same populations, oftentimes in the same people. This clustering means that they share some of the same risk factors. Hypertension (high blood pressure) is one factor[51, 57, 58]; another is high blood cholesterol.[53] Both of these, of course, can be controlled by diet.

A third risk factor is the amount of those nasty free radicals, which wreak havoc on brain function in our later years. Because free radical damage is so important to the process of cognitive dysfunction and dementia, researchers believe that consuming dietary antioxidants can shield our brains from this damage, as in other diseases. Animal-based foods lack antioxidant shields and tend to activate free radical production and cell damage, while plant-based foods, with their abundant antioxidants, tend to prevent such damage. It's the same dietary cause and effect that we saw with macular degeneration.

Of course, genetics plays a role, and specific genes have been identified that may increase the risk of cognitive decline.[52] But environmental factors also play a key role, most probably the dominant one.

In a recent study, it was found that Japanese American men living in Hawaii had a higher rate of Alzheimer's disease than Japanese living in Japan.[59] Another study found that native Africans had significantly lower rates of dementia and Alzheimer's than African Americans in Indiana.[60] Both of these findings clearly support the idea that environment plays an important role in cognitive disorders.

Worldwide, the prevalence patterns of cognitive disorders appear to be similar to other Western diseases. Rates of Alzheimer's are low in less developed areas.[61] A recent study compared Alzheimer's rates to dietary variables across eleven different countries and found that populations with a high fat intake and low cereal and grain intake had higher rates of the disease.[62, 63]

We seem to be on to something. Clearly, diet has an important voice in determining how well we think in our later years. But what exactly is good for us?

With regard to the more mild cognitive impairment condition, recent research has shown that high vitamin E levels in the blood are related to less memory loss.[64] Less memory loss also is associated with higher levels of vitamin C and selenium, both of which reduce free radical activity.[65] Vitamins E and C are antioxidants found almost exclusively in plant foods, while selenium is found in both animal- and plant-based foods.

In a study of 260 elderly people aged sixty-five to ninety years, it was reported that: "A diet with less fat, saturated fat and cholesterol, and more carbohydrate, fiber, vitamins (especially folate, vitamins C and E and beta-carotenes) and minerals (iron and zinc) may be advisable not only to improve the general health of the elderly but also to improve cognitive function."[66] This conclusion advocates plant-based foods and condemns animal-based foods for optimal brain function. Yet another study on several hundred older people found that scores on mental tests were higher among those people who consumed the most vitamin C and beta-carotene.[67] Other studies have also found that a low level of vitamin C in the blood is linked to poorer cognitive performance in old age,[68, 69] and some have found that B vitamins,[69] including beta-carotene,[70] are linked to better cognitive function.

The seven studies mentioned above all show that one or more nutrients found almost exclusively in plants are associated with a lower risk of cognitive decline in old age. Experimental animal studies have not only confirmed that plant foods are good for the brain, but they show the mechanisms by which these foods work.[71, 72] Although there are important variations in some of these study findings—for example, one study only finds an association for vitamin C, and another only finds an association for beta-carotene and not vitamin C—we shouldn't miss the forest by focusing on one or two trees. No study has ever found that consuming more dietary antioxidants increases memory loss. When associations are observed, it is always the other way around. Furthermore, the association appears to be significant, although more substantial research must be done before we can know exactly how much cognitive impairment is due to diet.

What about the more serious dementia caused by strokes (vascular dementia) and Alzheimer's? How does diet affect these diseases? The dementia that is caused by the same vascular problems that lead to stroke is clearly affected by diet. In a publication from the famous Framingham Study, researchers conclude that for every three additional servings of fruits and vegetables a day, the risk of stroke will be reduced by 22%.[73] Three servings of fruits and vegetables is less than you might think. The following examples count as one serving in this study: 1/2 cup peaches,

1/4 cup tomato sauce, 1/2 cup broccoli or one potato.[73] Half a cup is not much food. In fact, the men in this study who consumed the most fruits and vegetables consumed as many as nineteen servings a day. If every three servings lower the risk by 22%, the benefits can add up fast (risk reduction approaches but cannot exceed 100%).

This study provides evidence that the health of the arteries and vessels that transport blood to and from your brain is dependent on how well you eat. By extension, it is logical to assume that eating fruits and vegetables will protect against dementia caused by poor vascular health. Research again seems to prove the point. Scientists conducted mental health exams and assessed food intake for over 5,000 older people and monitored their health for over two years. They found that the people who consumed the most total fat and saturated fat had the highest risk of dementia due to vascular problems.[74]

Alzheimer's disease is also related to diet and is often found in conjunction with heart disease,[53] which suggests that they share the same causes. We know what causes heart disease, and we know what offers the best hope of reversing heart disease: diet. Experimental animal studies have convincingly shown that a high-cholesterol diet will promote the production of the beta-amyloid common to Alzheimer's.[53] In confirming these experimental animal results, a study of more than 5,000 people found that greater dietary fat and cholesterol intake tended to increase the risk of Alzheimer's disease specifically,[75] and all dementia in general.[74]

In another study on Alzheimer's,[76] the risk of getting the disease was 3.3 times greater among people whose blood folic acid levels were in the lowest one-third range and 4.5 times greater when blood homocysteine levels were in the highest one-third. What are folic acid and homocysteine? Folic acid is a compound derived exclusively from plant-based foods such as green and leafy vegetables. Homocysteine is an amino acid that is derived primarily from animal protein.[77] This study found that it was desirable to maintain low blood homocysteine and high blood folic acid. In other words, the combination of a diet high in animal-based foods and low in plant-based foods raises the risk of Alzheimer's disease.[78]

Mild cognitive impairment, the stuff jokes are made of, still permits the afflicted person to maintain an independent, functional life, but dementia and Alzheimer's are tragic, imposing almost impossibly heavy burdens on victims and their loved ones. Across this spectrum, from minor difficulties in keeping your thoughts in order to serious degeneration, the food you eat can drastically affect the likelihood of mental decline.

The diseases I've covered in this chapter take a heavy toll on most of us in our later years, even though they may not be fatal. Because they are not usually fatal, many people afflicted with these illnesses still live a long life. Their quality of life, however, deteriorates steadily, until the illness renders them largely dependent on others and unable to function in most capacities.

I've talked to so many people who say, "I may not live as long as you health nuts, but I sure am going to enjoy the time I have by eating steaks whenever I want, smoking if I so choose and doing anything else that I want." I grew up with these people, went to school with these people and made great friends with these people. Not long ago, one of my best friends suffered a difficult surgery for cancer and spent his last years paralyzed in a nursing home. During the many visits I made to the nursing home, I never failed to come away with a deep appreciation for the health I still possess in my old age. It was not uncommon for me to go to the nursing home to visit my friend and hear that one of the new patients in the home was someone whom my friend and I knew from our earlier days. Too often, they had Alzheimer's and were housed in a special section of the facility.

The enjoyment of life, especially the second half of life, is greatly compromised if we can't see, if we can't think, if our kidneys don't work or if our bones are broken or fragile. I, for one, hope that I am able to fully enjoy not only the time in the present, but also the time in the future, with good health and independence.

Part III
THE GOOD NUTRITION GUIDE

I WAS IN A RESTAURANT RECENTLY, looking at the menu, when I noticed a very peculiar "low-carb" meal option: a massive plate of pasta topped with vegetables, otherwise known as pasta primavera. The vast majority of calories in the meal clearly came from carbohydrates. How could it be "low-carb"? Was it a misprint? I didn't think so. At various other times I've noted that salads, breads and even cinnamon buns are labeled "low-carb," even though their ingredient lists demonstrate that, in fact, the bulk of calories are provided by carbohydrates. What's going on?

This "carb" mania is largely the result of the late Dr. Atkins and his dietary message. But recently *Dr. Atkins' New Diet Revolution* has been toppled and replaced by *The South Beach Diet* as the king of the diet books. The South Beach Diet is pitched as being more moderate, easier to follow and safer than Atkins, but from what I can tell, the weight-loss "wolf" has just put on a different set of sheep's clothing. Both of the diets are divided into three stages, both diets severely limit carbohydrate intake during the first phase, and both diets are heavily based on meat, dairy and eggs. The South Beach Diet, for example, prohibits bread, rice, potatoes, pasta, baked goods, sugar and even fruit during the first two weeks. After that, you can be weaned back onto carbohydrates until you are eating what appears to me to be a fairly typical American diet. Perhaps this is why *The South Beach Diet* is such a hot seller. According to *The South Beach Diet* Web site, *Newsweek* wrote, "the real value of the book is its sound nutritional advice. It retains the best part of the Atkins regime—meat—while losing the tenet that all carbs should be avoided."[1]

223

Who at *Newsweek* reviewed the literature to know whether this is sound nutritional advice or not? And if you have the Atkins Diet plus some "carbs," how different is this diet from the standard American diet, the toxic diet that has been shown to make us fat, give us heart disease, destroy our kidneys, make us blind and lead us to Alzheimer's, cancer and a host of other medical problems?

These are merely examples of the current state of nutrition awareness in the United States. Every day I am reminded that Americans are drowning in a flood of horrible nutrition information. I remember the adage told several decades ago: Americans love hogwash. Another one: Americans love to hear good things about their bad habits. It would appear from a quick glance that these two sayings are true. Or are they?

I have more faith in the average American. It's not true that Americans love hogwash—it's that hogwash inundates Americans, whether they want it or not! I know that some Americans want the truth, and just haven't been able to find it because it is drowned out by the hogwash. Very little of the nutrition information that makes it to the public consciousness is soundly based in science, and we pay a grave price. One day olive oil is terrible, the next it is heart healthy. One day eggs will clog your arteries, the next they are a good source of protein. One day potatoes and rice are great, the next they are the gravest threats to your weight you will ever face.

At the beginning of the book I said my goal was to redefine how we think of nutrition information—eliminate confusion, make health simple and base my claims on the evidence generated by peer-reviewed nutrition research published in peer-reviewed, professional publications. So far, you have seen a broad sample—and it's only a sample—of that evidence. You have seen that there is overwhelming scientific support for one, simple optimal diet—a whole foods, plant-based diet.

I want to condense the nutritional lessons learned from this broad range of evidence and from my experiences over the past forty-plus years into a simple guide to good nutrition. I have whittled my knowledge down to several core principles, principles that will illuminate how nutrition and health truly operate. Furthermore, I have translated the science into dietary recommendations that you can begin to incorporate into your own life. Not only will you gain a new understanding of nutrition and health, but you will also see exactly which foods you should eat and which foods you should avoid. What you decide to do with this information is up to you, but you can at least know that you, as a reader and a person, have finally been told something other than hogwash.

11

Eating Right: Eight Principles of Food and Health

THE BENEFITS OF A HEALTHY LIFESTYLE are enormous. I want you to know that you can:

- live longer
- look and feel younger
- have more energy
- lose weight
- lower your blood cholesterol
- prevent and even reverse heart disease
- lower your risk of prostate, breast and other cancers
- preserve your eyesight in your later years
- prevent and treat diabetes
- avoid surgery in many instances
- vastly decrease the need for pharmaceutical drugs
- keep your bones strong
- avoid impotence
- avoid stroke
- prevent kidney stones
- keep your baby from getting Type 1 diabetes
- alleviate constipation
- lower your blood pressure
- avoid Alzheimer's

- beat arthritis
- and more...

These are only some of the benefits, and all of them can be yours. The price? Simply changing your diet. I don't know that it has ever been so easy or so relatively effortless to achieve such profound benefits.

I have given you a sampling of the evidence and told you the journey that I have taken to come to my conclusions. Now I want to summarize the lessons about food, health and disease that I have learned along the way in the following eight principles. These principles should inform the way we do science, the way we treat the sick, the way we feed ourselves, the way we think about health and the way we perceive the world.

PRINCIPLE #1

Nutrition represents the combined activities of countless food substances. The whole is greater than the sum of its parts.

To illustrate this principle I only need to take you through the biochemical perspective of a meal. Let's say you prepare sautéed spinach with ginger and whole grain ravioli shells stuffed with butternut squash and spices, topped with a walnut tomato sauce.

The spinach alone is a cornucopia of various chemical components. Chart 11.1 is only a *partial list* of what you might find in your mouth after a bite of spinach.

As you can see, you've just introduced a bundle of nutrients into your body. In addition to this extremely complex mix, when you take a bite of that ravioli with its tomato sauce and squash filling, you get thousands and thousands of additional chemicals, all connected in different ways in each different food—truly a biochemical bonanza.

As soon as this food hits your saliva, your body begins working its magic, and the process of digestion starts. Each of these food chemicals interacts with the other food chemicals and your body's chemicals in very specific ways. It is an infinitely complex process, and it is literally impossible to understand precisely how each chemical interacts with every other chemical. We will never discover exactly how it all fits together.

CHART 11.1: NUTRIENTS IN SPINACH

Macronutrients	
Water	Fat (many kinds)
Calories	Carbohydrate
Protein (many kinds)	Fiber
Minerals	
Calcium	Sodium
Iron	Zinc
Magnesium	Copper
Phosphorus	Manganese
Potassium	Selenium
Vitamins	
C (Ascorbic Acid)	B-6 (Pyridoxine)
B-1 (Thiamin)	Folate
B-2 (Riboflavin)	A (as carotenoids)
B-3 (Niacin)	E (tocopherols)
Pantothenic acid	
Fatty Acids	
14:0 (Myristic acid)	18:1 (Oleic acid)
16:0 (Palmitic acid)	20:1 (Eicosenoic acid)
18:0 (Stearic acid)	18:2 (Linoleic acid)
16:1 (Palmitoleic acid)	18:3 (Linolenic acid)
Amino acids	
Tryptophan	Valine
Threonine	Arginine
Isoleucine	Histidine
Leucine	Alanine
Lysine	Aspartic acid
Methionine	Glutamic acid
Cystine	Glycine
Phenylalanine	Proline
Tyrosine	Serine
Phytosterols (many kinds)	

The main message I'm trying to get across is this: the chemicals we get from the foods we eat are engaged in a series of reactions that work in concert to produce good health. These chemicals are carefully orchestrated by intricate controls within our cells and all through our bodies, and these controls decide what nutrient goes where, how much of each nutrient is needed and when each reaction takes place.

Our bodies have evolved with this infinitely complex network of reactions in order to derive maximal benefit from whole foods, as they appear in nature. The misguided may trumpet the virtues of one specific nutrient or chemical, but this thinking is too simplistic. Our bodies have learned how to benefit from the chemicals in food as they are packaged together, discarding some and using others as they see fit. I cannot stress this enough, as it is the foundation of understanding what good nutrition means.

PRINCIPLE #2

Vitamin supplements are not a panacea for good health.

Because nutrition operates as an infinitely complex biochemical system involving thousands of chemicals and thousands of effects on your health, it makes little or no sense that isolated nutrients taken as supplements can substitute for whole foods. Supplements will not lead to long-lasting health and may cause unforeseen side effects. Furthermore, for those relying on supplements, beneficial and sustained diet change is postponed. The dangers of a Western diet cannot be overcome by consuming nutrient pills.

As I have watched the interest in nutrient supplements explode over the past twenty to thirty years, it has become abundantly clear why such a huge nutrient supplement industry has emerged. Huge profits are an excellent incentive, and new government regulations have paved the way for an expanded market. Furthermore, consumers want to continue eating their customary foods, and popping a few supplements makes people feel better about the potentially adverse health effects caused by their diet. Embracing supplements means the media can tell people what they want to hear and doctors have something to offer their patients. As a result, a multibillion-dollar supplement industry is now part of our nutritional landscape, and the majority of consumers have been duped into believing that they are buying health. This was the late Dr. Atkins's formula. He advocated a high-protein, high-fat diet—sacrificing long-term health for short-term gain—and then advocated taking his supplements to address what he called, in his own words, the "common dieters' problems" including constipation, sugar cravings, hunger, fluid retention, fatigue, nervousness and insomnia.[1]

This strategy of gaining and maintaining health with nutrient supplements, however, started to unravel in 1994–1996 with the large-scale investigation of the effects of beta-carotene (a precursor to vitamin A) supplements on lung cancer and other diseases.[2, 3] After four to eight years of supplement use, lung cancer had not decreased as expected; it had increased! No benefit was found from vitamins A and E for the prevention of heart disease either.

Since then, a large number of additional trials costing hundreds of millions of dollars have been conducted to determine if vitamins A, C and E prevent heart disease and cancer. Recently, two major reviews of these trials were published.[4, 5] The researchers, in their words, "could not determine the balance of benefits and harms of routine use of supplements of vitamins A, C or E; multivitamins with folic acid; or antioxidant combinations for the prevention of cancer or cardiovascular disease."[4] Indeed, they even recommended against the use of beta-carotene supplements.

It is not that these nutrients aren't important. They are—but only when consumed as food, not as supplements. Isolating nutrients and trying to get benefits equal to those of whole foods reveals an ignorance of how nutrition operates in the body. A recent special article in the *New York Times*[6] documents this failure of nutrient supplements to provide any proven health benefit. As time passes, I am confident that we will continue to "discover" that relying on the use of isolated nutrient supplements to maintain health, while consuming the usual Western diet, is not only a waste of money but is also potentially dangerous.

PRINCIPLE #3

There are virtually no nutrients in animal-based foods that are not better provided by plants.

Overall, it is fair to say that any plant-based food has many more similarities in terms of nutrient compositions to other plant-based foods than it does to animal-based foods. The same is true the other way around; all animal-based foods are more like other animal-based foods than they are to plant-based foods. For example, even though fish is significantly different from beef, fish has many more similarities to beef than it has to rice. Even the foods that are "exceptions" to these rules, such as nuts, seeds and processed low-fat animal products, remain in distinct plant and animal "nutrient" groups.

Eating animals is a markedly different nutritional experience from eating plants. The amounts and kinds of nutrients in these two types of foods, shown in Chart 11.2,[7, 8, 9] illustrate these striking nutritional differences.

CHART 11.2: NUTRIENT COMPOSITION OF PLANT AND ANIMAL-BASED FOODS (PER 500 CALORIES OF ENERGY)

Nutrient	Plant-Based Foods*	Animal-Based Foods**
Cholesterol (mg)	—	137
Fat (g)	4	36
Protein (g)	33	34
Beta-carotene (mcg)	29,919	17
Dietary Fiber (g)	31	—
Vitamin C (mg)	293	4
Folate (mcg)	1168	19
Vitamin E (mg_ATE)	11	0.5
Iron (mg)	20	2
Magnesium (mg)	548	51
Calcium (mg)	545	252

* Equal parts of tomatoes, spinach, lima beans, peas, potatoes

** Equal parts of beef, pork, chicken, whole milk

As you can see, plant foods have dramatically more antioxidants, fiber and minerals than animal foods. In fact, animal foods are almost completely devoid of several of these nutrients. Animal foods, on the other hand, have much more cholesterol and fat. They also have slightly more protein than plant foods, along with more B_{12} and vitamin D, although the vitamin D is largely due to artificial fortification in milk. Of course, there are some exceptions: some nuts and seeds are high in fat and protein (e.g., peanuts, sesame seeds) while some animal-based foods are low in fat, usually because they are stripped of their fat by artificial processing (e.g., skim milk). But if one looks a little more closely, the fat and the protein of nuts and seeds are different: they are more healthful than the fat and protein of animal foods. They also are accompanied by some interesting antioxidant substances. On the other hand, processed, low-fat, animal-based foods still have some cholesterol, lots of protein and very little or no antioxidants and dietary fiber, just like other animal-based foods. Since nutrients are primarily responsible for the healthful effects of foods and because of these major differences in nutrient composition between animal- and plant-based foods, isn't it therefore reasonable to assume that we should expect to see distinctly different effects on our bodies depending on which variety of foods we consume?

By definition, for a food chemical to be an essential nutrient, it must meet two requirements:

- the chemical is necessary for healthy human functioning
- the chemical must be something our bodies cannot make on their own, and therefore must be obtained from an outside source

One example of a chemical that is not essential is cholesterol, a component of animal-based food that is nonexistent in plant-based food. While cholesterol is essential for health, our bodies can make all that we require; so we do not need to consume any in food. Therefore, it is not an essential nutrient.

There are four nutrients which animal-based foods have that plant-based foods, for the most part, do not: cholesterol and vitamins A, D and B_{12}. Three of these are nonessential nutrients. As discussed above, cholesterol is made by our bodies naturally. Vitamin A can be readily made by our bodies from beta-carotene, and vitamin D can be readily made by our bodies simply by exposing our skin to about fifteen minutes of sunshine every couple days. Both of these vitamins are toxic if they are consumed in high amounts. This is one more indication that it is better to rely on the vitamin precursors, beta-carotene and sunshine, so that our bodies can readily control the timing and quantities of vitamins A and D that are needed.

Vitamin B_{12} is more problematic. Vitamin B_{12} is made by microorganisms found in the soil and by microorganisms in the intestines of animals, including our own. The amount made in our intestines is not adequately absorbed, so it is recommended that we consume B_{12} in food. Research has convincingly shown that plants grown in healthy soil that has a good concentration of vitamin B_{12} will readily absorb this nutrient.[10] However, plants grown in "lifeless" soil (non-organic soil) may be deficient in vitamin B_{12}. In the United States, most of our agriculture takes place on relatively lifeless soil, decimated from years of unnatural pesticide, herbicide and fertilizer use. So the plants grown in this soil and sold in our supermarkets lack B_{12}. In addition, we live in such a sanitized world that we rarely come into direct contact with the soilborne microorganisms that produce B_{12}. At one point in our history, we got B_{12} from vegetables that hadn't been scoured of all soil. Therefore, it is not unreasonable to assume that modern Americans who eat highly cleansed plant products and no animal products are unlikely to get enough vitamin B_{12}.

Though our society's obsession with nutrient supplements seriously detracts from other, far more important nutrition information, this is not to say that supplements should always be avoided. It is estimated that we hold a three-year store of vitamin B_{12} in our bodies. If you do not eat any animal products for three years or more, or are pregnant or breastfeeding, you should consider taking a small B_{12} supplement on occasion, or going to the doctor annually to check your blood levels of B vitamins and homocysteine. Likewise, if you never get sunshine exposure, especially during the winter months, you might want to take a vitamin D supplement. I would recommend taking the smallest dose you can find and making more of an effort to get outside.

I call these supplements "separation from nature pills," because a healthy diet of fresh, organic plant-based foods grown in rich soil and a lifestyle that regularly takes you outdoors is the best answer to these issues. Returning to our natural way of life in this small way provides innumerable other benefits, as well.

PRINCIPLE #4

Genes do not determine disease on their own. Genes function only by being activated, or expressed, and nutrition plays a critical role in determining which genes, good and bad, are expressed.

I can safely say that the origin of every single disease is genetic. Our genes are the code to everything in our bodies, good and bad. Without genes, there would be no cancer. Without genes, there would be no obesity, diabetes or heart disease. And without genes, there would be no life.

This might explain why we are spending hundreds of millions of dollars trying to figure out which gene causes which disease and how we can silence the dangerous genes. This also explains why some perfectly healthy young women have had their breasts removed simply because they were found to carry genes that are linked to breast cancer. This explains why the bulk of resources in science and health in the past decade has shifted to genetic research. At Cornell University alone $500 million is being raised to create a "Life Sciences Initiative." This initiative promises to "forever change the way life-science research is conducted and taught at the university." What is one of the main thrusts of the program? Integrating each scientific discipline into the all-encompassing umbrella of genetic research. It is the largest scientific effort in Cornell's history.[11]

Much of this focus on genes, however, misses a simple but crucial point: not all genes are fully expressed all the time. If they aren't activated, or expressed, they remain biochemically dormant. Dormant genes do not have any effect on our health. This is obvious to most scientists, and many laypeople, but the significance of this idea is seldom understood. What happens to cause some genes to remain dormant, and others to express themselves? The answer: environment, especially diet.

To reuse a previous analogy, it is useful to think of genes as seeds. As any good gardener knows, seeds will not grow into plants unless they have nutrient-rich soil, water and sunshine. Neither will genes be expressed unless they have the proper environment. In our body, nutrition is the environmental factor that determines the activity of genes. As we saw in chapter three, the genes that cause cancer were profoundly impacted by the consumption of protein. In my research group, we learned that we could turn the bad genes on and off simply by adjusting animal protein intake.

Furthermore, our China research findings showed that people of roughly the same ethnic background have hugely varying disease rates. These are people said to have similar genes, and yet they get different diseases depending on their environment. Dozens of studies have documented that as people migrate, they assume the disease risk of the country to which they move. They do not change their genes, and yet they fall prey to diseases and illnesses at rates that are rare in their homeland population.

Furthermore, we have seen disease rates change over time so drastically that it is biologically impossible to put the blame on genes. In twenty-five years, the percentage of our population that is obese has doubled, from 15% to 30%. In addition, diabetes, heart disease and many other diseases of affluence were rare until recent history, and our genetic code simply could not have changed significantly in the past 25, 100 or even 500 years.

So while we can say that genes are crucial to every biological process, we have some very convincing evidence that gene expression is far more important, and gene expression is controlled by environment, especially nutrition.

A further folly of this genetic research is assuming that understanding our genes is simple. It is not. Recently, for example, researchers studied genetic regulation of weight in a tiny worm species.[12] The scientists went through 16,757 genes, turning each one off, and observed the effect on weight. They discovered 417 genes that affect weight. How these hundreds of genes interact over the long term with each other and their ever-changing environment to alter weight gain or loss is an incredibly complex mystery. Goethe once said, "We know accurately only when we know little; with knowledge doubt increases."[13]

Expression of our genetic code represents a universe of biochemical interactions of almost infinite complexity. This biochemical "universe" interacts with many different systems, including nutrition, which itself represents whole systems of complex biochemistry. With genetic research, I suspect we are embarking on a massive quest to shortcut nature only to end up worse off than when we started.

Does all this mean I think that genes don't matter? Of course not. If you take two Americans living in the same environment and feed them exactly the same meaty food every day for their entire lives, I would not be surprised if one died of a heart attack at age fifty-four, and the other died of cancer at the age of eighty. What explains the difference? Genes. Genes give us our predispositions. We all have different disease risks due to our different genes. But while we will never know exactly which risks we are predisposed to, we do know how to control those risks. Regardless of our genes, we can all optimize our chances of expressing the right genes by providing our bodies with the best possible environment—that is, the best possible nutrition. Even though the two Americans in the example above succumbed to different diseases at different ages, it is entirely possible that both could have lived many more years with a higher quality of life if they would have practiced optimal nutrition.

PRINCIPLE #5

Nutrition can substantially control the adverse effects of noxious chemicals.

Stories of cancer-causing chemicals regularly appear in the press. Acrylamide, artificial sweeteners, nitrosamines, nitrites, Alar, heterocyclic amines and aflatoxin have all been linked to cancer in experimental studies.

There is a widely held perception that cancer is caused by toxic chemicals that make their way into our bodies in a sinister way. For example, people often cite health concerns to justify their opposition to pumping antibiotics and hormones into farm animals. The assumption is that the meat would be safe to eat if it didn't have those unnatural chemicals in it. The real danger of the meat, however, is the nutrient imbalances, regardless of the presence or absence of those nasty chemicals. Long before modern chemicals were introduced into our food, people still began to experience more cancer and more heart disease when they started to eat more animal-based foods.

A great example of a misunderstood "public health concern" regarding chemicals is the lengthy, $30 million investigation of minimally higher rates of breast cancer in Long Island, New York, referred to in chapter eight. Here, it seemed that chemical contaminants from certain industrial sites were creating breast cancer for women who lived nearby. But this ill-conceived story has proven to have no merit.

Another chemical carcinogen concern surrounds acrylamide, which is primarily found in processed or fried foods like potato chips. The implication is that if we could effectively remove this chemical from potato chips, they would be safe to eat, even though they continue to be highly unhealthy, processed slices of potatoes drenched with fat and salt.

So many of us seem to want a scapegoat. We do not want to hear that our favorite foods are a problem simply because of their nutritional content.

In chapter three, we saw that the potential effects of aflatoxin, a chemical touted as being highly carcinogenic, could be entirely controlled by nutrition. Even with large doses of aflatoxin, rats could be healthy, active and cancer-free if they were fed low-protein diets. We also saw how small findings can make big news every time cancer is mentioned. For example, if experimental animals have an increased incidence of cancer after gargantuan exposures, the chemical agent is trumpeted as a cause of cancer, as was the case for NSAR (see chapter three) and nitrites. However, like genes, the activities of these chemical carcinogens are primarily controlled by the nutrients that we eat.

So what do these examples tell us? In practical terms, you aren't doing yourself much good by eating organic beef instead of conventional beef that's been pumped full of chemicals. The organic beef might be marginally healthier, but I would never say that it was a safe choice. Both types of beef have a similar nutrient profile.

It is useful to think of this principle in another way: a chronic disease like cancer takes years to develop. Those chemicals that initiate cancer are often the ones that make headlines. What does not make headlines, however, is the fact that the disease process continues long after initiation, and can be accelerated or repressed during its promotion stage by nutrition. In other words, nutrition primarily determines whether the disease will ever do its damage.

PRINCIPLE #6

The same nutrition that prevents disease in its early stages (before diagnosis) can also halt or reverse disease in its later stages (after diagnosis).

It is worth repeating that chronic diseases take several years to develop. For example, there is a general thought that breast cancer can be initiated in adolescence and not become detectable until after menopause! *So we very well may have lots of middle-aged women walking around with breast cancer initiated during their teens that will not be detectable until after menopause.*[14] For many people this translates into the fatalistic notion that little can be done later in life. Does this mean that these women should start smoking and eating more chicken-fried steak because they're doomed anyway? What do we do, given that many of us may already have an initiated chronic disease lurking in our bodies, waiting to explode decades from now?

As we saw in chapter three, cancer that is already initiated and growing in experimental animals can be slowed, halted or even reversed by good nutrition. Luckily for us, *the same good nutrition maximizes health at every stage of a disease.* In humans, we have seen research findings showing that a whole foods, plant-based diet reverses advanced heart disease, helps obese people lose weight and helps diabetics get off their medication and return to a more normal, pre-diabetes life. Research has also shown that advanced melanoma, the deadly form of skin cancer, might be attenuated or reversed by lifestyle changes.[15]

Some diseases, of course, appear to be irreversible. The autoimmune diseases are perhaps most frightening because once the body turns against itself, it may become unstoppable. And yet, amazingly, even some of these diseases may be slowed or attenuated by diet. Recall the research showing that even Type 1 diabetics can lower their medication requirements by eating the right food. Evidence also shows that rheumatoid arthritis can be slowed by diet,[16] as can multiple sclerosis.[17, 18]

I believe that an ounce of prevention does equal a pound of cure, and the earlier in life good foods are eaten, the better one's health will be. But for those who already face the burden of disease, we must not forget that nutrition still can play a vital role.

PRINCIPLE #7

Nutrition that is truly beneficial for one chronic disease will support health across the board.

When I was trying to get this book published, I had a meeting with an editor at a major publishing house, and described to her my intent to create disease-specific chapters that related diet to specific ailments or groups of ailments. The editor asked, in effect, "Can you make specific diet plans for each disease, so that every chapter doesn't have the same recommendations?" In other words, could I tell people to eat a specific way for heart disease and a different way for diabetes? The implication, of course, was that the same eating plan for multiple diseases simply wasn't catchy enough, wasn't sufficiently "marketable."

Although this might be good marketing, it is not good science. As I have come to understand more about the biochemical processes of various diseases, I have also come to see how these diseases have much in common. Because of these impressive commonalities, it only makes sense that the same good nutrition will generate health and prevent diseases *across the board*. Even if a whole foods, plant-based diet is more effective at treating heart disease than brain cancer, you can be sure that this diet will not promote one disease while it stops another. It will never be "bad" for you. This one good diet can only help across the board.

So I'm afraid I don't have a different, catchy formula for each disease. I only have one dietary prescription. But rather than be forlorn about its effect on my book sales, I'd prefer to remain excited about telling you how simple food and health really is. It is a chance to clear away much of the incredible public confusion. *Quite simply, you can maximize health for diseases across the board with one simple diet.*

PRINCIPLE #8

Good nutrition creates health in all areas of our existence. All parts are interconnected.

Much has been made of "holistic" health in recent times. This concept can mean a variety of things to different people. Many people lump all of the "alternative" medicines and activities into this concept, so holistic health comes to mean acupressure, acupuncture, herbal medicines, meditation, vitamin supplements, chiropractic care, yoga, aromatherapy, Feng Shui, massage and even sound therapy.

Conceptually, I believe in holistic health, but not as a catchphrase for every unconventional and oftentimes unproven medicine around. Food and nutrition, for example, are of primary importance to our health. The process of eating is perhaps the most intimate encounter we have with our world; it is a process in which what we eat becomes part of our body. But other experiences also are important, such as physical activity, emotional and mental health and the well-being of our environment. Incorporating these various spheres into our concept of health is important because they are all interconnected. Indeed, this is a holistic concept.

These expanding interconnections became apparent to me through experimentation with animals. The rats fed the low-protein diets were not only spared liver cancer, but they also had lower blood cholesterol, noticeably more energy and voluntarily exercised twice as much as the high-protein rats. The evidence regarding increased energy levels was supported by an enormous amount of anecdotal evidence I have encountered over the years: people have more energy when they eat well. This synergy between nutrition and physical activity is extremely important, and is evidence that these two parts of life are not isolated from each other. Good nutrition and regular exercise combine to offer more health per person than the sum of each part alone.

We also know that physical activity has an effect on emotional and mental well-being. Much has been said about the effect physical activity has on various chemicals in our bodies, which in turn affect our moods and our concentration. And experiencing the rewards of feeling better emotionally and being more mentally alert provides the confidence and motivation to treat ourselves to optimal nutrition, which reinforces the entire cycle. Those who feel good about themselves are more likely to respect their health by practicing good nutrition.

Sometimes people try to play these different parts of their lives against each other. People wonder if they can erase bad eating habits by being a runner. The answer to this is no. The benefits and risks of diet are crucially important, and more sizable, than the benefits and risks of other activities. Besides, why would anyone want to try and balance benefits and risks when they could have all the benefits, working together? People also wonder whether a perceived health benefit is because of the exercise or because of a good diet. In the end, that's simply an academic question. The fact is that these two spheres of our lives are intimately interconnected, and what's important is that it *all works together to promote or derail health.*

Furthermore, it turns out that if we eat the way that promotes the best health for ourselves, we promote the best health for the planet. By eating a whole foods, plant-based diet, we use less water, less land, fewer resources and produce less pollution and less suffering for our farm animals. John Robbins has done more than any other person to bring this issue to the front of American consciousness, and I strongly recommend reading his most recent book, *The Food Revolution.*

Our food choices have an incredible impact not only on our metabolism, but also on the initiation, promotion and even reversal of disease, on our energy, on our physical activity, on our emotional and mental well-being and on our world environment. *All of these seemingly separate spheres are intimately interconnected.*

I have mentioned the wisdom of nature at various points in this book, and I have come to see the power of the workings of the natural world. It is a wondrous web of health, from molecules, to people, to other animals, to forests, to oceans, to the air we breathe. This is nature at work, from the microscopic to the macroscopic.

WHO CARES, ANYWAY?

The principles outlined in this chapter began, for me, with a narrowly focused question on diet and cancer in rats, then grew into an ever-expanding universe of questions about human and societal health around the world. In large measure, the principles in this chapter are the answers to the far-reaching questions that I could not help but ask during my career.

The applicability of these principles should not be underestimated. Most importantly, they can help to reduce public confusion regarding food and health. The latest fads, the newest headlines and the most recent study results are put into a useful context. We need not leap from our seats every time a chemical is called a carcinogen, every time a new diet book hits the shelf or every time a headline screams about solving disease through genetic research.

Simply put, we can relax. We can take a much-needed deep breath and sit back. Moreover, we can do science more intelligently, and ask better questions because we have a sound framework relating nutrition to health. In effect, we can interpret new findings with a broader context in mind. With these newly interpreted findings, we can enrich or modify our original framework and invest our money and resources where they matter to increase our society's health. The benefits of understanding these principles are wide-ranging and profound for individuals, societies, our fellow animals and our planet.

12
How to Eat

WHEN MY YOUNGEST SON and collaborator on this book, Tom, was thirteen years old, our family was in the final stages of a slow shift to becoming vegetarian. One Sunday morning, Tom came home from a sleepover at a close friend's house and told us a story I still remember.

The night before, Tom was being grilled, in a friendly way, on his eating habits. The sister of Tom's friend had asked him, rather incredulously, "You don't eat meat?" My son had never justified his eating habits; he had just gotten used to eating what was on the dinner table. As a consequence, Tom was not practiced at answering such a question. So he simply answered, "No, I don't," without offering any explanations.

The girl probed a bit more, "So what do you eat?" My son answered, with a few shrugs, "I guess just...plants." She said, "Oh," and that was the end of that.

The reason I enjoy this story is because my son's response, "plants," was so simple. It was a truthful answer, but couched in an entirely un-traditional manner. When someone asks for the glazed ham across the table, she doesn't say, "Pass the flesh of the pig's butt, please," and when someone tells his children to finish their peas and carrots, he doesn't say, "Finish your plants." But since my family and I changed our eating habits, I've come to enjoy thinking of food as either plants or animals. It fits well into my philosophy of keeping the information on food and health as simple as possible.

Food and health are anything but simple in our country. I often marvel at the complexity of various weight-loss plans. Although the writers always advertise their plan's ease of use, in reality it's never easy. Followers of these diets have to count calories, points, servings or nutrients or eat specific amounts of certain foods based on specific, mathematical ratios. There are tools to be used, supplements to be taken and worksheets to be completed. It is no wonder that dieting seldom succeeds.

Eating should be an enjoyable and worry-free experience, and shouldn't rely on deprivation. Keeping it simple is essential if we are to enjoy our food.

One of the most fortunate findings from the mountain of nutritional research I've encountered is that good food and good health is simple. The biology of the relationship of food and health is exceptionally complex, but the message is still simple. The recommendations coming from the published literature are so simple that I can state them in one sentence: eat a whole foods, plant-based diet, while minimizing the consumption of refined foods, added salt and added fats. (See table on page 243.)

SUPPLEMENTS

Daily supplements of vitamin B_{12}, and perhaps vitamin D for people who spend most of their time indoors and/or live in the northern climates are encouraged. For vitamin D, you shouldn't exceed RDA recommendations.

That's it. That's the diet science has found to be consistent with the greatest health and the lowest incidence of heart disease, cancer, obesity and many other Western diseases.

WHAT DOES MINIMIZE MEAN?
SHOULD YOU ELIMINATE MEAT COMPLETELY?

The findings from the China Study indicate that the lower the percentage of animal-based foods that are consumed, the greater the health benefits—even when that percentage declines from 10% to 0% of calories. So it's not unreasonable to assume that the optimum percentage of animal-based products is zero, at least for anyone with a predisposition for a degenerative disease.

But this has not been absolutely proven. Certainly it is true that most of the health benefits are realized at very low but non-zero levels of animal-based foods.

My advice is to try to eliminate all animal-based products from your diet, but not obsess over it. If a tasty vegetable soup has a chicken stock base, or if a hearty loaf of whole wheat bread includes a tiny amount of

**EAT ALL YOU WANT (WHILE GETTING LOTS OF VARIETY)
OF ANY WHOLE, UNREFINED PLANT-BASED FOOD**

General Category		Specific Examples
Fruits		orange, okra, kiwi, red pepper, apple, cucumber, tomato, avocado, zucchini, blueberries, strawberries, green pepper, raspberries, butternut squash, pumpkin, blackberries, mangoes, eggplant, pear, watermelon, cranberries, acorn squash, papaya, grapefruit, peach
Vegetables		
	Flowers	broccoli, cauliflower (not many of the huge variety of edible flowers are commonly eaten)
	Stems and Leaves	spinach, artichokes, kale, lettuce (all varieties), cabbage, Swiss chard, collard greens, celery, asparagus, mustard greens, brussels sprouts, turnip greens, beet greens, bok choi, arugula, Belgian endive, basil, cilantro, parsley, rhubarb, seaweed
	Roots	potatoes (all varieties), beets, carrots, turnips, onions, garlic, ginger, leeks, radish, rutabaga
	Legumes (seed-bearing nitrogen-fixing plants)	green beans, soybeans, peas, peanuts, adzuki beans, black beans, black-eye peas, cannellini beans, garbanzo beans, kidney beans, lentils, pinto beans, white beans
	Mushrooms	white button, baby bella, cremini, Portobello, shiitake, oyster
	Nuts	walnuts, almonds, macadamia, pecans, cashew, hazelnut, pistachio
Whole grains (in breads, pastas, etc)		wheat, rice, corn, millet, sorghum, rye, oats, barley, teff, buckwheat, amaranth, quinoa, kamut, spelt
Minimize		
Refined carbohydrates		pastas (except whole grain varieties), white bread, crackers, sugars and most cakes and pastries
Added vegetable oils		corn oil, peanut oil, olive oil
Fish		salmon, tuna, cod
Avoid		
Meat		steak, hamburger, lard
Poultry		chicken, turkey
Dairy		cheese, milk, yogurt
Eggs		eggs & products with a high egg content (i.e. mayonnaise)

egg, don't worry about it. These quantities, very likely, are nutritionally unimportant. Even more importantly, the ability to relax about very minor quantities of animal-based foods makes applying this diet much easier—especially when eating out or buying already-prepared foods.

While I recommend that you not worry about small quantities of animal products in your food, I am not suggesting that you deliberately plan to incorporate small portions of meat into your daily diet. My recommendation is that you try to avoid all animal-based products.

There are three excellent reasons to go all the way. First, following this diet requires a radical shift in your thinking about food. It's more work to just do it halfway. If you plan for animal-based products, you'll eat them—and you'll almost certainly eat more than you should. Second, you'll feel deprived. Instead of viewing your new food habit as being able to eat all the plant-based food you want, you'll be seeing it in terms of having to limit yourself, which is not conducive to staying on the diet long-term.

If your friend had been a smoker all of his or her life and looked to you for advice, would you tell them to cut down to only two cigarettes a day, or would you tell them to quit smoking all together? It's in this way that I'm telling you that moderation, even with the best intentions, sometimes makes it more difficult to succeed.

CAN YOU DO THIS?

For most Americans, the idea of giving up virtually all meat products—including beef, chicken, fish, cheese, milk and eggs—seems impossible. You might as well ask Americans to stop breathing. The whole idea seems strange, fanatical or fantastic.

This is the biggest obstacle to the adoption of a plant-based diet: most people who hear about it don't seriously consider it, despite the truly impressive health benefits.

If you are one of these people—if you are curious about these findings but know in your heart that you will never be able to give up meat–then I know that no amount of talk will ever convince you to change your mind.

You have to try it.

Give it one month. You've been eating cheeseburgers your whole life; a month without them won't kill you.

A month isn't enough time to give you any long-term benefits, but it is long enough for you to discover four things:

1. There are some great foods you can eat in a plant-based diet that
   you otherwise may never have discovered. You may not be eating everything you want (desire for meat may last longer than a
   month), but you will be eating lots of great, delicious foods.
2. It's not all that bad. Some people take to this diet quite quickly
   and love it. Many take months to fully adjust to it. But almost
   everyone will find that it's a lot easier than they thought.
3. You'll feel better. Even after only a month, most people will feel
   better and likely lose some weight, too. Try having your blood
   work done both before and after. Odds are, you'll see significant
   improvement in even that period of time.
4. Most importantly, you'll discover that it's possible. You may love
   the diet, or you may not, but at the very least you'll come away
   from your one-month trial knowing that it's possible. *You can do
   it, if you choose to.* All the health benefits discussed in this book
   are not just for Tibetan monks and fanatical spartans. You can
   have them too. It's your choice.

The first month can be challenging (more on this shortly), but it gets
much easier after that. And for many, it becomes a great pleasure.

I know this is hard to believe until you experience it for yourself, but
your tastes change when you are on a plant-based diet. You not only
lose your taste for meat, you begin to discover new flavors in much of
your food, flavors that were dulled when you ate a primarily animal-
based diet. A friend of mine once described it as like being dragged to an
independent film when you wanted to go to the latest Hollywood action
flick. You go in muttering, but you discover, to your surprise, that the
film is great—and much more fulfilling than the "shoot 'em up" movie
would have been.

THE TRANSITION

If you take me up on my suggestion of trying a plant-based diet for one
month, there are five main challenges you'll likely face:

- In the first week, you may have some stomach upset as your digestive system adjusts. This is natural; it is nothing to worry about
  and doesn't usually last long.
- You'll need to put some time into this. Don't begrudge this time—
  heart disease and cancer take time too. Specifically, you'll need to
  learn some new recipes, be willing to try new dishes, discover new

restaurants. You'll need to pay attention to your tastes and come up with meals that you really enjoy. This is key.

- You'll need to adjust psychologically. No matter how full the plate is, many of us were trained to think that without meat, it's not a real meal—especially at dinner. You'll need to overcome this prejudice.
- You may not be able to go to the same restaurants you used to go to, and if you can, you certainly won't be able to order the same things. This takes some adjustment.
- Your friends, family and colleagues may not be supportive. For whatever reasons, many people will find it threatening that you are now a vegetarian or vegan. Perhaps it's because, deep down, they know their diet isn't very healthy and find it threatening that someone else is able to give up unhealthy eating habits when they cannot.

I'd also like to offer you a few pieces of advice for your first month:

- In the long term, plant-based eating is cheaper than an animal-based diet, but as you learn you may spend a little extra money trying things. Do it. It's worth it.
- Eat well. If you eat out, try lots of restaurants to find some great vegan dishes. Often, ethnic restaurants not only offer the most options for plant-based meals, but the unique tastes are exquisite. Learn what's out there.
- Eat enough. One of your health goals may be to lose weight. That's fine, and on a plant-based diet you almost certainly will. But don't hold back—whatever you do, don't go hungry.
- Eat a variety. Mixing it up is important both for getting all the necessary nutrients and for maintaining your interest in the diet.

The bottom line is that you can eat a plant-based diet with great pleasure and satisfaction. But making the transition is a challenge. There are psychological barriers and practical ones. It takes time and effort. You may not get support from your friends and family. But the benefits are nothing short of miraculous. And you'll be amazed at how easy it becomes once you form new habits.

Take the one-month challenge. You'll not only do great things for yourself, you'll be part of the vanguard working toward moving America into a healthier, leaner future.

Glenn is an associate of mine who, until recently, was a dedicated meat-eater. In fact, he was recently on the Atkins diet, lost some weight, but dropped off it when his cholesterol went through the roof. He's forty-two and overweight. I gave him a draft of the manuscript for the China Study and he agreed to take the one-month challenge. Here are a few of his observations:

GLENN'S TIPS

The first week is quite challenging. It's hard to figure out what to eat. I'm not much of a cook, so I got some recipe books out and tried creating some vegan dishes. As someone who would swing through McDonald's or heat up a frozen dinner, I found it annoying to have to cook meals each evening. At least half of them were a disaster and had to be thrown out. But over time I found a few that were fantastic. My sister gave me a recipe for West African peanut stew that was incredible and like nothing I ever tasted. My mom gave me a vegetarian chili recipe that was great. And I stumbled on a great whole wheat spaghetti dish with lots of vegetables and a faux meat sauce (made from soy) that was amazing. I challenge anyone to know that this was a vegan dish. But all of this does take time.

I'm rediscovering fruit. I've always loved fruit, but for some reason I don't really eat much of it. Maybe it's not eating meat, but I'm finding that I'm enjoying fruit more than ever. I now cut up a grapefruit and eat it as a snack. I really like it! I would have never done that before; I actually think my tastes are getting more sensitive.

I was avoiding eating out—something I used to do constantly—for fear of not having a vegan option. But I'm getting more adventurous now. I've found some new restaurants that have some great vegan side dishes, including a wonderful local Vietnamese place (I know that most Vietnamese food isn't strictly vegan, since they use a fish sauce in many dishes, but for nutritional purposes it's very close). The other day I got dragged into a pizza place with a large group; there was nothing I could do, and I was starved. I ordered a cheese-less pizza with lots of vegetables. They even made it with a whole wheat crust. I was prepared to choke it down but actually it was surprisingly good. I've brought that home a few times since.

I'm finding that cravings for meat products are pretty much gone, particularly if I don't let myself get hungry. And, honestly, I'm eating like a pig. Being overweight, I've always been self-conscious about what I eat. Now I eat like a madman, and feel virtuous to boot. I can honestly say I'm enjoying the food I'm eating now a lot more than before, partly because I'm fussier now in what I eat. I only eat foods I really like.

The first month went by quicker than I thought it would. I've lost eight pounds and my cholesterol has dropped dramatically. I'm spending a lot less time on this now, particularly since I've found so many restaurants I can eat at, plus I cook huge meals and then freeze them. My freezer is stocked with vegan goodies.

The experiment is over but I stopped thinking of it as an experiment weeks ago. I can't imagine why I would go back to my old eating patterns.

Part IV

WHY HAVEN'T YOU HEARD THIS BEFORE?

OFTEN WHEN PEOPLE HEAR of scientific information that justifies a radical shift in diet to plant foods, they can't believe their ears. "If all that you say is true," they wonder, "why haven't I heard it before? In fact, why do I usually hear the opposite of what you say: that milk is good for us, that we need meat to get protein and that cancer and heart disease are all in the genes?" These are legitimate questions, and the answers are a crucial part of this story. In order to get to these answers, however, I believe that it is essential for us to know how information is created and how it reaches the public consciousness.

As you will come to see, much is governed by the Golden Rule: he who has the gold makes the rules. There are powerful, influential and enormously wealthy industries that stand to lose a vast amount of money if Americans start shifting to a plant-based diet. Their financial health depends on controlling what the public knows about nutrition and health. Like any good business enterprise, these industries do everything in their power to protect their profits and their shareholders.

You might be inclined to think that industry pays scientists under the table to "cook the data," bribes government officials or conducts illegal activities. Many people love a sensational story. But the powerful interests that maintain the status quo do not usually conduct illegal business. As far as I know, they do not pay scientists to "cook the data." They do not bribe elected officials or make sordid underhanded deals.

The situation is much worse.

The entire system—government, science, medicine, industry and media—promotes profits over health, technology over food and confusion over clarity. Most, but not all, of the confusion about nutrition is created in legal, fully disclosed ways and is disseminated by unsuspecting, well-intentioned people, whether they are researchers, politicians or journalists. The most damaging aspect of the system is not sensational, nor is it likely to create much of a stir upon its discovery. It is a silent enemy that few people see and understand.

My experiences within the scientific community illustrate how the entire system generates confusing information and why you haven't heard the message of this book before. In the following chapters, I have divided the "system" of problems into the entities of science, government, industry and medicine, but, as you will come to see, there are instances where it is nearly impossible to distinguish science from industry, government from science or government from industry.

13
Science—The Dark Side

WHEN I WAS LIVING IN A MOUNTAIN VALLEY outside of Blacksburg, Virginia, my family enjoyed visiting a retired farmer down the road, Mr. Kinsey, who always had a funny story to tell. We used to look forward to evenings listening to his stories on his front porch. One of my favorites was the great potato bug scam.

He told us of his farm days before pesticides, and recounted that when a potato crop became infested with potato bugs, the bugs had to be removed and killed, one by one, by hand. One day, Mr. Kinsey noticed an advertisement in a farm magazine for a great potato bug killer, on sale for five dollars. Although five dollars was no small sum of money in those days, Mr. Kinsey figured the bugs were enough of a hassle to warrant the investment. A short while later, when he received the great potato bug killer, he opened the package and found two blocks of wood and a short list of three instructions:

- Pick up one block of wood.
- Place the potato bug on the flat face of the wood.
- Pick up the second block of wood and press firmly onto the potato bug.

Scams, tricks and outright deception for personal gain are as old as history itself, and perhaps no discipline in our society has suffered more from this affliction than the discipline of health. Very few experiences are as personal and as powerful as those of people who have lost their health prematurely. Understandably, they are willing to believe and try just about anything that might help. They are a highly vulnerable group of consumers.

In the mid-1970s, along came a prime example of a health scam, at least according to the medical establishment. It concerned an alternative cancer treatment called Laetrile, a natural compound made largely from apricot pits. If you had cancer and had been unsuccessfully treated by your regular doctors here in the United States, you may have considered heading to Tijuana, Mexico. *Washington Post Magazine* documented the story of Sylvia Dutton, a fifty-three-year-old woman from Florida, who had done just that as a last attempt to thwart a cancer that had already spread from her ovaries to her lymph system.[1] Friends and fellow churchgoers had told her and her husband about the Laetrile treatment and its ability to cure advanced cancer. In the magazine article,[1] Sylvia's husband said, "There are at least a dozen people in this area who were told they were going to be dead from cancer who used Laetrile and now they're out playing tennis."

The catch, however, was that Laetrile was a highly contentious treatment. Some people in the medical establishment argued that animal studies had repeatedly shown Laetrile to have no effect on tumors.[1] Because of this, the U.S. Food and Drug Administration had decided to suppress the use of Laetrile, which gave rise to the popular clinics south of the border. One famous hospital in Tijuana treated "as many as 20,000 American patients a year."[1] One of those patients was Sylvia Dutton, for whom Laetrile unfortunately did not work.

But Laetrile was only one of many alternative health products. By the end of the 1970s, Americans were spending $1 billion a year on various supplements and potions that promised magical benefits.[2] These included pangamic acid, which was touted as a previously undiscovered vitamin with virtually unlimited powers, various bee concoctions and other supplement products including garlic and zinc.[2]

At the same time in the scientific community, more and more health information, specifically nutrition information, was being generated at a furious pace. In 1976, Senator George McGovern had convened a committee that drafted dietary goals recommending decreased consumption of fatty animal foods and increased consumption of fruits and vegetables because of their effects on heart disease. The first draft of this report, linking heart disease and food, caused such an uproar that a major revision was required before it was released for publication. In a personal conversation McGovern told me that he and five other powerful senators from agricultural states lost their respective elections in 1980 in part because they had dared to take on the animal foods industry.

At the end of the 1970s, the McGovern report succeeded in prodding the government to produce its first-ever dietary guidelines, which were rumored to promote a message similar to that of McGovern's committee. At about the same time, there were widely publicized government debates about whether food additives were safe, and whether saccharin caused cancer.

PLAYING MY PART

In the late 1970s I found myself in the middle of this rapidly changing environment. By 1975 my program in the Philippines had ended, and I was well into my experimental laboratory work here in the United States, after having accepted a full professorship with tenure at Cornell University. Some of my early work on aflatoxin and liver cancer in the Philippines (chapter two) had garnered widespread interest, and my subsequent laboratory work investigating nutritional factors, carcinogens and cancer (chapter three) was attracting national attention. At that time, I had one of only two or three laboratories in the country doing basic research on nutrition and cancer. It was a novel endeavor.

From 1978 to 1979 I took a year-long sabbatical leave from Cornell to go to the epicenter of national nutritional activity, Bethesda, Maryland. The organization that I was working with was the Federation of American Societies for Experimental Biology and Medicine, or FASEB. Six individual research societies made up the federation, representing pathology, biochemistry, pharmacology, nutrition, immunology and physiology. The FASEB sponsored the annual joint meetings of all six societies, and upwards of more than 20,000 scientists attended. I was a member of two of these societies, nutrition and pharmacology, and was particularly active in the American Institution of Nutrition (now named the American Society for Nutritional Sciences). My principle work was to chair, under contract to the Food and Drug Administration, a committee of scientists investigating potential hazards of using nutrient supplements.

While there, I also was invited to be on a public affairs committee that served as liaison between the FASEB and Congress. The committee's charge was to stay on top of congressional activity and represent our societies' interests in dealings with lawmakers. We reviewed policies, budgets and position statements, met with congressional staffs, and held meetings around big, impressive "boardroom" tables in distinguished, august meeting rooms. I often got the feeling I was in the citadel of science.

As a prerequisite to representing my nutrition society on this public affairs committee, I first had to decide, for myself, how nutrition is best defined. It's a far more difficult question than you may think. We had scientists who were interested in applied nutrition, which involves people and communities. We had medical doctors interested in isolated food compounds as pharmacological drugs and research scientists who only worked with isolated cells and well-identified chemicals in the laboratory. We even had people who thought nutrition studies should focus on livestock as well as people. The concept of nutrition was far from clear; clarification was critical. The average American's view of nutrition was even more varied and confused. Consumers were constantly being duped by fads, yet remained intensely interested in nutrient supplements and dietary advice coming from any source, whether that source was a diet book or a government official.

One day in late spring of 1979, while doing my more routine work, I got a call from the director of the public affairs office at the FASEB who coordinated the work of our congressional "liaison" committee.

Ellis informed me that there was yet another new committee being formed within one of the FASEB Societies, the American Institute of Nutrition, that might interest me.

"It's being called the Public Nutrition Information Committee," he told me, "and one of its responsibilities will be to decide what is sound nutritional advice to give to the public.

"Obviously," he said, "there's a big overlap between what this new committee wants to do and what we do on the public affairs committee."

I agreed.

"If you're interested, I would like to have you join this new committee as a representative of the public affairs office," he said.

The proposal sounded good to me because it was early in my career and it meant getting a chance to hear the scholarly views of some of the "big name" nutrition researchers. It also was a committee, according to its organizers, that could evolve into a "supreme court" of public nutrition information. It might serve, for example, to identify nutrition quackery.

A BIG SURPRISE

At the time that this new Public Nutrition Information Committee was being formed, a maelstrom was developing across town at the prestigious National Academy of Sciences (NAS). A public dispute was taking place between the NAS president, Phil Handler, and the internal NAS Food and Nutrition Board. Handler wanted to bring in a group of distinguished scientists from outside of the NAS organization to deliberate on the subject of diet, nutrition and cancer and to write a report. This did not please his internal Food and Nutrition Board, which wanted control over this project. Handler's NAS was being offered funding, from Congress, to produce a report on a subject that had not been previously considered in this way.

Within the scientific community it was widely known that the NAS Food and Nutrition Board was strongly influenced by the meat, dairy and egg industries. Two of its leaders, Bob Olson and Alf Harper, had strong connections to these industries. Olson was a well-paid consultant to the egg industry, and Harper acknowledged that 10% of his income came from offering his services to food companies, including large dairy corporations.[3]

Ultimately Handler, as president of the NAS, went around his Food and Nutrition Board and arranged for a panel of expert scientists from outside of his organization to write the 1982 report *Diet, Nutrition, and Cancer.*[4] As it turned out, I was one of thirteen scientists chosen to be on the panel to write the report.

As could be expected, Alf Harper, Bob Olson and their Food and Nutrition Board colleagues were not happy about losing control of this landmark report. They knew that the report could greatly influence national opinion about diet and disease. Mostly, they feared that the great American diet was going to be challenged, perhaps even called a possible cause of cancer.

James S. Turner, chairman of a related Consumer Liaison Panel within the NAS, was critical of the Food and Nutrition Board and wrote, "We can only conclude that the [Food and Nutrition] Board is dominated by a group of change-resistant scientists who share a rather isolated view about diet and disease."[3]

After being denied control of this promising new report on diet, nutrition and cancer, the pro-industry Board needed to do some damage control. An alternate group was quickly established elsewhere: the new Public Nutrition Information Committee. Who were the leaders of the new Public Nutrition Information Committee? Bob Olson, Alfred Harper and Tom Jukes, a long-time industry scientist, each of whom held a university faculty position. I was initially innocent of the group's purpose, but by our first meeting in the spring of 1980, I had discovered that, of the eighteen members on that committee, I was the only individual who did not have ties to the commercial world of food and drug companies and their coalitions.

This committee was a stacked deck; its members were entrenched in the status quo. Their professional associations, their friends, the people they fraternized with, were all pro-industry. They enjoyed the meaty American diet themselves and were unwilling to consider the possibility that their views were wrong. In addition, some of them enjoyed handsome benefits, including first-class travel expenses and nice consulting fees, paid by animal foods companies. Although there was nothing illegal about any of these activities, it certainly laid bare a serious conflict of interest that put most of the committee members at odds with the public interest.

This is analogous to the situation, as it unfolded, surrounding cigarettes and health. When scientific evidence first emerged to show that cigarettes were dangerous, there were hordes of health professionals who vigorously defended smoking. For example, the *Journal of the American Medical Association* continued to advertise tobacco products, and many others played their part to staunchly defend tobacco use. In many cases, these scientists were motivated by understandable caution. But there were quite a few others, particularly as the evidence against tobacco mounted, whose motivations were clearly personal bias and greed.

So there I was, on a committee that was to judge the merit of nutrition information, a committee that was comprised of some of the most powerful pro-industry scientists. I was the only one not hand-picked by the industry cronies, as I was there at the behest of the director of the FASEB public affairs office. At that point in my career, I had not formed any particularly strong views for or against the standard American diet. More than anything, I was interested in promoting honest, open debate—something that would immediately put me at odds with this new organization.

THE FIRST MEETING

From the first moment of the first meeting in April 1980, I knew I was the chicken who had wandered into a fox's den, although I went in with high hopes and an open, though naïve, mind. After all, lots of scientists, myself included, have consulted with companies while working to maintain an objective mind in the best interest of the public health.

In the second session of our first committee meeting the chairman, Tom Jukes, passed around a proposed news release, handwritten by himself, regarding the mission of the committee. In addition to announcing our formation, the news release listed examples of the kind of nutrition frauds that our committee intended to expose.

As I scanned the list of so-called frauds, I was stunned to see the 1977 McGovern dietary goals[5] on the list. First drafted in 1976, these relatively modest goals suggested that less meat and fat consumption and more fruit and vegetable consumption might prevent heart disease. In this proposed news release, they were described as nothing more than simple quackery, just like the widely condemned Laetrile and pangamic acid preparations. In essence, the recommendation to shift our eating habits to more fruits and vegetables and whole grains was a fraud. This was the committee's attempt to demonstrate their ability to be the supreme arbiter of reliable scientific information!

Having looked forward to my membership on this new committee, I was shocked to see what was emerging. Although I had no particular predilection toward any one type of diet at the time, I knew that the landmark diet, nutrition and cancer panel that I was on at the National Academy of Sciences would likely recommend something similar to McGovern's goals, this time citing cancer research instead of heart disease research. The scientific results with which I was familiar very clearly seemed to justify the moderate recommendations made by McGovern's dietary goals committee.

Sitting next to me at our first meeting was Alf Harper, whom I had held in high esteem since our days at MIT where he was the General Foods Professor of Nutritional Sciences. Early in the meeting, when this handwritten proposed news release was passed out to the committee members, I leaned over to Harper and pointed to the place where it listed McGovern's dietary goals amongst other common scams and whispered incredulously, "Do you see this?"

Harper could sense my unease, even disbelief, and so quickly spoke up. In a patronizing tone, he said to the group, "There are honorable people in our society who may not necessarily agree with this list. Perhaps we should put it on hold." A reluctant discussion ensued, and they decided to forgo the proposed press release.

With the conclusion of the news release issue, the meeting came to an end. As far as I was concerned, it was a dubious beginning, at best.

A couple of weeks later, back in upstate New York, I turned on a morning TV news show and Tom Brokaw appeared on the screen and started talking about nutrition with Bob Olson, of all people. They were discussing a recent report that Olson and friends had produced at the National Academy of Sciences called "Toward Healthful Diets." This report, which was one of the briefest, most superficial reports on health ever produced by the NAS, extolled the virtues of the high-fat, high-meat American diet and basically confirmed that all was well with how America was eating.

From a scientific point of view, the message was a doozy. I remember one exchange where Tom Brokaw asked about fast food, and Olson confidently stated that McDonald's hamburgers were fine. With millions of viewers watching this "expert" praise the health value of McDonald's hamburgers, it's no wonder that consumers around the country were confused. Only a handful of insiders could possibly know that his views did not even come close to reflecting the best understanding of the science at the time.

THE SECOND MEETING

We were back for round two in Atlantic City at our annual meeting in late spring of 1981. From our correspondence over the past year, the committee already had an informal agenda in place. First, we were to establish the proposition that nutrition scams were eroding the public's trust in the nutrition research community. Second, we needed to publicize the idea that advocating more vegetable and fruit consumption and less meat and high-fat foods was, itself, a scam. Third, we intended to position our committee as a permanent, standing organization. Up to this point, our group had only served in a temporary capacity, as an exploratory committee. Now it was time to get on with our job of becoming the permanent, principle source of reliable nutrition information in the U.S.

Within the first few days of arriving at the convention, a fellow member of the committee, Howard Applebaum, told me of the developing gossip. "Did you hear?" he whispered. "Olson's decided that they're going to reconstitute the committee and you are going to be removed." At that time, Olson was still serving his one-year term as president of the parent society, the American Institute of Nutrition, and had the power to do such things.

I remember thinking that this news was neither surprising nor disappointing. I knew I was the black sheep of the committee and had already stepped out of line at our inaugural meeting the previous year. My continued involvement in this particular group was going to amount to nothing more than trying to swim up Niagara Falls. The only reason I was involved in the first place was because the director of the public affairs office at the FASEB had secured me the spot.

I had thought the first year's committee meeting was dubious, but I ran into an even more bizarre beginning at that second meeting a year later, before Olson had the chance to remove me. When the proposal to become a permanent organization within our society was put forth, I was the only one to challenge the idea. I expressed concern that this committee and its activities reeked of McCarthyism, which had no place in a scientific research society. What I was saying made the chair of the committee intensely angry and physically hostile, and I decided it was best to just leave the room. I was clearly a threat to everything the committee members wanted to achieve.

After relating the whole ordeal to the newly-elected incoming president of the society, Professor Doris Calloway of UC Berkeley, the committee was abolished and reformed, with me as the chair. Fortunately, I persuaded our six-member committee to disband after less than a year, and the whole sorry affair came to an end.

To stay and "fight the good fight," so to speak, was not an option. It was early in my career and the awesome power wielded by the seniors in my society was stark and intellectually brutal. For many of these characters, searching for a truth that promoted public health over the status quo was not an option. I am absolutely convinced that had I busied myself with tackling these issues so early in my career, I would not be writing this book. Research funding and publications would have been difficult if not impossible to obtain.

Meanwhile, Bob Olson and some of his colleagues turned their attention elsewhere, focusing on a relatively new organization founded in 1978 called the American Council on Science and Health (ACSH). Headquartered in New York City, the ACSH bills itself, still today, as a "consumer education consortium concerned with issues related to food, nutrition, chemicals, pharmaceuticals, lifestyle, the environment and health." The group also claims to be an "independent, nonprofit, tax-exempt organization,"[6] but they receive 76% of their funding from corporations and corporate donors, according to the National Environmental Trust who cite the Congressional Quarterly's Public Interest Profiles.[7]

According to the National Environmental Trust,[7] the ACSH has claimed, in their reports, that cholesterol is not related to coronary heart disease, "the unpopularity of food irradiation... is not based in science," "endocrine disruptors" (e.g., PCBs, dioxins, etc.) are not a human health problem, saccharin is not carcinogenic and implementation of fossil-fuel restrictions to control global warming should not be implemented. Searching for a serious critique of the food industry from the ACSH is like searching for a needle in a haystack. Although I believe that some of their arguments may have merit, I seriously question their claim to be an objective broker of "consumer education."

FALLING ON MY PETARD

During the entire experience with the Public Nutrition Information Committee, I continued to work on the National Academy of Sciences report on diet, nutrition and cancer, which was released in June 1982.[4] As might have been expected, when this report was published all hell broke loose. Being the first such report on diet and cancer, it received extensive publicity, fast becoming the most sought-after report in NAS history. It was establishing high-profile goals for the dietary prevention of cancer which were very similar to those of the 1976 McGovern Committee report on diet and heart disease. Principally, we were encouraging the consumption of fruits, vegetables and whole grain cereal products, while decreasing total fat intake. The fact that this report was concerned with cancer instead of heart disease, however, elevated emotions. The stakes were high and getting higher; cancer incites a far greater fear than heart disease.

Given the stakes, some powerful enemies came out of the woodwork. Within two weeks, the Council on Agriculture, Science and Technology (CAST), an influential lobbying group for the livestock-based farming industry, produced a report summarizing the views of fifty-six "experts" who were concerned about the effect of our NAS report on the agriculture and food industries. Olson, Jukes, Harper and their like-minded colleagues on the now defunct Public Nutrition Information Committee weighed in as experts. Their report was quickly published, then placed in the hands of all 535 U.S. congressional members. It was clear that the CAST was deeply concerned about the possible impact that our report might have on the public.

The CAST wasn't the only group that stepped up to criticize the report. In addition, there were the American Meat Institute, National Broiler Council, National Cattlemen's Association, National Livestock and Meat Board, National Meat Association, National Milk Producers Federation, National Pork Producers Council, National Turkey Federation and United Egg Producers.[3] I wouldn't presume to know how much cancer research the National Turkey Federation conducts, but I'm guessing that their criticism of our report was not born out of their desire for truth in science.

It was ironic that I had learned some of my most valuable lessons growing up on a dairy farm, and yet the work I was doing was portrayed as being at odds with agricultural interests. Of course, these mammoth corporate interests were far removed from the farmers I knew growing up—the hardworking, honest families that maintained small farms, just big enough to get by comfortably. I often have wondered whether these Washington agricultural interests truly represent America's great farming tradition, or whether they only represent agricultural conglomerates with operations worth tens of millions of dollars.

Alf Harper, who had written a strong letter of support for my first faculty position after leaving MIT, wrote me a stern personal letter in which he declared that I had "fallen on [my] own petard." A petard is a type of bomb or firecracker. Apparently, my involvement in the Public Nutrition Information Committee and the NAS *Diet, Nutrition and Cancer* report was finally too much for even him to bear.

Times were hot, to be sure. Congressional hearings, in which I testified, were held on the NAS report itself; *People* magazine featured me in a prominent article, and an endless series of news media reports continued over the next year.

AMERICAN INSTITUTE FOR CANCER RESEARCH

It seemed that for the first time in our history, the government was seriously thinking about what we eat as a means of controlling cancer. This was fertile territory for doing something new, and something new did indeed fall into my lap. I was invited to assist a new organization called the American Institute for Cancer Research (AICR) in Falls Church, Virginia. The founders of this organization were fund-raisers and had learned that it was possible to raise, through mailing campaigns, large sums of money for cancer research. It seemed that many people were interested in learning something new about cancer beyond the usual model of surgery, radiation and cytotoxic drugs.

This budding organization was well aware of our 1982 NAS report[4] that focused on diet and cancer, and so invited me to join them as their senior science advisor. I encouraged them to focus on diet because the nutrition connection with cancer was becoming an important area of research, yet was receiving very little, if any, support from the major funding agencies. I especially encouraged them to emphasize whole foods as a source of nutrition, not nutrient supplements, partly because this was the message of the NAS report.

As I began to work with the AICR, two challenges simultaneously arose. First, the AICR needed to get established as a credible organization to promote the message and to support research. Second, the NAS recommendations needed to be publicized. Therefore, I thought it made sense for the AICR to help publicize the NAS recommendations. Dr. Sushma Palmer, executive director of the NAS project,[4] and Harvard professor Mark Hegsted, who was the key advisor to the McGovern Committee, agreed to join me in endorsing this AICR project. Simultaneously, the AICR president, Marilyn Gentry, suggested that the AICR could publish the NAS report and send free copies to 50,000 physicians in the U.S. These projects, which seemed to me to be logical, useful and socially responsible, were also highly successful. The associations we were making and the exposure we were generating were aimed at increasing the public's health. As I was quick to find out, however, creating an organization focused on diet as a central link in cancer causation was seen as a threat to a great many people. It was clear that the AICR's projects were beginning to hit the mark because of the hostile feedback coming from the food, medical and drug industries. It seemed that every effort was being made to discredit them.

I was surprised that government interference was particularly harsh. National and state attorney general offices questioned the AICR's status and its fund-raising procedures. The U.S. Post Office joined in the fray, questioning whether the AICR could use the mail to spread "junk" information. We all had our suspicions as to who were encouraging these government offices to quash the dissemination of this diet and cancer information. Collectively, these public agencies were making life very difficult. Why were they attacking a nonprofit organization promoting cancer research? It all came down to the fact that the AICR, like the NAS, was pushing an agenda that connected diet and cancer.

The American Cancer Society became an especially vigorous detractor. In its eyes, the AICR had two strikes against it: it might compete for the same funding donors, and it was trying to shift the cancer discussion toward diet. The American Cancer Society had not yet acknowledged that diet and nutrition were connected to cancer. (It wasn't until many years later in the early 1990s that it developed dietary recommendations to control cancer when the idea was receiving considerable currency with the public.) It was very much a medically-based organization invested in the conventional use of drugs, radiation and surgery. A short while before, the American Cancer Society had contacted our NAS committee about the possibility of our joining them to produce dietary recommendations to prevent cancer. As a committee, we declined, although a couple of the people on our committee did offer their individual services. The American Cancer Society seemed to sense a big story on the horizon and didn't like the idea that another organization, the AICR, might get the credit.

MISINFORMATION

It may seem that I am coming down a tad harshly on an organization that most people regard as purely benevolent, but the American Cancer Society acted differently behind the scenes than it did in public.

On one occasion, I traveled to an upstate New York town where I had been invited to give a lecture to the local chapter of the American Cancer Society, as I had done elsewhere. During my lecture, I showed a slide that made reference to the new AICR organization. I did not mention my personal association, so the audience was not aware that I was their senior science advisor.

After the lecture, I took questions and my host asked me, "Do you know that AICR is an organization of quacks?"

"No," I said, "I don't." I'm afraid I didn't do such a good job of hiding my skepticism of her comment, because she felt obliged to explain, "That organization is being run by a group of quacks and discredited doctors. Some of them have even served time in prison."

Prison time? This was news to me!

Again, without revealing my association with the AICR, I asked, "How do you know that?" She said she saw a memo that had been circulated to local American Cancer Society offices around the country.

Before leaving, I arranged for her to send me a copy of the memo she was referring to, and, in a day or so, she did.

The memo had been sent from the office of the national president of the American Cancer Society, who also was a senior executive of the prestigious Roswell Park Memorial Institute for Cancer Research in Buffalo. This memo alleged that the scientific "chair" of the organization, without naming me, was heading up a group of "eight or nine" discredited physicians, several of whom had spent time in prison. It was total fabrication. I didn't even recognize the names of these discredited physicians and had no idea how something so vicious could have gotten started.

After snooping around a little more, I discovered the person in the American Cancer Society office in Buffalo who was responsible for the memo. I phoned him. Not surprisingly, he was evasive and only said that he had gotten this information from an unnamed reporter. It was impossible to trace the original source. The one thing I do know for sure was that this memo was distributed by the office of the American Cancer Society's president.

I also learned that the National Dairy Council, a powerful industry lobbying group, had obtained a copy of the same memo and proceeded to distribute a notice of its own to its local offices around the country. The smear campaign against the AICR was widespread. The food, pharmaceutical and medical industries through and/or parallel to the American Cancer Society and the National Dairy Council were showing their true colors. Prevention of cancer with low-cost, low-profit plant foods was not welcomed by the food and pharmaco-medical industries. With support from a trusting media, their combined power to influence the public was overwhelming.

PERSONAL CONSEQUENCES

The ending of this story, however, is a happy one. Although the AICR's first couple of years were turbulent and difficult for me both personally and professionally, the smear campaigns finally started to wane. No longer considered "on the fringe," the AICR has now expanded to England (the World Cancer Research Fund, WCRF, in London) and elsewhere. For over twenty years now, the AICR has run a program that funds research and education projects on the link between diet and cancer. I initially organized and chaired that grant program, and then continued as the AICR's senior science advisor for several years, in a few different stints, after its initial founding.

One more unfortunate affair, however, bears mention. I was informed by my nutrition society's Board of Directors that two society members (Bob Olson and Alf Harper) had proposed to have me expelled from the society, supposedly because of my association with the AICR. It would have been the first expulsion in the history of the society. I had to go to Washington to be "interviewed" by the president of the society and the director of nutrition at the FDA. Most of their questions concerned the AICR.

The whole ordeal proved stranger than fiction. Expel a prominent society member—shortly after I was nominated to be the organization's president—for being involved with a cancer research organization? Later, I found myself reflecting on the whole ordeal with a colleague who knew the inner workings of our society, Professor Sam Tove of North Carolina State University. He, of course, knew all about the investigation, as well as other shenanigans. In our discussion, I told him about AICR being a worthy organization with good intentions. His response has resonated with me ever since. "It's not about AICR," he said. "It's about what you did on the National Academy of Sciences report on diet, nutrition and cancer."

When the NAS's report concluded in June 1982 that a lower intake of fat and a higher intake of fruits, vegetables and whole grain products would make for a healthier diet, I had betrayed, in the eyes of some, the nutrition research community. Supposedly, as one of the two diet and cancer experimental researchers on the panel, it was my job to protect the reputation of the American diet as it was. After my failure to do so, my subsequent involvement with the AICR and its promotion of the NAS report only made matters worse.

Luckily, reason prevailed in this whole farcical encounter. A board meeting was held to vote on whether I should be expelled from my society, and I handily survived the vote (6–0, with two abstentions).

It was hard not to take all of this personally, but there's a larger point here, and it's not personal. In the world of nutrition and health, scientists are not free to pursue their research wherever it leads. Coming to the "wrong" conclusions, even through first-rate science, can damage your career. Trying to disseminate these "wrong" conclusions to the public, for the sake of public health, can destroy your career. Mine was not destroyed—I was lucky, and some good people stood up for me. But it could have gone much worse.

After all of these numerous ordeals, I have a better understanding of why my society did the things it did. The awards funded by Mead John-son Nutritionals, Lederle Laboratories, BioServe Biotechnologies and previously Procter and Gamble and the Dannon Institute—all food and drug outfits—represented a strange marriage between industry and my society.[8] Do you believe that these "friends" of the society are interested in pursuing scientific investigation, no matter what the conclusions may be?

CONSEQUENCES FOR THE PUBLIC

Ultimately, the lessons I learned in my career had little to do with specific names or specific institutions. These lessons have more to do with what goes on behind the scenes of any large institution. What happens behind the scenes during national policy discussions, wheth-er it happens in scientific societies, the government or in industry boardrooms, is supremely important for our health as a nation. The personal experiences I have talked about in this chapter—only a sam-ple of such experiences—have consequences far greater than personal aggravation and damage to my career. These experiences illustrate the dark side of science, the side that harms not just individual research-ers who get in the way, but all of society. It does this by systematically attempting to conceal, defeat and destroy viewpoints that oppose the status quo.

There are some people in very influential government and university positions who operate under the guise of being scientific "experts," whose real jobs are to stifle open and honest scientific debate. Perhaps they receive significant personal compensation for attending to the in-terests of powerful food and drug companies, or perhaps they merely have an honest personal bias toward a company-friendly viewpoint. Personal bias is stronger than you may think. I know scientists with family members who died from cancer and it angers them to entertain the possibility that personal choices, like diet, could have played a role in the death of their loved ones. Likewise, there are scientists for whom the high-fat, high animal-based food diet they eat every day is simply what they learned was healthy at a young age; they love the habit, and they don't want to change.

The vast majority of scientists are honorable, intelligent and dedicated to the search for the common good rather than personal gain. However, there are a few scientists who are willing to sell their souls to the high-est bidder. They may not be many in number, but their influence can be vast. They can corrupt the good name of institutions of which they are a part and, most importantly, they can create vast confusion among the public, which often cannot know who is who. You might turn on the TV one day to see an expert praising McDonald's hamburgers, and then read a magazine the same day that you should eat less high-fat red meat to protect yourself against cancer. Who is to be believed?

Institutions also are part of the dark side of science. Committees like the Public Nutrition Information Committee and the American Council on Science and Health generate lopsided panels and committees and institutions that are far more interested in promoting their point of view than debating scientific research with an open mind. If a Public Nutrition Information Committee report says that low-fat diets are fraudulent scams, and a National Academy of Sciences report says the opposite, which one is right?

In addition, this closed-mindedness in science spreads across entire systems. The American Cancer Society was not the only health institution that worked to make life difficult for the AICR. The National Cancer Institute public information office, Harvard Medical School and a few other universities with medical schools were highly skeptical of the AICR and, in some cases, outright hostile. The hostility of medical schools first surprised me, but when the American Cancer Society, a very traditional medical institution, also joined the fray, it became obvious that there really was a "Medical Establishment." The behemoth did not take kindly to the idea of a serious connection between diet and cancer or, for that matter, virtually any other disease. Big Medicine in America is in the business of treating disease with drugs and surgery after symptoms appear. This means that you might have turned on the TV to see that the American Cancer Society gives almost no credence to the idea that diet is linked to cancer, and then opened the paper to see that the American Institute for Cancer Research says what you eat impacts your risk of getting cancer. Who do you trust?

Only someone familiar with the inside of the system can distinguish between sincere positions based in science and insincere, self-serving positions. I was on the inside of the system for many years, working at the very top levels, and saw enough to be able to say that science is not always the honest search for truth that so many believe it to be. It far too often involves money, power, ego and protection of personal interests above the common good. Very few, if any, illegal acts need to occur. It doesn't involve large payoffs being delivered to secret bank accounts or to private investigators in smoky hotel lobbies. It's not a Hollywood story; it's just day-to-day government, science and industry in the United States.

14
Scientific Reductionism

WHEN OUR NATIONAL ACADEMY OF SCIENCES (NAS) Diet, Nutrition and Cancer Committee was deciding how to summarize the research on diet and cancer, we included chapters on individual nutrients and nutrient groups. This was the way research had been done, one nutrient at a time. For example, the chapter on vitamins included information on the relationships between cancer and vitamins A, C, E and some B vitamins. However, in the report summary, we recommended getting these nutrients from foods, not pills or supplements. We explicitly stated that "These recommendations apply only to foods as sources of nutrients— not to dietary supplements of individual nutrients."[1]

The report quickly found its way to the corporate world, which saw a major money-making opportunity. They ignored our cautionary message distinguishing foods from pills and began advertising vitamin pills as products that could prevent cancer, arrogantly citing our report as justification. This was a great opening to a vast new market—commercial vitamin supplements.

General Nutrition, Inc., the company with thousands of General Nutrition Centers, started selling a product called "Healthy Greens," a multivitamin supplement of vitamins A, C and E, beta-carotene, selenium and a miniscule half-gram of dehydrated vegetables. Then they advertised their product by making the following claims[2]:

> [The *Diet, Nutrition and Cancer* report] recommended we increase among other things our amounts of specific vegetables to help safeguard our bodies against the risk of certain forms of cancer.

269

These vegetables recommended by the [National Academy of Sciences report] . . . are the ones we should increase[:] cabbages, Brussels sprouts, cauliflower, broccoli, carrots and spinach. . . . Mom was right!

Research scientists and technicians at General Nutrition Labs, realizing the importance of the research, instantly went to work to harness all of the vegetables and combined all of them into a natural, easy to take potent tablet.

[T]he result is Health Greens [sic], a new potent breakthrough in nutrition that millions of people can now help safeguard their well-being with . . . the greens that the [National Academy of Sciences Committee] recommends we eat more of!

GNC was advertising an untested product and improperly using a government document to support its sensational claims. So the Federal Trade Commission went to court to bar the company from making these claims. It was a battle that lasted years, a battle that was rumored to cost General Nutrition, Inc. about $7 million. The National Academy of Sciences recommended me as their expert witness because of my co-authorship of the report in question and because of my harping on this point during our committee deliberations.

A research associate in my group, Dr. Tom O'Connor, and I spent three intellectually stimulating years working on this project, including my three full days on the witness stand. In 1988, General Nutrition, Inc., settled the false advertising charges relating to Healthy Greens and other food supplements by agreeing to pay $600,000, divided equally, to three different health organizations.[3] This was a small price for the company to pay, considering the ultimate revenues that were generated by the exploding nutrient supplement market.

FOCUS ON FAT

The focus on individual nutrients instead of whole foods has become commonplace in the past two decades, and part of the blame can be put on our 1982 report. As mentioned before, our committee organized the scientific information on diet and cancer by nutrients, with a separate chapter for each nutrient or class of nutrients. There were individual chapters for fat, protein, carbohydrate, vitamins and minerals. I am convinced it was a great mistake on our part. We did not stress enough that our recommendations were concerned with *whole* foods because many people still regarded the report as cataloging the specific effects of individual nutrients.

The nutrient that our committee focused on the most was fat. The first guideline in the report explicitly stated that high fat consumption is linked to cancer, and recommended reducing our fat intake from 40% to 30% of calories, although this goal of 30% was an arbitrary cutoff point. The accompanying text said, "[T]he data could be used to justify an even greater reduction. However, in the judgment of the committee, the suggested reduction is a moderate and practical target, and is likely to be beneficial." One of the committee members, the director of the United States Department of Agriculture (USDA) Nutrition Laboratory, told us that if we went below 30%, consumers would be required to reduce animal food intake and that would be the death of the report.

At the time of this report, all of the human-based studies showing fat to be related to cancer (mostly breast and large bowel) were actually showing that the populations with more cancer consumed not just more fat, but also more animal-based foods and less plant-based foods (see chapter four). This meant that these cancers could just as easily be caused by animal protein, dietary cholesterol, something else exclusively found in animal-based foods, or a lack of plant-based foods (discussed in chapters four and eight). But rather than wagging the finger at animal-based foods in these studies, dietary fat was given as the main culprit. I argued against putting the emphasis on specific nutrients in the committee meetings, but only with modest success. (It was this point of view that landed me the expert witness opportunity at the FTC hearings.)

This mistake of characterizing whole foods by the health effects of specific nutrients is what I call reductionism. For example, the health effect of a hamburger cannot be simply attributed to the effect of a few grams of saturated fat in the meat. Saturated fat is merely one ingredient. Hamburgers also include other types of fat, in addition to cholesterol, protein and very small amounts of vitamins and minerals. Even if you change the level of saturated fat in the meat, all of the other nutrients are still present and may still have harmful effects on health. It is a case of the whole (the hamburger) being greater than the sum of its parts (the saturated fat, the cholesterol, etc.).

One scientist especially took note[4] of our focused critique of dietary fat, and decided to test the hypothesis that fat causes breast cancer in a large group of American women. He was Dr. Walter Willett of the

Harvard School of Public Health, and the study he used is the famous Nurses' Health Study.

Starting in 1976, researchers at the Harvard School of Public Health had enrolled over 120,000 nurses from around the country for a study that was intended to investigate the relationship between various diseases and oral contraceptives, post-menopausal hormones, cigarettes and other factors, such as hair dyes.[5] Beginning in 1980, Professor Willett added a dietary questionnaire to the study and four years later, in 1984, expanded the dietary questionnaire to include more food items. This expanded dietary questionnaire was mailed to nurses again in 1986 and 1990.

Data now have been collected for over two decades. The Nurses' Health Study is widely known as the longest-running, premier study on women's health.[6] It has spawned three satellite studies, all together costing $4–5 million per year.[6] When I give lectures to health conscious audiences, upwards of 70% of the people have heard of the Nurses' Health Study.

The scientific community has followed this study closely. The researchers in charge of the study have produced hundreds of scientific articles in the best peer-reviewed journals. The design of the study makes it a prospective cohort study, which means it follows a group of people, a cohort, and records information on diets before disease events are diagnosed, making the study "prospective." Many regard a prospective cohort study as the best experimental design for human studies.

The question of whether diets high in fat are linked to breast cancer was a natural outgrowth of the fierce discussion going on in the mid-1970s and the early 1980s. High-fat diets not only were associated with heart disease (the McGovern dietary goals), but also with cancer (the *Diet, Nutrition and Cancer* report). What better study to answer this question than the Nurses' Health Study? It has a good design, massive numbers of women, top-flight researchers and a long follow-up period. Sounds perfect, right? *Wrong.*

The Nurses' Health Study suffers from flaws that seriously doom its results. It is the premier example of how reductionism in science can create massive amounts of confusion and misinformation, even when the scientists involved are honest, well intentioned and positioned at the top institutions in the world. Hardly any study has done more damage to the nutritional landscape than the Nurses' Health Study, and it should serve as a warning for the rest of science for what not to do.

CARNIVOROUS NURSES

In order to understand my rather harsh criticism, it is necessary to obtain some perspective on the American diet itself, especially when compared with the international studies that gave impetus to the dietary fat hypothesis.[7] Americans eat a lot of meat and fat compared to developing countries. We eat more total protein, and even more significantly, 70% of our protein comes from animal sources. The fact that 70% of our total protein comes from animal sources means only one thing: we are consuming very few fruits and vegetables. To make matters worse, when we do eat plant-based foods, we eat a large amount of highly processed products that often have more added fat, sugar and salt. For example, the United States Department of Agriculture (USDA) national school lunch program counts French fried potatoes as a vegetable!

In contrast, people in rural China eat very little animal foods; they provide only about 10% of their total protein intake. The striking difference between the two dietary patterns is shown in two ways in Chart 14.1.[8]

These distinctions are typical of the dietary differences between Western cultures and traditional cultures. In general, people in Western countries are mostly meat eaters, and people in traditional countries are mostly plant eaters.

So what about the women in the Nurses' Health Study? As you might guess, virtually all of these women consume a diet very rich in animal-based foods, even richer than the average American. Their average protein intake (as % of calories) is around 19%, compared with a U.S.

CHART 14.1: PROTEIN INTAKE IN THE U.S. AND RURAL CHINA[8]

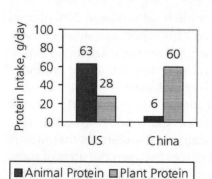
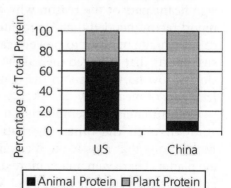

CHART 14.2: PERCENTAGE OF TOTAL PROTEIN
THAT COMES FROM ANIMAL FOOD

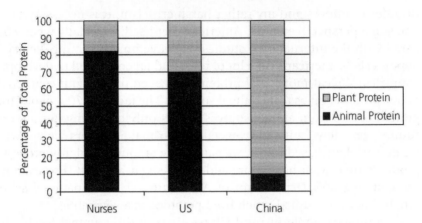

average of about 15–16%. To give these figures some perspective, the recommended daily allowance (RDA) for protein is only about 9–10%.

But even more importantly, *of the protein consumed by the nurses in this study, between 78% and 86% comes from animal-based foods,*[9] as shown in Chart 14.2.[8, 9] Even in the group of nurses that eat the lowest amount of total protein, 79% of it comes from animal-based foods.[9] *In other words, virtually all of these nurses are more carnivorous than an average American woman.* They consume very few whole, plant-based foods.

This is a crucially important point. To get further perspective, I must return to the 1975 international comparison by Ken Carroll shown earlier in Charts 4.7 to 4.9. Chart 4.7 is reproduced here in Chart 14.3.

This chart became one of the most influential observations on diet and chronic disease of the last fifty years. Like other studies, it was a significant part of the reason why the 1982 *Diet, Nutrition and Cancer* report recommended that Americans cut their fat intake to 30% of total caloric intake in order to prevent cancer. This report and other consensus reports that followed thereafter eventually set the stage for an explosion of low-fat products in the marketplace ("low-fat" dairy products, lean cuts of meat, "low-fat" sweets and snack foods).

Unfortunately, the emphasis on fat alone was misguided. Carroll's study, like all the other international comparisons, was comparing populations that mostly ate meat and dairy to populations that mostly ate plants. There were many more differences between the diets of these countries than just the fat intake! What Carroll's graph really shows is

CHART 14.3: FAT INTAKE AND BREAST CANCER MORTALITY

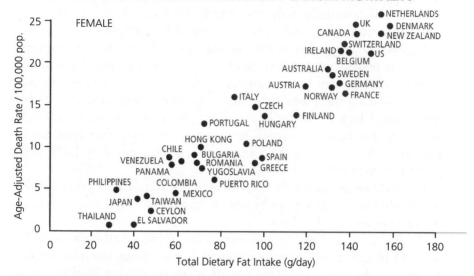

that the closer a population gets to consuming a plant-based diet, the lower its risk of breast cancer.

But because the women in the Nurses' Health Study are so far from a plant-based diet, *there is no way to study the diet and breast cancer relationship originally suggested by the international studies*. There are virtually no nurses that eat a diet typical of the countries at the bottom of this graph. Make no mistake about it: virtually this entire cohort of nurses is consuming a high-risk diet. Most people who look at the Nurses' Health Study miss this flaw because, as Harvard researchers will point out, there is a wide range of fat intake among the nurses.

The group of nurses who consume the least fat eat 20–25% of their calories as fat, and the group of nurses who consume the most fat eat 50–55% of their calories as fat.[10] At a casual glance, this range appears to indicate substantial differences in their diets, but this is just not true, as almost all women uniformly eat a diet very rich in animal-based foods. That begs the question, how can their fat intake vary dramatically while they all uniformly consume large amounts of animal-based foods?

Ever since "low-fat" became synonymous with "healthy," technology has created many of the same foods that you know and love, without the fat. You can now have all kinds of low-fat or no-fat dairy products, low-fat processed meats, low-fat dressings and sauces, low-fat crackers, low-fat candies and low-fat "junk food," like chips and cookies. In other words, you can eat mostly the same foods as you did twenty-five years ago, while substantially reducing your fat intake. But you still retain the same proportion of animal- and plant-based food intakes.

In practical terms this means that beef, pork, lamb and veal consumption is decreasing while lower-fat chicken, turkey and fish consumption is increasing. In fact, by consuming more poultry and fish, people have been increasing their total meat intake to record-high amounts,[11] while trying (and largely failing[12]) to reduce their fat intake. In addition, whole milk is being consumed less, but low-fat and skim milk are being consumed more. Cheese consumption has increased by 150% in the past thirty years.[13]

Overall, we are as carnivorous now as we were thirty years ago, but we are able to selectively lower our fat intake if we so desire, due to the wonders of food technology.

To illustrate, we need only to look at two typical American meals.[14, 15] Meal #1 is served in a health-conscious home, where the main grocery shopper in the family reads the nutrition labels on every food item he or she buys. The result: a low-fat dining experience.

Meal #2 is served in a home where the standard American fare is everyone's favorite. When they cook at home, they make the meal "rich." The result: a high-fat dining experience.

CHART 14.4: LOW-FAT AND HIGH-FAT AMERICAN DINNERS (ONE PERSON'S DINNER)

	Low-Fat Meal #1	**High-Fat Meal #2**
Dinner	8 oz. roasted turkey	4.5 oz. pan-seared steak
	Low-fat gravy	Green beans almondine
	Golden roasted potatoes	Herb-seasoned potato pockets
Beverage	1 cup skim milk	Water
Dessert	Nonfat yogurt	Apple crisp
	Reduced-fat cheesecake	

Both meals provide roughly 1,000 calories, but are markedly different in their fat content. The low-fat meal (#1) contains about twenty-five grams of fat, and the high-fat meal (#2) contains just over sixty grams of fat. In the low-fat meal, 22% of the total calories come from fat, and in the high-fat meal, 54% of the calories come from fat.

The health-conscious home has managed to create a meal that is much lower in fat than the average American dinner, but they've done it without adjusting their proportionate intakes of animal- and plant-based foods. Both meals are centered on animal-based foods. In fact, the low-fat meal actually has more animal-based foods than the high-fat meal. In effect, this is how the nurses in the Nurses' Health Study achieved such a wide variation in fat intake. Some nurses simply are more diligent about choosing low-fat animal products.

Many people would consider the low-fat meal to be a triumph of healthy meal planning, but what about the other nutrients in these meals? What about protein and cholesterol? *As it turns out, the low-fat meal contains more than double the protein of the high-fat meal, and almost all of it comes from animal-based foods. In addition, the low-fat meal contains almost twice as much cholesterol* (Chart 14.5).[14, 15]

CHART 14.5: NUTRIENT CONTENTS OF TWO SAMPLE MEALS

	Low-Fat Meal #1	**High-Fat Meal #2**
Fat (percent of total calories)	22%	54%
Protein (percent of total calories)	36%	16%
Percentage of total protein derived from animal-based foods	93%	86%
Cholesterol	307	165

An overwhelming amount of scientific information suggests that diets high in animal-based protein can have unfavorable health consequences, as can diets high in cholesterol. In the low-fat meal, the amount of both of these unhealthy nutrients is significantly *higher.*

FAT VERSUS ANIMAL FOOD

When women in America, such as those in the Nurses' Health Study and the billion-dollar[4] Women's Health Trial,[16–19] reduce their fat intake, they *do not* do it by reducing their consumption of animal-based foods. Instead, they use low-fat and nonfat animal products, along with less fat during cooking and at the table. Thus, they are *not* adopting the diets that were shown, in the international correlation studies and in our rural China study, to be associated with low breast cancer rates.

This is a very important discrepancy, and is illustrated by the correlation between the consumption of dietary animal protein and dietary fat for a group of countries (Chart 14.6).[8, 9, 18, 20–22] The most reliable comparison was published in 1975[20]; it showed a highly convincing correlation of more than 90%. This means that as fat intake goes up in various countries, animal protein intake increases in an almost perfectly parallel manner. Likewise, in the China Study, the intakes of fat and animal protein also show a similar correlation of 84%.[8, 21]

In the Nurses' Health Study, this is not the case. The correlation between animal protein and total fat intakes is only about 16%.[9] In the Women's Health Trial, also including American women, it is even worse, at −17%[18, 21, 22]; as fat goes down, animal protein goes up. This practice is typical of American women who have been led to believe that, by decreasing their fat intake, they are changing to a healthier diet. A nurse consuming a "low-fat" diet in the Harvard study, like American women everywhere, is likely to continue eating large amounts of animal protein, as shown in meal #1 (Chart 14.4).

Sadly, this evidence on the effects of animal-based food on cancer and other diseases of affluence has been ignored, even maligned, as we continue to focus on fat and other nutrients in isolation. Because of this, the Nurses' Health Study and virtually every other human epidemiological study published to date have been seriously shortchanged in their in-

CHART 14.6: PERCENT CORRELATIONS OF TOTAL FAT AND ANIMAL PROTEIN CONSUMPTION

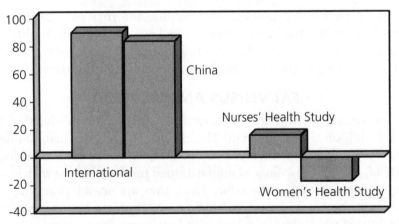

vestigations of diet and disease associations. Virtually all the subjects under study consume the very diet that causes diseases of affluence. If one kind of animal-based food is substituted for another, then the adverse health effects of both foods, when compared to plant-based food, are easily missed. To make matters worse, these studies often focus on the consumption of just one nutrient, such as fat. Because of these very serious flaws, these studies have been a virtual disaster for discovering the really significant effects of diet on these diseases.

THE $100(+) MILLION RESULTS

So now that you know how I interpret the Nurses' Health Study and its flaws, we should take a look at its conclusions. After more than $100 million and decades of work, there is no shortage of results. So what are they? The logical place to start is, of course, the question of whether fat intake really is linked to breast cancer. Here are some of the findings, cited verbatim:

- "these data provide evidence against both an adverse influence of fat intake and a protective effect of fiber consumption by middle-aged women on breast cancer incidence over eight years"[23]

  Translation: The Nurses' Health Study did not detect a relationship between dietary fat and fiber and breast cancer risk.

- "we found no evidence that lower intake of total fat or specific major types of fat was associated with decreased risk of breast cancer"[10]

  Translation: The Nurses' Health Study did not detect a relationship between reducing fat, whether it be total fat or certain kinds of fat, and breast cancer risk.

- "existing data, however, provide little support for the hypothesis that reduction in dietary fat composition, even to 20% of energy during adulthood, will lead to a substantial reduction in breast cancer in Western cultures"[24]

  Translation: The Nurses' Health Study did not detect a breast cancer association with fat even when women reduced their fat consumption all the way down to 20% of calories.

- "relative risks for...monounsaturated and polyunsaturated fat... were close to unity"[25]

  Translation: The Nurses' Health Study did not detect a relationship between these "good" fats and breast cancer risk.

- "we found no significant associations between intake of meat and dairy products and risk of breast cancer"[26]

  Translation: The Nurses' Heath Study did not detect a relationship between meat and dairy consumption and breast cancer risk.

- "our findings do not support a link between physical activity, in late adolescence or in the recent past, and breast cancer risk among young adult women"[27]

  Translation: The Nurses' Health Study did not detect a relationship between exercise and breast cancer risk.

- "these data are suggestive of only a weak positive association with substitution of saturated fat for carbohydrate consumption; none of the other types of fat examined was significantly associated with breast cancer risk relative to an equivalent reduction in carbohydrate consumption"[28]

  Translation: The Nurses' Health Study detected little or no effect on breast cancer when women substituted fat for carbohydrates.

- "selenium intake later in life is not likely to be an important factor in the etiology of breast cancer"[29]

  Translation: The Nurses' Health Study did not detect a protective effect of selenium on breast cancer risk.

- "these results suggest that fruit and vegetable consumption during adulthood is not significantly associated with reduced breast cancer risk"[30]

  Translation: The Nurses' Health Study did not detect a relationship between fruits and vegetables and breast cancer risk.

So there it is, readers. Breast cancer risk does not rise with increased intakes of fat, meat, dairy or saturated fat. Breast cancer is not prevented by increased intakes of fruits and vegetables, or reduced by exercise (either during the teenage years or during adulthood), dietary fiber, monounsaturated fats or polyunsaturated fats. Also, the mineral selenium, long considered to be protective of certain cancers, has no effect on breast cancer. *In other words, we might as well conclude that diet is completely unrelated to breast cancer.*

I can understand the frustration of Professor Meir Stampfer, one of the leading researchers in this group, when he was quoted as saying, "This has been our greatest failure and disappointment—that we have not learned more about what people can do to lower their risk."[6] He was making his comment in response to an opinion that "the single biggest challenge for the future [is] sorting out the mess of contradictory findings and lack of information on breast cancer."[6] I applaud Professor Stampfer for his candor, but it's unfortunate that so much money has been spent to learn so little. Perhaps the most rewarding finding, ironically, was the demonstration that tinkering with one nutrient at a time, while maintaining the same overall dietary patterns, does not lead to better health or to better health information.

Yet Harvard researchers have been steadily cranking out their findings, despite these challenges. From their slew of studies, here are some findings that I would consider as very troubling contradictions when comparing disease risks for men versus women:

- Men who consume alcohol three or four times a week have a lower heart attack risk.[31]
- Men with Type 2 diabetes who consume a moderate amount of alcohol have a lower risk of coronary heart disease.[32]

And yet...

- Alcohol consumption increases breast cancer incidence by 41% for women consuming 30–60 g/day of alcohol compared to non-drinking women.[33]

Apparently alcohol is good for heart disease and bad for breast cancer. The husband can have a drink with dinner but should never share it with his wife. Is this a difference between men and women, or is this a difference in response between heart disease and cancer? Do you feel more informed or more confused?

Then there are those wonderful omega-3 fatty acids. Some types of fish contain relatively large amounts of these fats and have been getting their share of positive press these days. If you've heard anything about omega-3 fatty acids, it's that you need more of them to be healthy. Again, more Harvard findings:

- "...contrary to the predominant hypothesis, we found an increased risk of breast cancer associated with omega-3 fat from fish" (This increased risk was statistically significant and was associated with an increase of only 0.1% of the total dietary energy.)[10]
- "our findings suggest that eating fish once per month or more can reduce the risk of ischemic stroke in men"[34]
- "data suggest that consumption of fish at least once per week may reduce the risk of sudden cardiac death in men [but not reduce the] risk of total myocardial infarction, non-sudden cardiac death or total cardiovascular mortality"[35] (In other words, fish may prevent some aspects of heart disease but ultimately has no effect on mortality from heart disease, or even heart attack risk.)

Is this yet another question of deciding which disease you fear the least? Or is this another man versus woman difference?

Here's an even older story: We have been warned for a long time to cut down on our cholesterol intake, and it was largely for this reason that consumption of eggs was brought into question. One egg has a whopping 200 mg or more of cholesterol,[36] which takes up a large proportion of our 300 mg recommended daily limit. So, what do the Harvard studies tell us on this timeworn issue?

...consumption of up to one egg per day is unlikely to have substantial overall impact on the risk of CHD or stroke among healthy men and women[37]

But, for breast cancer,

Our findings [representing eight prospective studies] suggest a possible modest increase in [breast cancer] risk with egg consumption.... breast cancer risk was found to increase by 22% with every 100-g per day increment of egg consumption [about 2 eggs][26] [There was a 67% increase in risk for the Nurses' Health Study.][26]

But earlier, the Harvard researchers took a slightly different position:

...among healthy men and women, moderate egg consumption can be part of a nutritious and balanced diet[38]

Most recently, the Nurses' Health Study is cited as having come up with an even more powerful endorsement for eggs. A recent news item stated:

Eating eggs during adolescence could protect women against breast cancer....[39]

The article goes on to quote a Harvard researcher as saying:

Women who had, during adolescence, a higher consumption of eggs...had a lower risk of breast cancer....[39]

Most people who read this news article will likely say that eggs are back in favor—even when they don't know how many eggs per day are okay or whether there are exceptions to this generalization. Eggs will only seem to be more healthful when the henhouse industry adds their words of wisdom. But wait a minute—evidence says egg consumption for teenage girls is okay, maybe even good, but evidence also says more egg consumption overall increases breast cancer risk. By the way, here's something else to think about. Multiple studies have rather consistently shown that egg consumption can increase colon cancer risk, more so for women than for men.[40]

What are we to believe? One minute alcohol intake can reduce our disease risks, the next minute it can increase them. One minute fish consumption can help to reduce our disease risks, the next minute it can hurt. One minute eggs are bad, the next minute they can be healthy. It seems to me that what is missing here is the larger context. What you have without that context is just a lot of confusion.

UNRAVELING DIET AND CANCER

In addition to stating that diet and exercise are unrelated to breast cancer, the Harvard researchers have been chipping away at other popular notions regarding diet and cancer. For example, the Harvard studies have not been able to detect any association between colorectal cancer and fiber or fruit and vegetable intake.[4, 41, 42]

Dietary fiber, of course, only comes from plant-based foods, thus these findings put a dent in the idea that fiber or fruits, vegetables and cereals prevent large bowel cancer. Keep in mind that the Harvard studies are dealing with uniformly carnivorous populations, almost none of which are using a whole foods, plant-based diet that is naturally low in fat and high in fiber. It is likely that the potential protective effect of fiber or fruits and vegetables does not kick in against colorectal cancer until there is a complete dietary shift away from an animal-based diet.

Between the colon cancer and breast cancer findings, the Nurses' Health Study has done much to confuse, if not discredit, the idea that diet is related to cancer. After these decades of work, Professor Walt Willett says:

> . . . increasing fruits and vegetables overall appears to be less promising as a way to substantially reduce cancer risk. . . . the benefits [of these foods] appear greater for cardiovascular disease than for cancer[4]

This statement sounds a bit ominous. Colon cancer, historically one of the first cancers said to be prevented by a plant-based diet,[43-45] now is being said to be unrelated to diet? And low-fat diets don't prevent breast cancer? With results like these, it's only a matter of time before the hypothesis of a dietary connection to cancer starts falling apart. In fact, I have already heard people within the scientific community beginning to say that diet may have no effect on cancer.

These are the reasons that I believe that the Nurses' Health Study has done considerable damage to the nutrition landscape. It has virtually nullified many of the advances that have been made over the past fifty years without actually posing a scientifically reliable challenge to earlier findings regarding diet and cancer.

This problem of studying a population that uniformly consumes a high-risk diet and looking at the differences in consumption of one nutrient at a time is not unique to the Nurses' Health Study. It is common to virtually all studies using Western subjects. Furthermore, there is little or no value to pooling the results of many large studies for analysis in order to get a more reliable result if all the studies have the same flaw. A pooling strategy is often used for identifying cause-and-effect associations that are more subtle and uncertain within single studies. This is a reliable assumption when each study is properly done, but obviously it is not when all the studies are similarly flawed. The combined results only give a more reliable picture of the flaw.

The Harvard researchers have done several of these multi-study pooled analyses. One such pooled analysis concerned the question of whether meat and dairy foods had any effect on breast cancer.[26] A previous 1993 pooling of nineteen studies[46] had shown a modest, statistically significant 18% increase in breast cancer risk with increased meat intake and 17% increase with increased milk intake.[46] The Harvard researchers therefore summarized in 2002 a more recent group of studies, this time including eight large prospective studies where dietary information was thought to be more reliable and where a much larger group of women was included. The researchers concluded:

> We found no significant association between intake of meat or dairy products and risk of breast cancer.[26]

Most people would say, "Well, that's it. There is no convincing evidence that meat and dairy foods are associated with breast cancer risk." But let's take another look at this supposedly more sophisticated analysis.

All eight of these studies represented diets that had a high proportion of animal-based foods. In effect, each study in this pool was subject to the same flaw from which the Nurses' Health Study suffered. It makes no sense, and does no good, to combine them. In spite of there being 351,041 women and 7,379 breast cancer cases in this mega-database, these results cannot detect the true effect of diets rich in meat and dairy on breast cancer risk. This would be true even if there were a few million subjects in the study. Like the Nurses' Health Study, these studies all involved typical Western diets highly skewed toward the consumption of animal-based foods, where people are tinkering with the intake of only one nutrient or one food at a time. Every study failed to take into account a broader range of dietary choices—including those which demonstrated positive effects on breast cancer risk in the past.

IGNORING MY CRITIQUE

Once, after reading a publication on animal protein and heart disease in the Nurses' Health Study,[9] I published a critique[47] summarizing some of the same points that I am making in this chapter, including the inability of the Nurses' Health Study to advance our understanding of the original international correlation studies. They responded, and our exchange is as follows.

First, my comment:

> Within a dietary range [so rich in animal-based foods], it makes no sense to me that it is possible to reliably detect the so-called independent associations of the individual constituents of this group when it can be expected that they share the same disease outcomes

and when there are so many difficult-to-measure and interacting risk factor exposures. When will it be understood that it is the total diet and the aggregate and comprehensive effects of large food groups that make the greatest contribution to the maintenance of health and prevention of disease? The sort of reductionism embodied in the interpretation of data from this [Nurses' Health Study] cohort runs the risk of severely misleading discourse on meaningful public health and public policy programs.[47]

Then the response from Dr. Hu and Professor Willett:

Although we agree that overall dietary patterns are also important in determining disease risk (ref. cited), we believe that identification of associations with individual nutrients should be the first step because it is the specific compounds or groups of compounds that are fundamentally related to the [disease process]. Specific components of diet can be modified, and individuals and the food industry are actively doing so. Understanding the health effects of specific dietary changes, which Campbell refers to as "reductionism," is therefore an important undertaking.[48]

I agree that studying the independent effects of individual food substances (their identities, functions, mechanisms) is worthwhile, but Willett and I sharply disagree with how to interpret and use these findings.

I strongly reject the implications in Willett's argument that "specific components of the diet can be modified" to the benefit of one's health. This is precisely what is wrong with this area of research. In fact, if the Nurses' Health Study shows nothing else, it demonstrates that modifying the intake of one nutrient at a time, without questioning whole dietary patterns, does not confer significant health benefits. Women who tinker with fat, while maintaining a near-carnivorous diet, do not have a lower breast cancer risk.

This gets to the heart of reductionism in science. As long as scientists study highly isolated chemicals and food components, and take the information out of context to make sweeping assumptions about complex diet and disease relationships, confusion will result. Misleading news headlines about this or that food chemical and this or that disease will be the norm. The more impressive message about the benefits of broad dietary change will be muted as long as we focus on relatively trivial details.

On occasions, when our paths have crossed, Professor Willett and I have had discussions about the findings on fat as they relate to the China Study and the Nurses' Health Study. I have always made the same point: whole foods, plant-based diets, naturally low in fat, are not included in the Nurses' Health Study cohort, and that it is these types of diets that are the most beneficial for our health. Professor Willett has said to me, in response, on more than one occasion, "You may be right, Colin, but people don't want to go there." This comment has disturbing implications.

Scientists should not be ignoring ideas just because we perceive that the public does not want to hear them. Too often during my career, I have heard comments that seem to be more of an attempt to please the public than to engage in an open, honest debate, wherever it may take us. This is wrong. The role of science in a society is to observe, to ask questions, to form and test hypotheses and to interpret the findings without bias—not to kowtow to people's perceived desires. Consumers have the ultimate choice of whether to integrate our findings into their lifestyles, but we owe it to them to give them the best information possible with which to make that decision and not decide for them. It is they who paid for this research and it is only they who have the right to decide what to do with it.

The perception in the scientific community that the public only wants magic bullets and simple dietary tinkering is overrated. I have learned in my public lectures that there is more interest in diet/lifestyle change than the academic community is willing to admit.

This method of investigating details out of context, what I call reductionism, and trying to judge complex relationships from the results is deadly. It is even more damaging than the misbehavior of the small minority of scientists I discussed in chapter thirteen. Unfortunately, this flawed way of investigating nutrition has become the norm. As a consequence, honest, hardworking, well-intentioned scientists around the world are forced to make judgments about whole dietary effects on the basis of narrowly focused studies on individual nutrients. The greatest danger is that reductionism science, standing naked from its larger environment, has come to be the gold standard. Indeed, I know many researchers who would even say that this is what defines "good" science.

These problems are especially egregious in the investigation of vitamin supplements. As I noted at the beginning of the chapter, I spent over three years during the early history of the nutrient supplement business developing testimony for the Federal Trade Commission and the National Academy of Sciences in their court case against General Nutrition, Inc. I argued that specific health benefits for chronic diseases could not be claimed for isolated vitamins and minerals in supplement form. For this, I took a lot of heat from my colleagues who believed otherwise. Now, more than fifteen years later, after hundreds of millions of dollars of research funding and billions of dollars of consumer spending, we now have this conclusion from a recent survey of the evidence:

> The U.S. Preventive Services Task Force (USPSTF) concludes that the evidence is insufficient to recommend for or against the use of supplements of A, C or E; multivitamins with folic acid; or antioxidant combinations for the prevention of cancer or cardiovascular disease.[49, 50]

How many more billions of dollars must be spent before we understand the limitations of reductionist research? Scientific investigations of the effects of single nutrients on complex diseases have little or no meaning when the main dietary effect is due to the consumption of an extraordinary collection of nutrients and other substances found in whole foods. This is especially true when no subjects in the study population consume a whole foods, plant-based diet when it is this diet that is most consistent with the biologically-based evidence, supported by the most impressive array of professional literature, consonant with the extremely low disease rates seen in the international studies, far more harmonious with a sustainable environment, possessed of the power to heal advanced disease, and has the potential, without parallel, for supporting a new, low-cost health care system. I categorically reject the idea of doing reductionism research in this field without seeking or understanding the larger context. The endless stream of confusion generated by misinterpreted reductionism undermines not only the entire science of nutrition, but also the health of America.

15

The "Science" of Industry

WHAT DOES EVERY AMERICAN SPEND money on several times a day? Eating. After a lifetime of eating, what do we all do? Die—a process that usually involves large costs as we try to postpone it for as long as possible. We're all customers of hunger and death, so there's a lot of money to be spent and made.

Because of this, the food and health industries in America are among the most influential organizations in the world. The revenue generated by the companies that produce food and health products is staggering. Many individual food companies have over $10 billion in annual revenues. Kraft has revenues of roughly $30 billion a year. The Danone Group, an international dairy company based in France, operates the Dannon brand and has revenues of $15 billion a year. And of course, there are the large fast food companies. McDonald's has revenues in excess of $15 billion a year, and Wendy's International generates almost $3 billion a year. *Total food expenditures, including food bought by individuals, government and business, exceed $700 billion a year.*[1]

The massive drug company Pfizer had $32 billion in revenue in 2002, while Eli Lilly & Co. chalked up over $11 billion. Johnson and Johnson collected over $36 billion from selling their products. It's not an overstatement to say over a trillion dollars every year is riding on what we choose to eat and how we choose to treat sickness and promote health. That's a lot of money.

There are powerful players that compete for your food and health dollars. Individual companies, of course, do what they can to sell more of their products, but also there are industry groups that work to increase general demand for their products. The National Dairy Council, National Dairy Promotion and Research Board, National Fluid Milk Processor Promotion Board, International Sprout Growers Association, American Meat Institute, Florida Citrus Processors Association, and United Egg Producers are examples of such industry groups. These organizations, operating independently of any single company, wield significant influence—the most powerful among them have yearly budgets in the hundreds of millions of dollars.

These food companies and associations use whatever methods they can to enhance their products' appeal and grow their market. One way to accomplish this is to claim nutritional benefits for the food products they sell. At the same time, these companies and associations must protect their products from being considered unhealthy. If a product is linked to cancer or some other disease, profits and revenue will evaporate. So food business interests need to claim that their product is good for you, or, at least, that it's not bad for you. In this process, the "science" of nutrition becomes the "business" of marketing.

THE AIRPORT CLUB

While I was getting the China Study off the ground, I learned of a committee of seven prominent research scientists who had been retained by the animal-based foods industry (the National Dairy Council and the American Meat Institute) to keep tabs on any research projects in the U.S. likely to cause harm to their industry. I knew six of the seven members, four of them quite well. A graduate student of mine was visiting with one of these scientists and was given a file on the committee activity. I have never learned exactly why the file passed hands. Perhaps the scientist's conscience was getting the better of him. In any case, the file was ultimately given to me.

The file contained minutes of committee meetings, the latest being held at Chicago's O'Hare Airport. From then on, I have called this group of scientists "The Airport Club." It was run by Professors E. M. Foster and Michael Pariza, faculty members of the University of Wisconsin (where Alf Harper was located), and was funded by the meat and dairy industry. This committee's main objective was to have members observe projects that might do "harm" to their industry. With such surveillance, the industry could more effectively respond to unexpected discoveries from researchers that might make otherwise unanticipated news. I had learned well that, when the stakes are high, industry was not averse to putting its own spin on a story.

They listed about nine potentially damaging projects, and I had the dubious distinction of being the only researcher responsible for two of the projects. I was named once for the China Study, which one of the members was assigned to watch over, and once for my association with the American Institute for Cancer Research (AICR), especially my chairing of the review panel that decided which research applications on diet and cancer got funded. Another panel member had the task of keeping an eye on the AICR activity.

After learning of The Airport Club, and of the individual assigned to watch over me at the AICR grant meetings, I was in a position to see how his spying was going to unfold. I went into the first AICR review panel meeting after learning of the Club with an eye on the spy who was keeping an eye on me!

One might argue that this industry-funded "spying" was not illegal, and that it is prudent for a business to keep tabs on potentially damaging information that might affect its future. I agree completely, even if it was disconcerting to find myself on the list of those being spied on. But industry does more than just keep tabs on "dangerous" research. It actively markets its version, regardless of potentially disastrous health effects, and corrupts the integrity of the science to do so. This is especially troubling when academic scientists do the spying and hide their intentions.

POWERFUL GROUPS

The dairy industry, one of the sponsors of The Airport Club, is particularly powerful in this country. Founded in 1915, the well-organized, well-funded National Dairy Council has been promoting milk for almost a hundred years.[2] In 1995, two major milk industry groups put a new face on their old establishment, renaming it Dairy Management, Inc. The purpose of this new group was "to do one thing: increase demand for U.S.-produced dairy products," to cite their Web site.[3] They had a 2003 marketing budget of more than $165 million to do it.[4] In comparison, the National Watermelon Promotion Board has a budget of $1.6 million.[5] A Dairy Management, Inc., press release includes the following items[4]:

Rosemont, Illinois—National, state and regional dairy producer directors have approved a budget of $165.7 million for a 2003 Unified Marketing Plan (UMP) designed to help increase dairy demand....

...Major program areas include:

Fluid Milk: In addition to key ongoing activities in advertising, promotion and public relations efforts targeted to children ages six to twelve and their mothers, 2003 dairy checkoff efforts will focus on developing and extending partnerships with major food marketers, including Kellogg's®, Kraft foods® and McDonald's®....

...School Marketing: As part of an effort to guide school-age children to become life-long consumers of dairy products, 2003 activities will target students, parents, educators and school foodservice professionals. Programs are underway in both the classroom and the lunchroom, where dairy checkoff organizations look to widen the success of last year's School Milk Pilot Test....

...Dairy Image/Confidence: This ongoing program area aims to protect and enhance consumer confidence in dairy products and the dairy industry. A major component involves conducting and communicating the results of dairy nutrition research showing the healthfulness of dairy products, as well as issues and crisis management....

If I may paraphrase the dairy industry's efforts: their goals are to 1) market to young children and their mothers; 2) use schools as a channel to young customers; 3) conduct and publicize research favorable to the industry.

Many people are not aware of the dairy industry's presence in our schools. But make no mistake: on nutrition information, the dairy industry reaches young children more effectively than any other industry.

The dairy industry has enlisted the public education system as the primary vehicle for increasing demand for its products. The 2001 Dairy Management, Inc., annual report stated[6]:

As the best avenue to increase fluid milk consumption long-term, children are without a doubt the future of dairy consumption. That's why the dairy checkoff continues to implement school milk marketing programs as one way to help increase kids' fluid milk consumption.

Dairy producers...launched two groundbreaking initiatives in 2001. A yearlong school milk research program that began in the fall of 2001 examines how improved packaging, additional flavors, coolers with merchandising and better temperature regulation can affect fluid milk consumption and kids' attitudes toward milk both in and out of school. The study concludes at the end of the 2001–02 school year. Also, dairy producers and processors worked together to conduct a five-month vending study in middle and high schools in five major U.S. markets. The study revealed that many students would choose milk over competitive beverages if it were available when, where and how they wanted.

Many other successful school programs continue to encourage children to drink milk. Nutrition education programs, such as "Pyramid Explorations" and "Pyramid Café," teach students that dairy products are a key part of a healthy diet; the "Cold Is Cool" program teaches school cafeteria managers how to keep milk cold, just how kids like it; and the checkoff is helping expand dairy-friendly school breakfast programs. In addition, the popular "got milk" campaign continues to reach children at school and through such kid-focused media outlets as Nickelodeon and the Cartoon Network.

These activities are far from small-scale; in 1999, "Chef Combo's Fantastic Adventures," an "educational" (marketing) set of lesson plans produced by the dairy industry, "was placed in 76% of preschool kindergarten sites nationally."[7] According to a dairy industry report to Congress,[8] the dairy industry's "nutrition education" programs are doing quite well:

"Pyramid Cafe®" and "Pyramid Explorations™," targeted to second and fourth grades, reach over 12 million students with messages that milk and dairy products are a key part of a healthy diet. Survey results continue to show a very high utilization rate for these two programs, currently at over 70% of the instructors that have the programs.

America is entrusting the important task of educating our children about nutrition and health to the dairy industry. In addition to ubiquitous nutrition lesson plans and "educational" kits, the industry supplies high schools with videos, posters and teaching guides regarding nutrition; it runs special promotions in cafeterias to increase milk consumption in thousands of schools; it distributes information to principals at national conferences; it runs back-to-school promotions with over 20,000 schools; and it runs sports promotions targeted toward youth.

Should we be worried? In a word, yes. If you are curious as to what kind of "education" is being taught by the dairy industry, take a look at their Web site.[9] When I visited the site in July 2003, one of the first bits of information to greet me was, "July is National Ice Cream Month." Upon clicking for more information on National Ice Cream Month, I read, "If you're wondering if you can have your ice cream and good nutrition too, the answer is 'yes'!"[9] Great. So much for combating childhood obesity and diabetes!

The Web site is divided up into three sections, one for educators, one for parents and one for food service professionals. When I looked at the Web site in July 2003 (the Web site regularly changes its content), in the educator portion of the site, teachers could download lesson plans to teach nutrition to their classrooms. Lesson plans included making hand puppets of cows and dairy foods and doing a finger play. Once the puppets are made, the teacher should "[t]ell the students they're going to meet five special friends, and these friends want boys and girls to grow up to be strong and healthy."[9] Another lesson was "Dairy Treat Day," where each child gets to taste cheese, pudding, yogurt, cottage cheese and ice cream.[9] Or teachers could lead their classes in making "Moo Masks."[9] For the more advanced fourth grader, teachers could do a lesson plan from Pyramid Explorations in which students explore the five food groups, and their health benefits, as follows[9]:

Milk Group (Build strong bones and teeth.)
Meat Group (Build strong muscles.)
Vegetable Group (Help you see in the dark.)
Fruit Group (Help heal cuts and bruises.)
Grain Group (Give us energy.)

Based on the evidence presented in the previous chapters, you know that if this is what our children are learning about nutrition and health then we are in for a painful journey, courtesy of Dairy Management, Inc. Obviously neither kids nor their parents are learning about how milk has been linked to Type 1 diabetes, prostate cancer, osteoporosis, multiple sclerosis or other autoimmune diseases, and how casein, the main protein in dairy foods, has been shown to experimentally promote cancer and increase blood cholesterol and atherosclerotic plaque.

In 2002, this marketing Web site delivered *over 70,000 lesson plans* to educators.[8] The dairy industry truly is teaching its version of nutrition to the next generation of Americans.

The industry has been doing this for decades, and it has been successful. I have encountered many people who, when they hear about the potential adverse effects of dairy foods, immediately say, "Milk can't be bad." Usually these people don't have any evidence to support their position; they just have a feeling that milk is good. They've always known it to be that way, and they like it that way. You can trace some of their opinions back to their school days, when they learned that there are seven continents, two plus two equals four, and milk is healthy. If you think about it this way, you will understand why the dairy industry has had such exceptional influence in this country by using education for its marketing purposes.

If this marketing program weren't such a widespread threat to our children's health, it would be downright laughable that an industry group would try to peddle its food product under such a thinly-veiled "education" plan. Don't people wonder what's going on when almost every single children's book advertised in the "Nutrition Bookshelf" portion of this Web site revolved around either milk, cheese or ice cream, with such titles as *Ice Cream: Great Moments in Ice Cream History*?[9] After all, during July 2003 there were no vegetable books anywhere to be found on this "Nutrition Bookshelf"! Aren't they healthy?

At least when the dairy industry describes all of these school-related activities in the official reports to Congress and in industry press releases, it rightly refers to them as "marketing" activities.

CONJUGATED LINOLEIC ACID

The dairy industry doesn't stop with kids. For adults, the industry puts a heavy emphasis on "science" and the communication of research results that might be construed as showing health benefits from eating dairy foods. The dairy industry spends $4 to $5 million a year to fund research towards the goal of finding something healthy to talk about.[7, 10] In addition, the dairy industry promoters employ a Medical Advisory Board made up of doctors, academics and other health professionals. These scientists are the ones who appear as medical professionals in the media, providing science-based statements supporting the health benefits of milk.

The Airport Club was a good example of industry efforts to maintain favorable product image and "confidence." In addition to keeping an eye on potentially damaging projects, the Club was trying to generate research that might show that cancer could be prevented by drinking cow's milk. What a coup that would be! At that time, the industry was getting quite edgy about the growing evidence showing that the consumption of animal-based foods is associated with cancer and related ailments.

Their hook for this research was an unusual group of fatty acids produced by bacteria in the cow's rumen (the biggest of the four stomachs). These fatty acids were collectively called conjugated linoleic acid (CLA), which is produced from the linoleic acid commonly found in corn that the cow eats. From the cow's rumen, CLA is then absorbed and gets stored in the meat and milk of the animal, eventually to be consumed by humans.

The big payday for The Airport Club was when initial tests on experimental mice suggested that CLA might help to block the formation of stomach tumors produced by a weak chemical carcinogen called benzo(a)pyrene.[11, 12] But there was a catch in this research. The catch was that researchers gave CLA to the mice first, and then gave the carcinogen benzo(a)pyrene. The ordering of these chemical feedings was backwards. In the body there is an enzyme system that works to minimize the amount of cancer caused by a carcinogen. When a chemical such as CLA is initially consumed, it "excites" that enzyme system so that it has increased activity. So the trick was to administer CLA first, to excite the enzyme system, and then administer the carcinogen. In this order, the enzyme system excited by CLA would be more effective at getting rid of the carcinogen. As a result, CLA could be called an anticarcinogen.

Let me give you an analogous situation. Let's say you have a bag of a potent pesticide in your garage. The pesticide bag says, "Do not swallow! In case of ingestion, contact your local poison control health authorities," or some such warning. But let's say you're hungry and you eat a handful of pesticide anyway. That pesticide in your body will "rev up" the enzyme systems in all of your cells that are responsible for eliminating nasty things. If you then go inside and eat a handful of peanuts dripping with aflatoxin, your body's enzyme systems will be primed to deal with the aflatoxin, and you'll end up with fewer aflatoxin-induced tumors. So, the pesticide, which will ultimately do all sorts of nasty things in your body, is an anticarcinogen! This scenario is obviously absurd, and the research on mice that initially showed CLA to be an anticarcinogen was similarly absurd. However, the end results of the mice research sounded pretty good to people who don't know this methodology (including most scientists).

Airport Club member Michael Pariza headed the research that studied CLA in some detail.[13-15] Later, at Roswell Park Memorial Institute for Cancer Research in Buffalo, a very good researcher and his group extended the research still further and demonstrated that it did more than merely block the first step in the formation of tumors. CLA also appeared to slow down subsequent tumor growth[16, 17] when fed after the carcinogen. This was a more convincing finding of the anticancer properties of CLA than the initial studies,[11, 12] which showed only an inhibition of tumor initiation.

Regardless of how promising these mouse and cow studies were becoming, this research remained two major steps removed from human cancer. First, it had not been shown that cow's milk containing CLA, as a whole food (as opposed to the isolated chemical CLA), prevents cancer in mice. Second, even if such an effect existed in mice, it would need to be confirmed in humans. In fact, as has been discussed earlier in this book, if cow's milk has any effect at all, it has been shown to increase, not decrease, cancer. The far more significant nutrient in milk is protein, whose potent cancer-promoting properties are consistent with the human data.

In other words, to make any health claims regarding CLA in milk and its effect on human cancer would require unreasonably large leaps of faith. But never doubt the tenacity (i.e., money) of those who would like to have the public believe that cow's milk prevents cancer. Lo and behold, a recent front-page headline in our local newspaper, the *Ithaca Journal*, stated "Changing Cows' Diets Elevates Milk's Cancer-Fighting."[18] This article concerned the studies of a Cornell professor who was instrumental in the development of bovine growth hormone now fed to cows. He showed that he could increase CLA in cow's milk by feeding the animals more corn oil.

The *Ithaca Journal* article, although only in a local, hometown newspaper, really was a dream come true for the sponsors of The Airport Club. The headline delivers a powerful but very simple message to the public: drinking milk reduces cancer risk. I know that media people like punchy statements so, initially, I suspected that the reporter had made claims beyond what the researchers had said. But in the article the enthusiasm expressed by Professor Bauman for the implications for this research equaled that of the headline. The study cited in this article only showed that CLA is higher in the milk of cows fed corn oil. That's a long way from having any relevance to human cancer. No studies had yet shown that humans or even mice drinking cow's milk had a lower risk of cancer—of any kind. Yet Bauman, who is a technically competent researcher, was quoted as saying that these findings have "good potential because CLA happens to be [a] very potent [anticarcinogen]." The journalist went on to say "CLA has been shown to suppress carcinogens and inhibit the spread of colon, prostate, ovarian and breast cancers and leukemia," and concluded that "all indications are that CLA is effective in humans even in low concentrations." According to the article, Bauman says that this "research represents the new focus on designing foods to enhance their nutritional and health qualities." These claims could not be more dramatic, considering the absence of the necessary human research.

Bauman, Pariza and their many other colleagues[19] have vigorously pursued this line of research for fifteen years and have published a large number of research papers. Although additional beneficial effects of CLA are said to exist, the key research still has not been done, namely, testing whether the consumption of milk from cows fed high-corn oil diets really will reduce human cancer risk.

More recently, Bauman and his colleagues have attempted to take a step toward finding this essential connection. They have shown that the milk fat of cows fed high amounts of corn oil (i.e., linoleic acid, the parent of CLA), like synthetic CLA, was able to decrease tumors in rats treated with a carcinogen.[20] But again, they used the tricky experimental method. They administered the milk fat *before*, not *after* the carcinogen. Yet their claims will be as dramatic as ever, because this is the first time that CLA, as present in food (i.e., the fat), is shown to be as anticarcinogenic as the isolated chemical. Translated: eat butter from cows fed corn oil—it prevents cancer!

THE SCIENCE OF INDUSTRY

The CLA story is a good example of how industry uses science to increase demand for its product in order to make more money. At the very least, industry science often leads to public confusion (Are eggs good? Are they bad?), and at its worst, industry science leads unsuspecting consumers to foods that are actually bad for them, all in the name of better health.

Conflicts of interest abound in this science of industry. The CLA research was created with special interest money and has grown and been sustained with special interest money. The National Dairy Council,[20-22] Kraft Foods, Inc.,[20] the Northeast Dairy Foods Research Center,[20, 21] the Cattlemen's Beef Board[23] and the Cattlemen's Beef Association[23] are groups that have frequently funded these studies.

Corporate influence in the academic research world can take many forms, ranging from flagrant abuses of personal power to conflicts of interest, all hidden from public view. This influence does not need to be a crass payoff to researchers to fabricate data. That sort of behavior is rare. The more significant way for corporate interests to influence academic research is much more sophisticated and effective. As illustrated by the CLA example, scientists investigate a detail out of context that can be construed as a favorable message and industry exploits it for all it's worth. Almost no one knows where the CLA hypothesis started and who originally funded it.

Few people really question such research if it is published in the best journals. Very few people, especially among the public, know which studies are "benefiting" from direct corporate funding. Very few people are able to sort out the technical details and recognize the missing information that would otherwise establish context. Almost everyone, however, understands that headline in my local newspaper.

I could play this game, too. If I wanted to hurt the dairy industry and be a little wild in my interpretation of study results, I could produce another headline to say, "New birth control chemical discovered in cow's milk." Recent research, for example, showed that CLA dramatically kills chick embryos.[13] Also, CLA increases the tissue level of saturated fats that could (using our dramatic method of interpretation) exacerbate heart disease risk. Of course, I have taken these two unrelated effects grossly out of context in my example. I don't really know whether these CLA effects actually translate into less fertility and more heart disease for humans, but if I were playing the game the way industry enthusiasts do, I wouldn't mind. It would make a great headline, and that can go a long way.

I recently met with one of the members of The Airport Club, a scientist who has been involved in the CLA effort, and he confessed that the CLA effect will never be anything more than a drug effect. However, you can bet that what is known in private will not be told in public.

INDUSTRY'S LOVE OF TINKERING

Much of The Airport Club and the CLA story is a story about the "dark side" of science, which I detailed in chapter thirteen. But the CLA story is also about the dangers of reductionism, of taking details out of context and making claims about diet and health, which I discussed in the previous chapter. Like academia, industry is also an essential player in the system of scientific reductionism that undermines the knowledge we have about dietary patterns and disease. Industry, you see, loves to tinker. Securing patents based on details leads to marketing claims and, ultimately, to greater revenues.

In a recent paper[20] by several CLA researchers (including Professor Dale Bauman, a long-time friend of the animal foods industry), the following sentence appeared, revealing much about how some industry enthusiasts feel as we "tinker" our way to health:

> The concept of CLA-enriched foods could be particularly appealing to people who desire a diet-based approach to cancer prevention without making radical changes in their eating habits.[20]

I know that, for Bauman and others, "making radical changes in...eating habits" means consuming a diet rich in plant-based foods. Rather than avoiding bad foods altogether, these researchers are suggesting that we tinker with the existing, but problematic, foods to correct the problem. Instead of working with nature to maintain health, they want us to rely on technology—their technology.

This faith in technological tinkering, in man over nature, is ever-present. It is not limited to the dairy industry, or the meat industry, or the processed foods industry. It has become part of every single food and health industry in the country, from oranges to tomatoes, from cereals to vitamin supplements.

The plant food industry got carried away recently when another carotenoid was "discovered." You've probably heard of it. It is called lycopene, and it provides the red color in tomatoes. In 1995, it was reported that people who ate more tomatoes, including whole tomatoes and tomato-containing foods like pasta sauces, had a lower risk for prostate cancer,[24] supporting an earlier report.[25]

For those companies that make foods with tomato products, this was a gift from above. Marketing people in the corporate world quickly got the message. But what they zeroed in on was lycopene, not tomatoes.

The media, willing to oblige, rose to the occasion. It was lycopene time! Suddenly lycopene became widely known as something to eat more of if you don't want prostate cancer. The scientific world, investigating details, escalated its efforts to decipher the "lycopene magic." As of this writing, there now are 1,361(!) scientific publications on lycopene cited by the National Library of Medicine.[26] A major market is developing, with trade names like Lycopene 10 Cold Water Dispersion and LycoVit 10% to be used as food supplements.[27] Judging by the health claims, we might be on the way to bringing prostate cancer, a leading cancer among men, under control.

There are, though, a couple of disquieting thoughts. First, after spending millions of research and development dollars, there is some doubt whether lycopene, as an isolated chemical, can prevent prostate cancer. According to a more recent publication, six studies now have shown a statistically significant decrease in prostate cancer risk with increased lycopene intake; three non-statistically significant studies agree; and seven studies do not show any association.[28] But these studies measured lycopene intake from *whole foods*, namely tomatoes. So, while these studies certainly indicate that the tomato is still a healthy food,[28] does that mean we can assume that lycopene, by itself, reduces prostate cancer risk? There are hundreds, even thousands, of chemicals in tomatoes. Do we have evidence that isolated lycopene will do what tomatoes do, especially for those who don't like tomatoes? The answer is no.[29]

There is no evidence for a lycopene-specific effect on prostate cancer, and I seriously doubt whether we will ever have convincing evidence. Nonetheless the lycopene business is up and running. In-depth studies are underway to determine the most effective dose of lycopene as well as to determine whether commercial lycopene preparations are safe (when tested in rats and rabbits, that is).[27] Also, consideration is being given to the possibility of genetically modifying plants for higher levels of lycopene and other carotenoids.[30] It is a real stretch to call this series of lycopene reports legitimate science. In my book, this is what I call technological tinkering and marketing, not science.

Five years before the latest "discovery" of lycopene, a graduate student of mine, Youping He, compared four different carotenoids (beta-carotene, lycopene from tomatoes, canthaxanthin from carrots and cryptoxanthin from oranges) regarding their ability to prevent cancer in experimental animals.[31, 32] Depending on what we were testing and how we did the test, single carotenoids could have widely ranging potencies. While one carotenoid is potent in one reaction, the same carotenoid is far less potent for another reaction. This variation manifests itself in countless ways involving hundreds of antioxidants and thousands of different reactions, forming a nearly indecipherable network. Consuming one carotenoid at a time in the form of a pill will never be the same as eating the whole food, which provides the natural network of health-supporting nutrients.

Five years after our rather obscure work on these antioxidants,[32] a Harvard study[33] effectively kicked off the lycopene campaign. In my opinion, lycopene, as a cancer fighter, is headed for an already over-crowded magic bullet graveyard, leaving behind a trail of deep confusion.

FRUIT CLAIMS

The fruit industry plays this game just like everyone else. For example, when you think of vitamin C, what food product comes to mind? If you don't think of oranges and orange juice, you are unusual. Most of us have heard ad nauseum that oranges are a good source of vitamin C.

This belief, however, is just another result of good marketing. How much do you know, for example, about vitamin C's relationship to diet and disease? Let's start with the basics. Although you probably know that oranges are a good source of vitamin C, you may be surprised to know that many other plant foods have considerably more. One cup of peppers, strawberries, broccoli or peas all have more. One papaya has as much as four times more vitamin C than one orange.[34]

Beyond the fact that many other foods are better sources of vitamin C, what can we say about the vitamin C that is in oranges? This concerns the ability of the vitamin to act as an antioxidant. How much of the total antioxidant activity in an orange is actually contributed by its vitamin C? Probably not more than 1–2%.[35] Furthermore, measuring antioxidant activity by using "test tube" studies does not represent the same vitamin C activity that takes place in our bodies.

Most of our impressions about vitamin C and oranges are a mixture of conjectures and assumptions about out-of-context evidence. Who first established these assumptions? Orange merchants. Did they justify their assumptions on the basis of careful research? Of course not. Did these assumptions (presented as fact) sound good to the marketing people? Of course they did. Would I eat an orange to get my vitamin

C? No. Would I eat an orange because it is a healthy plant food with a complex network of chemicals that almost certainly offer health benefits? Absolutely.

I played a small role in this story a couple of decades ago. In the 1970s and 1980s, I appeared in a television ad for citrus fruits. A New York public relations firm for the Florida Citrus Commission had earlier interviewed me about fruit, nutrition and health. This interview, unknown to me at the time, was the source of my presence on the ad. I had not seen the ad and I did not get paid for it, but, nonetheless, I was one of the talking heads that helped the Florida Citrus Commission build its case for the vitamin C content of oranges. Why did I do the interview? At that point in my career, I probably thought that the vitamin C in oranges was important, and, regardless of vitamin C, oranges were very healthy foods to eat.

It is very easy for scientists to get caught in the reductionism web of thinking, even if they have other intentions. It has not been until recently, after a lifetime of research, that I have come to realize how damaging it is to take details out of context and to make subsequent claims about diet and health. Industry uses these details extremely well, and the result is public confusion. Every year, it seems, some new product is being touted as the key to good health. The situation is so bad that "health" sections of grocery stores are often stocked more with supplements and special preparations of seemingly magic ingredients than they are with real food. Don't be tricked: the healthiest section of any store is the place where they sell whole fruits and vegetables—the produce section.

Perhaps worst of all, industry corrupts scientific evidence even when its product has been linked to serious health problems. Our kids are often the most coveted targets of their marketing. The American government has passed legislation preventing cigarette and alcohol companies from marketing their products to children. Why have we ignored food? Even though it is accepted that food plays a major role in many chronic diseases, we allow food industries not only to market directly to children, but also to use our publicly-funded school systems to do it. The long-term burden of our short-sighted indiscretion is incalculable.

16

Government:
Is It for the People?

DURING THE PAST TWO TO THREE DECADES, we have acquired substantial evidence that most chronic diseases in America can be partially attributed to bad nutrition. Expert government panels have said it, the surgeon general has said it and academic scientists have said it. More people die because of the way they eat than by tobacco use, accidents or any other lifestyle or environmental factor. We know that the incidence of obesity and diabetes is skyrocketing and that Americans' health is slipping away, and we know what to blame: diet. So shouldn't the government be leading us to better nutrition? There is nothing better the government could do that would prevent more pain and suffering in this country than telling Americans unequivocally to eat less animal products, less highly-refined plant products and more whole, plant-based foods. It is a message soundly based on the breadth and depth of scientific evidence, and the government could make this clear, as it did with cigarettes. Cigarettes kill, and so do these bad foods. *But instead of doing this, the government is saying that animal products, dairy and meat, refined sugar and fat in your diet are good for you!* The government is turning a blind eye to the evidence as well as to the millions of Americans who suffer from nutrition-related illnesses. The covenant of trust between the U.S. government and the American citizen has been broken. The United

305

States government is not only failing to put out our fires, it is actively fanning the flames.

DIETARY RANGES: THE LATEST ASSAULT

The Food and Nutrition Board (FNB), as part of the Institute of Medicine (IOM) of the National Academy of Sciences, has the responsibility every five years or so to review and update the recommended consumption of individual nutrients. The FNB has been making nutrient recommendations since 1943 when it established a plan for the U.S. Armed Forces wherein it recommended daily allowances (RDAs) for each individual nutrient.

In the most recent FNB report,[1] published in 2002, nutrient recommendations are presented as ranges instead of single numbers, as was the practice until 2002. For good health, we are now advised to consume from 45% to 65% of our calories as carbohydrates. There are ranges for fat and protein as well.

A few quotes from the news release announcing this massive 900+ page report say it all. Here is the first sentence in the news release[2]:

> To meet the body's daily energy and nutritional needs while minimizing risk for chronic disease, adults should get 45% to 65% of their calories from carbohydrates, 20% to 35% from fat and 10% to 35% from protein....

Further, we find:

> ...added sugars should comprise no more than 25% of total calories consumed....added sugars are those incorporated into foods and beverages during production [and] major sources include candy, soft drinks, fruit drinks, pastries and other sweets.[2]

Let's take a closer look. What are these recommendations really saying? Remember, the news release starts off by stating the report's objective of "minimizing risk for chronic disease."[2] This report says that we can consume a diet containing up to 35% of calories as fat; this is up from the 30% limit of previous reports. It also recommends that we can consume up to 35% of calories as protein; this number is far higher than the suggestion of any other responsible authority.

The last recommendation puts the frosting on the cake, so to speak. We can consume up to 25% of calories as added sugars. Remember, sugars are the most refined type of carbohydrates. In effect, although the report advises that we need a minimum of 45% of calories as car-bohydrates, more than half of this amount (i.e., 25%) can be the sugars present in candies, soft drinks and pastries. The critical assumption of this report is this: the American diet is not only the best there is, but you should now feel free to eat an even richer diet and still be confident that you are "minimizing risk for chronic disease." Forget any words of caution you may find in this report—with such a range of possibilities, virtually any diet can be advocated as minimizing disease risk.

You may have trouble getting your mind around what these figures mean in everyday terms, so I have prepared the following menu plan that supplies nutrients in accordance with these guidelines (Chart 16.1).[3, 4]

CHART 16.1: SAMPLE MENU THAT FITS INTO THE ACCEPTABLE NUTRIENT RANGES

Meal	Foods
Breakfast	1 cup Froot Loops 1 cup skim milk 1 package M&M milk chocolate candies Fiber and vitamin supplements
Lunch	Grilled cheddar cheeseburger
Dinner	3 slices pepperoni pizza, 1 16 oz. soda, 1 serving Archway sugar cookies

CHART 16.2: NUTRIENT PROFILE OF SAMPLE MENU PLAN AND REPORT RECOMMENDATIONS

Nutrient	Sample Menu Content	Recommended Ranges
Total Calories	~1800	Varies by height/weight
Protein (% of total calories)	~18%	10–35%
Fat (% of total calories)	~31%	20–35%
Carbohydrates (% of total calories)	~51%	45–65%
Sugars in Sweets, or Added Sugars (% of total calories)	~23%	Up to 25%

Folks, I'm not kidding. This disastrous menu plan fits the recommen-dations of the report and is supposedly consistent with "minimizing chronic disease."

What's amazing is that I could put together a variety of menus, all drenched in animal foods and added sugars, that conform to these recommended daily allowances. At this point in the book, I don't need to tell you that when we eat a diet like this day in and day out, we will be not just marching, but *sprinting* into the arms of chronic disease. In sad fact, this is what a large proportion of our population already does.

PROTEIN

Perhaps the most shocking figure is the upper limit on protein intake. Relative to total calorie intake, only 5–6% dietary protein is required to replace the protein regularly excreted by the body (as amino acids). About 9–10% protein, however, is the amount that has been recommended for the past fifty years to be assured that most people at least get their 5–6% "requirement." This 9–10% recommendation is equivalent to the well-known recommended daily allowance, or RDA.[5]

Almost all Americans exceed this 9–10% recommendation; we consume protein within the range of about 11–21%, with an average of about 15–16%.[6] The relatively few people consuming more than 21% protein mostly are those who "pump iron," recently joined by those on high-protein diets.

It is extremely puzzling that these new government-sponsored 2002 FNB recommendations now say that we should be able to consume protein up to the extraordinary level of 35% as a means of minimizing chronic diseases like cancer and heart disease. This is an unbelievable travesty, considering the scientific evidence. The evidence presented in this book shows that increasing dietary protein within the range of about 10–20% is associated with a broad array of health problems, especially when most of the protein is from animal sources.

As reviewed earlier in this book, diets with more animal-based protein will create higher blood cholesterol levels and higher risks of atherosclerosis, cancer, osteoporosis, Alzheimer's disease and kidney stones, to name just a few chronic diseases that the FNB committee mysteriously chooses to ignore.

Furthermore, the FNB panel had the audacity to say that this 10–35% recommendation range is the same as previous reports. Their press release clearly states, "protein intake recommendations are the same [as previous reports]." *I know of no report that has even remotely suggested a level as high as this.*

When I initially saw this protein recommendation, I honestly thought that it was a printing error. But, no, it was correct. I know several of the people on the panel who wrote this report and decided to give them a ring. The first panel member, a long-time acquaintance, said this was the first time he had even heard about the 35% protein limit! He suggested that this protein recommendation might have been drafted in the last days of preparing the report. He also told me that there was little discussion of the evidence on protein, for or against a high consumption level, although he recollected there being some pro-Atkins sympathy on the committee. He had not worked in the protein area, so he did not know the literature. In any event, this important recommendation slipped through the panel without much notice and made the first sentence of the FNB news release!

The second panel member, a long-time friend and colleague, was a subcommittee chair during the latter part of the panel's existence. He is not a nutritional scientist and also was surprised to hear my concerns about the upper limit for protein. He did not recall much discussion on the topic either. When I reminded him of some of the evidence linking high-animal protein diets to chronic disease, he initially was a little defensive. But with a little more persistence on my part about the evidence, he finally said, "Colin, you know that I really don't know anything about nutrition." How, then, was he a member—let alone the chair—of this important subcommittee? *And it gets worse.* The chair of the standing committee on the evaluation of these recommendations left the panel shortly before its completion for a senior executive position in a very large food company—a company that will salivate over these new recommendations.

A SUGARCOATED REPORT

The recommendation on added sugar is as outrageous as the one for protein. At about the time this FNB report was being released, an expert panel put together by the WHO (World Health Organization) and the FAO (Food and Agriculture Organization) was completing a new report on diet, nutrition and the prevention of chronic diseases. Professor Phillip James, another friend of mine, was a member of this panel and a panel spokesperson on the added sugar recommendation. Early rumors of the report's findings indicated that the WHO/FAO was on the verge of recommending an upper safe limit of 10% for added sugar, far lower than the 25% established by the American FNB group.

Politics, however, had early entered the discussion, as it had done in earlier reports on added sugars.[7] According to a news release from the director-general's office at the WHO,[8] the U.S.-based Sugar Association and the World Sugar Research Organization, who "represent the interests of the sugar growers and refiners, had mounted a strong lobbying campaign in an attempt to discredit the [WHO] report and suppress its release." They did not like setting the upper safe limit so low. According to the *Guardian* newspaper of London,[7] the U.S. sugar industry was threatening "to bring the World Health Organization to its knees" unless it abandoned these guidelines on added sugar. WHO people were describing the threat "as tantamount to blackmail and worse than any pressure exerted by the tobacco industry."[7] The U.S.-based group even publicly threatened to lobby the U.S. Congress to reduce the $406 million U.S. funding of the WHO if it persisted in keeping the upper limit so low at 10%! There were reports, after a letter was sent by the industry to Secretary of Health and Human Services Tommy Thompson, that the Bush administration was inclined to side with the sugar industry. I, and many other scientists, were being encouraged at that time to contact our congressional representatives to stop this outrageous strong-armed tactic by the U.S. sugar companies.

So, for added sugars, we now have two different upper "safe" limits: a 10% limit for the international community and a 25% limit for the U.S. Why such a huge difference? Did the sugar industry succeed in controlling the U.S.-based FNB report but fail with the WHO/FAO report? What does this say about the FNB scientists who also devised the new protein recommendation? These wildly different estimates are not a matter of scientific interpretation. This is nothing more than naked political muscle. Professor James and his colleagues at the WHO stood up to the pressure; the FNB group appears to have caved in. The U.S. panel received funding from the M&M Mars candy company and a consortium of soft drink companies. Is it possible that the U.S. group felt an obligation to these sugar companies? Incidentally, the sugar industry, in their fight against the WHO conclusion, has relied heavily[7] on the FNB report with its 25% limit. In other words, the FNB committee produces a friendly recommendation for the sugar industry which then turns around and uses this finding to support its claim against the WHO report.

THE INFLUENCE OF INDUSTRY

This discussion still leaves unanswered the question of how industry develops such extraordinary influence. Mostly, industry develops consultancies with a few publicly visible figures in academia, who then take leadership in policy positions outside of academia. However, these industry consultants continue to wear their academic hats. They organize symposia and workshops, write commissioned reviews, chair expert policy groups and/or become officers of key professional societies. They gravitate toward the leadership positions in science-based organizations that develop significant policy and publicity.

Once in these positions, these people then have the opportunity to assemble teams to their liking, by choosing committee members, symposia speakers, management staff, etc. The kinds of people most helpful to the team are either colleagues with similar prejudices and/or colleagues who are oblivious to who is "calling the shots." It's called "stacking the deck," and it really works.

In the case of the FNB, its panel was organized while under the chairmanship of an academic who had strong personal ties with the dairy industry. He helped in selecting the "right" people and helped in setting the agenda for the report, the most significant roles that anyone could have played. Is it surprising that the dairy industry, which must be ecstatic with the panel's findings, also helped to finance the report?

You might be surprised to learn that academic scientists can receive personal compensation from industry while simultaneously undertaking government-sponsored activities of considerable public importance. Ironically, they can even help set the agenda for the same government authorities who have long been restricted from such corporate associations. It is a huge "conflict-of-interest" loophole allowing industries to exercise their influence through the side door of academia. In effect, the entire system is essentially under the control of industry. The government and academic communities, playing their respective roles, mostly do as they are expected to do.

In addition to M&M Mars company, the corporate sponsors of the FNB report also included major food and drug companies that would benefit from higher protein and sugar allowances.[2] The Dannon Institute, a leading dairy-based consortium promoting its own brand of nutrition information, and the International Life Sciences Institute (ILSI), which is a front group for about fifty food, supplement and drug companies, both contributed funding for the FNB report. Corporate members include Coca-Cola, Taco Bell, Burger King, Nestlé, Pfizer and Roche Vitamins.[9] Some drug companies sponsored the report directly, in addition to their support through the International Life Sciences Institute. I don't recall private corporations providing financial support for the NAS expert panels that I served on.

It seems as if there is no end to this story. The chair of the FNB has been an important consultant to several major dairy-related companies (e.g., National Dairy Council, Mead Johnson Nutritionals, which is a major seller of dairy-based products, Nestlé Company and a Dannon yogurt affiliate).[10] Simultaneously, he was chair of the Dietary Guidelines Committee that establishes the Food Guide Pyramid and sets national nutrition policy affecting the National School Lunch and Breakfast programs, the Food Stamp Program and the Women, Infants and Children Supplemental Feeding Program (WIC).[1, 10] As chair of this latter committee, his personal financial associations with the food industry were not publicly revealed as required by federal law.[11] Eventually a court order, initiated by the Physician's Committee for Responsible Medicine,[12] was required to force him and his fellow colleagues to reveal their relationships with the food industry. Although the chair's industry associations were more substantial, *six of the eleven committee members also were shown to have ties to the dairy industry.*[10, 11]

The entire system of developing public nutrition information, as I originally saw with the Public Nutrition Information Committee that I once chaired (see chapter eleven), has been invaded and co-opted by industry sources that have the interest and resources to do so. They run the show. They buy a few academic hacks who have gained positions of power and who exercise considerable influence, both within academia and government.

It seems curious that while government scientists are not allowed to receive personal compensation from the private sector, their colleagues in academia can receive all that they can get. In turn, these conflicted individuals then run the show in collaboration with their government counterparts. However, restricting academics from receiving corporate consultancies is not the answer. That would only drive it underground. Rather, the situation would be best handled by making one's industry connections a matter of public disclosure. Everyone needs to know the full extent of each academic's associations with the private sector. Disclosure and full transparency is in everyone's interest. These associations should not be something we have to go to court to discover.

SETTING US BACK FOR YEARS

Lest you think that this Food and Nutrition Board report is merely a five-second news bite that then gets filed into a dusty old cabinet somewhere in Washington, let me assure you that tens of millions of people are directly affected by this panel's findings. According to the summary of the report itself,[13] the recommended levels of nutrient consumption that are set by this panel are

the basis for nutrition labeling of foods, for the Food Guide Pyramid and for other nutrition education programs ... [They are] used to determine the types and amounts of food:

- provided in the WIC (Women, Infants and Children) Supplemental Feeding Program and the Child Nutrition Programs such as School Lunch,
- served in hospitals and nursing homes for Medicare reimbursement,
- found in the food supply that should be fortified with specific nutrients,
- used in a host of other important federal and state programs and activities [such as establishing reference values used in food labeling][13]

The School Lunch Program feeds 28 million children every day. With officially recommended consumption patterns like these, we are at liberty to put any agricultural commodity we want into the hungry mouths of children already suffering from unprecedented levels of obesity and diabetes. By the way, the 2002 FNB report does make one special exception for children: it says that they can consume up to 40% of calories as fat, up from 35% for the rest of us, while minimizing the risk of chronic disease. The Women, Infants and Children Program affects the diets of another 7 million Americans, and the Medicare hospital programs feed millions of people every year. It is safe to say that the food provided by these government programs directly feeds at least 35 million Americans a month.

For people who are not directly fed by the government, this nutrient information still has significant consequences. From September 2002 onwards, nutrition education programs around the country have incorporated these new guidelines. This includes education in primary schools, universities, health professional programs and other community-based programs. Food labels also will be affected by these changes, as will the nutrition information that seeps into our lives via advertising.

Almost all of the wide-ranging effects of this 2002 FNB report will be profoundly harmful. In school, our children can be fed more fat, more meat, more milk, more animal protein and more sugar. They will also learn that this food is consistent with good health. The ramifications of this are serious, as a whole generation will walk the path of obesity, diabetes and other chronic illnesses, all the while believing that they are doing the right thing. Meanwhile, our government and its academic hacks can feel free to unload more meat, more fat, more animal protein and more sugar onto the neediest among us (e.g., the Women, Infants and Children (WIC) participants). I consider this to be an irresponsible and callous disregard for American citizens. Of course, these women and infants are not in a position to pay for research, donate to politicians, give academics special favors or fund government panels! For others concerned about nutrition, every time they see a dietitian, every time they see their doctor, every time they see a nutritionist and every time they go to a community health center, they may be told that a diet high in fat, animal protein, meat and dairy is consistent with good health, and they needn't worry about eating too many sweets. Posters that deck the bulletin boards of public institutions will now feature these new government guidelines as well.

In short, this 2002 FNB report, which represents the most sweeping, regressive nutrition policy statement I have ever seen, will either indirectly or directly promote sickness among Americans for many years to come. Having been a member of several diet and health policy-making expert panels over a twenty-year period I harbored the view that these panels were dedicated to the promotion of consumer health. I no longer believe this to be true.

UNFUNDED NUTRITION

Not only is the government failing to promote health through its recommendations and reports, it is squandering an opportunity to promote public health through scientific research. The U.S. National Institutes of Health (NIH) is responsible for funding at least 80–90% of all biomedical and nutrition-related research that is published in the scientific literature. To address various health topics, the NIH is comprised of twenty-seven separate institutes and centers, including its two largest, the National Cancer Institute (NCI) and the National Heart, Lung and Blood Institute.[14] With a proposed 2005 budget of almost $29 billion,[15] the NIH is the center of the government's gigantic medical research efforts.

In terms of nutrition research, however, something is amiss. None of these twenty-seven institutes and centers at the NIH is devoted to nutrition, despite the pivotal nature of nutrition in health, and despite the public interest in the subject. One of the arguments against having a separate institute for nutrition is that the existing institutes already concern themselves with nutrition. But this does not happen. Chart 16.3 shows the funding priorities for various health topics at the NIH.[16]

Of the $28 billion NIH budget proposed for 2004, only about 3.6% is designated for projects that are related in some way to nutrition[17] and 24% for projects that are related to prevention. That may not sound too bad. But these figures are seriously misleading.

Most of the prevention and nutrition budgets have absolutely nothing to do with prevention and nutrition, as I have written in this book.

**CHART 16.3: NIH 2004 ESTIMATED FUNDING
FOR DIFFERENT HEALTH TOPICS[17]**

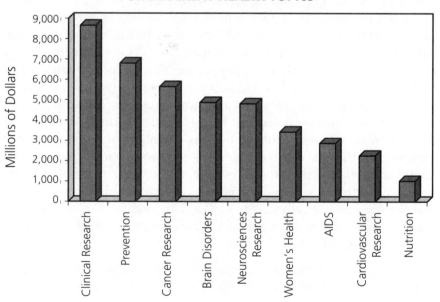

We won't be hearing about exciting research on dietary patterns, nor will there be serious efforts to tell the public how diet affects health. Instead, the prevention and nutrition budgets will be designated for developing drugs and nutrient supplements. A few years ago, the director of the NCI, the oldest of the NIH institutes, described prevention as "efforts to directly prevent and/or inhibit malignant transformation, to identify, characterize and manipulate factors that might be effective in achieving that inhibition and attempts to promote preventative measures."[18] This so-called prevention is all about manipulation of isolated chemicals. "Identifying, characterizing and manipulating factors" is a not-so-secret code for drug discovery.

Considered from another perspective, the NCI (of the NIH), in 1999, had a budget of $2.93 billion.[19] In a "major" 5-A-Day dietary program, it was spending $500,000 to $1 million to educate the public to consume five or more servings of fruits and vegetables per day.[18] This is only *three hundredths of one percent* (0.0256%) of its budget. That's $2.56 for every $10,000! If it calls this a major campaign, I pity its minor campaigns.

The NCI also has been funding a couple of multi-year large studies, including the Nurses' Health Study at Harvard (discussed in chapter twelve) and the Women's Health Initiative, mostly devoted to the testing of hormone replacement therapy, vitamin D and calcium supplementation, and the effect of a moderately low-fat diet on prevention of breast and colon cancer. These rare nutrition-related studies unfortunately suffer from the same experimental flaws described in chapter fourteen. Almost always, these studies are designed to tinker with one nutrient at a time, among an experimental population that uniformly consumes a high-risk, animal-based diet. These studies have a very high probability of creating some very expensive confusion that we hardly need.

If very few of our tax dollars are used to fund nutrition research, what do they fund? Almost all of the billions of dollars of taxpayer money expended by the NIH each year funds projects to develop drugs, supplements and mechanical devices. In essence, the vast bulk of biomedical research funded by you and me is basic research to discover products that the pharmaceutical industry can develop and market. In 2000, Dr. Marcia Angell, a former editor of the *New England Journal of Medicine*, summarized it well when she wrote[20]:

> ...the pharmaceutical industry enjoys extraordinary government protections and subsidies. Much of the early basic research that

may lead to drug development is funded by the National Institutes of Health (ref. cited). It is usually only later, when the research shows practical promise, that the drug companies become involved. The industry also enjoys great tax advantages. Not only are its research and development costs deductible, but so are its massive marketing expenses. The average tax rate of major U.S. industries from 1993 to 1996 was 27.3% of revenues. During the same period the pharmaceutical industry was reportedly taxed at a rate of only 16.2% (ref. cited). Most important, the drug companies enjoy seventeen-year government-granted monopolies on their new drugs—that is, patent protection. Once a drug is patented, no one else may sell it, and the drug company is free to charge whatever the traffic will bear.[20]

Our tax dollars are used to make the pharmaceutical industry more profitable. One could argue that this is justified by gains in public health, but the alarming fact is that this litany of research into drugs, genes, devices and technology research *will never cure our chronic diseases*. Our chronic diseases are largely the result of infinitely complex assaults on our bodies resulting from eating bad food. No single chemical intervention will ever equal the power of consuming the healthiest food. In addition, isolated chemicals in drug form can be very dangerous. The National Cancer Institute itself states, "What is clear is that most of our current treatments will produce some measure of adversity."[21] There is no danger to eating a healthy diet, and there are far more benefits, including massive cost savings both on the front end of preventing disease and on the back end of treating disease. So why is our government ignoring the abundant scientific research supporting a dietary approach in favor of largely ineffective, potentially dangerous drug and device interventions?

PERSONAL ACCOUNTS

In terms of public nutrition policy, I want to leave you with one short story that says so much about the government's priorities. One of my former graduate students at Cornell, Antonia Demas (now Dr. Antonia Demas), did her doctoral research in education by teaching a healthy food-and-nutrition-based curriculum[22] to elementary school kids and then integrating those healthy foods into the school lunch program. She had been doing this work as a volunteer mother in her children's schools for seventeen years prior to her graduate studies. I was her advisor for the nutrition part of her dissertation research.

The U.S. Department of Agriculture administers the school lunch program to 28 million children, largely relying on an inventory of government-subsidized foods. The government program, as it now stands, uses mostly animal-based products and even requires that participating schools make available cow's milk. At the local level, this usually means that consumption of milk is mandatory.

Dr. Demas's innovative research on the school lunch program was a great success; children loved the learning style and were excited to eat the healthy foods when they went through the lunch line. The children then convinced their parents to eat the healthy food at home. Dr. Demas's program won national awards for the "most creative implementation of the dietary guidelines" and "excellence in nutrition education." The program has proven to be of interest to more than 300 school lunch and behavioral rehabilitation programs around the U.S., including schools in areas as widely dispersed as Hawaii, Florida, Indiana, New England, California and New Mexico. In this effort, Dr. Demas has organized a nonprofit foundation (Food Studies Institute, Trumansburg, New York) and written a curriculum ("Food is Elementary"). And here's the kicker: Dr. Demas's program is entirely plant-based.

I had the opportunity to go to Washington and talk with Dr. Eileen Kennedy, who, at the time, was the director of the Center for Nutrition Policy and Promotion at the USDA. Dr. Kennedy was deeply involved both in the school lunch program and the dietary guidelines committee, on which it was revealed that she had ties to the dairy industry. She is now the Deputy Undersecretary for the USDA's Research, Education and Economics division. The topic of our discussion was Dr. Demas's innovative school lunch program and how it was garnering national attention. At the end of this discussion, I said to her, "You know, that program is entirely plant-based." She looked at me, wagged her finger as if I were being a bad boy, and said, "We can't have that."

I have come to the conclusion that when it comes to health, government is not for the people; it is for the food industry and the pharmaceutical industry at the expense of the people. It is a systemic problem where industry, academia and government combine to determine the health of this country. Industry provides funding for public health reports, and academic leaders with industry ties play key roles in developing them. A revolving door exists between government jobs and industry jobs, and government research funding goes to the development of drugs and devices instead of healthy nutrition. It is a system built by people who play their isolated parts, oftentimes unaware of the top decision makers and their ulterior motivations. The system is a waste of taxpayer money and is profoundly damaging to our health.

17

Big Medicine: Whose Health Are They Protecting?

WHEN IS THE LAST TIME that you went to the doctor and he or she told you what to eat or what not to eat? You've probably never had that experience. But the vast majority of Americans will fall prey to one of the chronic diseases of affluence discussed in Part II, and, as you have seen, there is a wealth of published research that suggests these diseases are a result of poor nutrition, not poor genes or bad luck. So why doesn't the medical system take nutrition seriously?

Four words: money, ego, power and control. While it is unfair to generalize about individual doctors, it is safe to say that the system they work in, the system that currently takes responsibility for promoting the health of Americans, is failing us. No one knows this better than the tiny minority of doctors who treat their patients from a nutritional perspective. Two of the most prominent doctors in this minority have spent many years emphasizing diet and health, both in public within their profession and in private with their patients. They have had exceptionally impressive results protecting their patients' health. These two doctors are Caldwell B. Esselstyn, Jr., whose work I discussed in chapter five, and John McDougall, an internist. My son Tom and I sat down with these men recently to discuss their experience advocating a whole foods, plant-based diet in the medical setting.

DR. SPROUTS

Long before our country was founded, Dutch pioneers had settled in the Hudson Valley north of New York City. One of these settler families were the Esselstyns. They started farming a plot of land in 1675. Nine generations later, that farm still belongs to the Esselstyn family. Dr. Esselstyn and his wife Ann own the several-hundred-acre Hudson Valley farm, just over two hours north of New York City. They spent the summer of 2003 living in the country, working the farm, growing a garden, hosting their kids and grandkids and enjoying a more relaxed life than what they're used to in Cleveland, Ohio.

Ess and Ann have a modest house: a large, rectangular, converted storage building. The simplicity of it belies the fact that this is one of the oldest family farms in America. Only upon closer inspection does it become apparent that there is something unusual about this place. Hanging on the wall is a framed certificate from New York State given to the Esselstyn family in recognition of their family farm, a farm that has now seen parts of five different centuries. Nearby an oar hangs on the wall. It is the oar Ess used in 1955 as an oarsman at Yale, when Yale beat Harvard by five seconds. Ess explains he has three other oars: two from beating Harvard in other years, and one for winning the gold medal in the Olympics with the Yale crew in 1956.

Downstairs, there is an exceptionally old photograph of Ess's great great grandfather on the farm. Around the corner there's an impressive-looking museum-style schematic of the Esselstyn family tree, and on the other end of the hall, there's a large black and white picture of Ess's father standing in front of a microphone, exchanging comments with John F. Kennedy during a White House address. Despite its humble appearance, it is very clear that this is a place with a distinguished history.

After touring the farm on a tractor, we sat down with Ess and asked him about his past. After graduating from Yale, he was trained as a surgeon at the Cleveland Clinic and at St. George's Hospital in London. He remembers fondly some of his most influential mentors: Dr. George Crile, Jr., Dr. Turnbull and Dr. Brook. Dr. Crile, a giant at the Cleveland Clinic, eventually became Ess's father-in-law upon Ess's marriage to Ann. Dr. Crile was a man of exceptional accomplishment, playing a courageous, leading role in questioning the macabre surgery called "radical mastectomy."[1] Dr. Turnbull and Dr. Brook were also renowned surgeons. In addition, Ess's own father was a distinguished physician with a national reputation. But, as Ess remembers, despite being "health experts," all four of these men were "ravaged by cardiovascular disease." His own father had a heart attack at age forty-two and Dr. Brook had a heart attack at age fifty-two.

These were the men he looked up to, and when it came to cardiovascular disease, all of them were helpless. Shaking his head, Ess said, "You can't escape this disease. These people, who were giants in the prime of their years, just *withered.*" As he took a moment to remember his father, he said, "It was the last year or two of my dad's life, and we were just strolling along one day. He was saying, 'We are going to have to show people how to lead healthier lives.' *He was right on it.* He was intensely interested in preventive medicine, but he didn't have any information." His father's interest has been a driving influence in Ess's life.

Following in these men's footsteps, Ess went on to amass an extraordinarily impressive list of awards and credentials: an Olympic gold medal in rowing; a Bronze Star for military service in Vietnam; President of the Staff, member of the Board of Governors, chairman of the Breast Cancer Task Force, and head of the Section of Thyroid and Parathyroid Surgery at the Cleveland Clinic, one of the top-ranked medical institutions in the world; president of the American Association of Endocrine Surgeons; over 100 professional scientific articles; and inclusion on a list in 1994–95 of the best doctors in America.[2] He remembers, "For about a ten- to fifteen-year period I was the top earner in the department of general surgery. As Dr. Crile's son-in-law, I was panicked about not pulling my weight. I didn't get home until late at night, but I had a position that was secure." When the then-president of the American Medical Association needed thyroid surgery, he wanted Ess to be the one to operate.

But despite the accolades, the titles and the awards, something was not right. *So often, Ess's patients did not regain their health, even after his best efforts.* As Ess described it, he had "this haunting feeling that was really beginning to bother me. I kept looking at how the patients were doing after these operations." Slightly exasperated, he said, "What is the survival rate for cancer of the colon? It's not so great!" He recounted the operation for colon cancer on one of his best friends. During surgery, they saw that the cancer had spread throughout the intestines. Ess lowered his voice ever so slightly in remembering this, saying, "You get there after the horse has left the barn." In thinking about all the breast surgery he had done, the lumpectomies and mastectomies, he expressed disgust at the idea of "disfiguring somebody when you know that you haven't changed their chances for recovery."

He began to do some soul searching. "What is my epitaph going to be? Five thousand mastectomies! You've disfigured more women than anybody else in Ohio!" Dropping the sarcasm, he said with sincerity, "I think everybody likes to leave the planet thinking that maybe...maybe you've helped a little."

Dr. Esselstyn began studying the literature on the diseases he commonly treated. He read some of the popular work of Dr. John McDougall, who had just written a best-selling diet and health book called *The McDougall Plan*.[3] He read the scientific literature that compared international disease rates and lifestyle choices, and a study by a University of Chicago pathologist showing that a low-fat, low-cholesterol diet fed to nonhuman primates could reverse atherosclerosis. He came to the realization that the diseases that so often plagued his patients were due to a diet rich in meat, fat and highly refined foods.

As mentioned in chapter five, he got the idea to treat heart patients with a low-fat, plant-based diet, and in 1985 went to the head of the Cleveland Clinic to discuss his study. She said that nobody had ever shown that heart disease in humans could be reversed by using dietary treatment. Still, Ess knew he was on the right track and went about quietly conducting his study over the next several years. The study he published, of eighteen patients with heart disease, demonstrated the most dramatic reversal of heart disease in the history of medicine, simply by using a low-fat, plant-based diet and a minimal amount of cholesterol-reducing medication.

Esselstyn has become a champion of dietary treatment of disease, and he has the data to prove his case. But it hasn't been easy. Rather than recognizing him as a hero, some in the medical establishment would rather he disappear. Somewhere in this transition from top-ranked, self-described "macho, hard-ass surgeon" to dietary advocate, he has become known, behind his back, as Dr. Sprouts.

A DAUNTING TASK

What's interesting about this story is that a man who had reached the pinnacle of a highly respected profession dared to try something different, succeeded, and then quickly found himself on the outside of the establishment looking in. He had threatened the status quo by his circumvention of standard treatments.

Some of Ess's colleagues have disparaged his treatment as being too "extreme." Some doctors have dismissed it by saying, "I think the research in this area is pretty soft," which is an absurd comment considering the breadth and depth of the international studies, the animal studies and the intervention studies. Some doctors have said to Ess, "Yeah okay, but nobody is going to eat like that. I can't even get my patients to stop smoking." Ess's response was, "Well, you really have no training in this. This requires just as much expertise as doing a bypass. It takes three hours for me to counsel a patient," not to mention the diligence required for the constant follow-up and monitoring of the patient's health. One patient told his cardiologist that he wanted to see Ess and commit to a dietary program to reverse his heart disease. The cardiologist responded, "Now you listen to me. There is no way to reverse this disease." You'd think that doctors would be more excited about healing their patients!

In talking about doctors and their unwillingness to embrace a whole foods, plant-based diet, Ess says, "You can't get frustrated. These aren't evil people. There are sixty cardiologists [at the Cleveland Clinic], any number of whom are closet believers in what I do, but they're a little afraid because of the power structure."

For Ess, however, it has been impossible to avoid his share of frustration. Early on, when he was first suggesting dietary treatment of heart disease, colleagues greeted the idea with caution. Ess figured that their attitude was born out of the fact that scientific research showing effective dietary intervention of heart disease in humans wasn't yet strong enough. But later, scientific results of unparalleled success, including Esselstyn's, were published. The data have been strong, consistent and deep, yet Ess still encountered reluctance to embrace this idea:

> You take a cardiologist and he's learned all about beta blockers, he's learned about calcium antagonists, he's learned about how to run this catheter up into your heart and blow up balloons or laser it or stent it without killing you and it's very sophisticated. And there's all these nurses and there's lights out and there's drama. I mean it's just, oh my god, the doctor blows up the balloon in his head. The ego of these people is enormous. And then someone comes along and says, "You know, I think we can cure this with brussels sprouts and broc-

coli." The doctor's response is, "WHAT? I learned all this crap, I'm making a freakin' fortune, and you want to take it all away?"

Then when that person comes along and actually cures patients with brussels sprouts and broccoli, as Esselstyn did, and gets better results than any other pill or procedure known, you've suddenly announced that something works, hands down, better than what 99% of the profession is doing. Summarizing his point, Ess says:

> Cardiologists are supposed to be expert in diseases of the heart— and yet they have no expertise in treating heart disease, and when that awareness strikes them, they get very defensive. They can treat the symptoms, they can take care of arrythmias, they can get you interventions, but they don't know how to treat the disease, which is a nutritional treatment.... Imagine a dietitian training a heart surgeon!

Esselstyn has found that merely saying that patients can have control over their own health is a challenge to many. These experts, after all, are built up to be the dispensers of health and healing. "Intellectually it's very challenging to think that the patient can do this with greater alacrity, dispatch, safety, and it's something that's going to endure." With all of the doctor's gadgets, technologies, training and knowledge, nothing is more effective than guiding the patient to make the right lifestyle choices.

But Ess is quick to point out that doctors are not malicious people engaged in a conspiracy:

> The only person that likes change is a newborn, and it's natural, it's human nature. Anywhere you go, 99% of the people are eating incorrectly. The numbers are against you, and it's very hard for those 99% to look at you in the 1% and say, "Yes, he's right, we are all wrong."

Another obstacle: lack of nutrition knowledge amongst physicians. Ess has had his share of interaction with ignorant doctors, and his impression is that "it's absolutely daunting, the lack of physician knowledge that there is about the fact that disease can be reversed. You wonder, what is the literature that these guys read?"

Physician knowledge often involves only the standard treatments: pills and procedures. "What does the twentieth century of medicine have to offer? We have pills and we have procedures. Right?" Esselstyn leans forward and, with a slight grin, as if he's about to tell us the emperor has no clothes, he says, "*But who ever says, 'Maybe we ought to stop disease'?*" In Dr. Esselstyn's experience, stopping disease does not figure prominently into the status quo.

LACK OF TRAINING

The medical status quo relies heavily on medication and surgery, at the exclusion of nutrition and lifestyle. Doctors have virtually *no training in nutrition and how it relates to health*. In 1985 the United States National Research Council funded an expert panel report that investigated the quantity and quality of nutrition education in U.S. medical schools.[4] The committee's findings were clear: "The committee concluded that nutrition education programs in U.S. medical schools are largely inadequate to meet the present and future demands of the medical profession."[4] But this finding was nothing new. The committee noted that in 1961 the "American Medical Association Council on Foods and Nutrition reported that nutrition in the U.S. medical schools received 'inadequate recognition, support and attention.'"[4, 5] In other words, over forty years ago, the doctors themselves said that their nutrition training was inadequate. Nothing had changed by 1985, and up to the present time, articles continue to be written documenting the lack of nutrition training in medical schools.[6, 7]

This situation is dangerous. Nutrition training of doctors is not merely inadequate; it is practically nonexistent. In 1985, the National Research Council report found that physicians receive, on average, only twenty-one classroom hours (about two credits) of nutrition training during their four years of medical school.[4] The majority of the schools surveyed actually taught less than twenty contact hours of nutrition, or one to two credit hours. By comparison, an undergraduate nutrition major at Cornell will receive twenty-five to forty credit hours of instruction, or about 250–500 contact hours; registered dietitians will have more than 500 contact hours.

It gets worse. The bulk of these nutrition hours are taught in the first year of medical school, as part of other basic science courses. Topics covered in a basic biochemistry course may include nutrient metabolism and/or biochemical reactions involving certain vitamins or minerals. *In other words, nutrition is often not taught in relation to public health problems, like obesity, cancer, diabetes, etc.* In conjunction with the 1985 government report, the president of the American Medical Students Association, William Kassler, writes[8]:

> Most nutrition in the formal curriculum is incorporated into other courses. Biochemistry, physiology and pharmacology are the courses most often alleged to contain some nutrition instruction. Too often in such courses, nutrition is touched on briefly, with the primary emphasis on the major discipline. *It is quite possible to finish such a course and not even realize that nutrition was covered* [my emphasis]. Nutrition taught by those whose interest and expertise lie elsewhere simply doesn't work.

It gets even worse! When nutrition education is provided in relation to public health problems, guess who is supplying the "educational" material? The Dannon Institute, Egg Nutrition Board, National Cattlemen's Beef Association, National Dairy Council, Nestlé Clinical Nutrition, Wyeth-Ayerst Laboratories, Bristol-Myers Squibb Company, Baxter Healthcare Corporation and others have all joined forces to produce a Nutrition in Medicine program and the Medical Nutrition Curriculum Initiative.[9, 10] Do you think that this all-star team of animal foods and drug industries representatives is going to objectively judge and promote optimal nutrition, which science has shown to be a whole foods, plant-based diet that minimizes the need for drugs? Or might they try to protect the meat-centered, Western diet where everyone expects to pop a pill for every sickness? This organization is creating nutrition curricula, involving CD-ROMS, and giving them away to medical schools for free. As of late 2003, 112 medical schools were using the curriculum.[11] According to their Web site, "Plans are underway for developing versions for undergraduate nutrition students, continuing medical education and other health professions audiences." (http://www.med.unc.edu/nutr/nim/FAQ.htm#anchor197343)

The dairy industry has also funded research investigations into nutrition education in medical schools[12] and has funded "prestigious" awards.[13, 14] These efforts show that industry is well prepared to promote its monetary interests whenever the opportunity presents itself.

You should not assume that your doctor has any more knowledge about food and its relation to health than your neighbors and coworkers. It's a situation in which nutritionally untrained doctors prescribe milk and sugar-based meal-replacement shakes for overweight diabetics, high-meat, high-fat diets for patients who ask how to lose weight and extra milk for patients who have osteoporosis. *The health damage that results from doctors' ignorance of nutrition is astounding.*

Apparently, there aren't enough "nutrition-oriented physician role models" in medical education. A recent survey found "a shortage of nutrition-oriented physician role models is probably the major constraint in teaching nutrition to residents."[12] I suspect that these medical programs lack nutrition-oriented physicians simply because they do not make it a priority to hire them. Nobody knows this better than Dr. John McDougall.

DR. MCDOUGALL'S CHALLENGE

Dr. John McDougall has been advocating a whole foods, plant-based approach to health longer than any practitioner I know. He has written ten books, including several that have sold over a half a million copies each. His nutrition and health knowledge is phenomenal, greater than any other doctor I've met and greater than any of my nutrition colleagues in academia. We met recently in his Northern California home, and one of the first things he showed me was his bank of four or five full- size metal file cabinets lined up along the back of his study. There can't be many people in the country with a collection of scientific literature on diet and disease that could rival John McDougall's, and, most importantly, John maintains a high level of familiarity with all of it. It is not unusual for him to spend a couple of hours a day on the Internet reviewing the latest journal articles. If anybody would be a perfect "nutrition-oriented physician role model" in an educational setting, it would be Dr. John McDougall.

Growing up, John ate a rich, Western diet. As he says, he had four feasts a day: Easter during breakfast, Thanksgiving at lunch, Christmas at dinner and a birthday party for dessert. It caught up to him, and at the age of eighteen, a few months into college, John had a stroke. After recovering with a new appreciation for life, he became a straight A student as an undergraduate and then completed medical school in Michigan and an internship in Hawaii. He chose to practice on the Big Island of Hawaii, where he cared for thousands of patients, some of whom had recently migrated from China or the Philippines, and some who were fourth generation Chinese or Filipino Americans.

It was there that John became an unhappy doctor. Many of his patients' health problems were a result of chronic illnesses, such as obesity, diabetes, cancer, heart disease and arthritis. John would treat them as he was taught, with the standard sets of pills and procedures, but very few of them became healthy. Their chronic diseases didn't go away, and John quickly realized that he had severe limitations as a doctor. He also started to learn something else from his patients: the first and second generation Americans from Asia, the ones who ate more traditional, Asian staple diets of rice and vegetables, were trim, fit and not afflicted with the chronic diseases that plagued John's other patients. The third and fourth generation Asian Americans, however, had fully adopted America's eating habits and suffered from obesity, diabetes and the whole host of other chronic diseases. It was from these people that John began to notice how important diet was for health.

Because John wasn't healing people, and the pills and procedures weren't working, he decided he needed more education and entered a graduate medical program (residency) at the Queens Medical Center in Honolulu. It was there that he began to understand the boundaries that the medical establishment had set and the way that medical education molds the way doctors are supposed to think.

John went into the program hoping to find out how to perfect the pills and procedures so that he could become a better doctor. But after observing experienced doctors treating their patients with pills and procedures, he realized that *these authoritative doctors didn't do any better than he did*. Their patients didn't just stay sick—they got worse. John realized something was wrong with the system, not him, so he began to read the scientific literature. Like Dr. Esselstyn, once he started reading the literature, John became convinced that a whole foods, plant-based diet had the potential not only to prevent these diseases that were plaguing patients, but also the potential to treat them. This idea, he was to find out, was not received kindly by his teachers and colleagues.

In this environment, diet was considered quackery. John would ask, "Doesn't diet have something to do with heart disease?" and his colleagues would tell him that the science was controversial. John continued to read the scientific research and to talk to his colleagues and only became even more baffled. "When I looked at the literature, I couldn't find the controversy. It was absolutely clear what the literature said." Through those years, John came to understand why so many physicians claimed diet was controversial: "The scientist is sitting down at the breakfast table and in the one hand he has a paper that says that cholesterol will rot your arteries and kill you, and in the other hand he has a fork shoveling bacon and eggs into his mouth, and he says, 'There's something confusing here. I'm confused.' And that's the controversy. That's all it is."

John tells a story about seeing a thirty-eight-year-old man and his wife after the man had suffered a second heart attack. As the attending resident (not their primary physician), he asked the patient what he was going to do to prevent a third, fatal heart attack. "You're thirty-eight years old with a beautiful young wife, five kids. What are you going to do to keep your wife from being a widow and your kids from becoming fatherless?" The man was despondent, frustrated and said, "There's nothing I can do. I don't drink. I don't smoke. I exercise, I follow the same diet the dietitian gave me after my last heart attack. There's nothing more I can do."

John told the couple what he had been learning about diet. He suggested that the man might reverse his disease if he ate the right way. The patient and his wife received the news with enthusiasm. John talked with them for quite a long time, left the room and felt great. He had finally helped someone; he had finally done his job.

That lasted for about two hours. He was called into the Chief of Medicine's office. The Chief of Medicine wields absolute authority over the residents. If he fires a resident, not only is that person out of his or her job, that person is out of his or her career. The excited couple had told their primary physician what they had just learned. The doctor replied that what they had been told wasn't true, and promptly reported John to the Chief of Medicine.

The Chief of Medicine had a serious conversation with John, who remembers being told that "I was stepping far beyond my duties as a resident. I should get serious about medicine and give up all this nonsense about food having anything to do with disease." The Chief of Medicine made it clear that on this point, John's job, and his subsequent career, was on the line. So John bit his tongue for the rest of his education.

On the day of John's graduation, he and the Chief of Medicine had a final talk. John remembers the man as being smart, with a good heart, but he was too entrenched in the status quo. The Chief of Medicine sat him down and said, "John, I think you're a good doctor. I want you to know that. I want you to know that I like your family. That's why I'm going to tell you this. I'm concerned that you're going to starve to death with all your crazy ideas about food. All you're going to do is collect a bunch of bums and hippies."

John paused to gather his thoughts, and then said, "That may be the case. Then I'll have to starve. I can't put people on drugs or surgeries that don't work. Besides, I think you're wrong. I don't think it will be bums and hippies. I think it will be successful people who have done well in life. They'll ask themselves, 'I'm such a big success, so how come I'm so fat?'" With that, John looked at the Chief's generous belly, and continued, "They'll ask, 'If I'm such a big success, why are my health and my future out of control?' They'll look at what I have to say, and they're going to buy it."

John finished his formal medical education having had only one hour of nutrition instruction, which involved learning which infant formulas to use. His experience confirms every study that has found nutrition training among physicians to be sorely inadequate.

HOOKED ON DRUGS

John touched on another important area where the medical profession has lost credibility: its ties with the drug industry. Medical education and drug companies are in bed together, and have been for quite some time. John talked some about the depth of the problem and how the educational system has been corrupted. He said:

> The problem with doctors starts with our education. The whole system is paid for by the drug industry, from education to research. The drug industry has bought the minds of the medical profession. It starts the day you enter medical school. All the way through medical school everything is supported by the drug industry.

John is not alone in criticizing the way in which the medical establishment has partnered with the drug industry. Many prominent scientists have published scathing observations showing how corrupt the system has become. Among the common observations are:

- The drug industry ingratiates itself with medical students with free gifts, including meals, entertainment and travel; educational events, including lectures, which are little more than drug advertisements; and conferences, which include speakers who are little more than drug spokespeople.[15–17]
- Graduate medical students (physician residents) and other physicians actually change their prescribing habits because of information provided by drug salespeople,[18–20] even though this information

is known to be "overly positive and prescribing habits are less appropriate as a result."[17, 21, 22]

- Research and academic medicine merely carry out the pharmaceutical industry's bidding. This can happen because: the drug companies, and not researchers, may design the research, which allows the company to "rig" the study[23, 24]; the researchers may have a direct financial stake in the drug company whose product they are studying[15, 25]; the drug company may be responsible for collecting and collating the raw data, and then only selectively allowing researchers to view the data[23, 26]; the drug company may retain veto power over whether the findings are published, and may retain editorial rights over any scientific publications resulting from the research[23, 25, 27]; the drug company may hire a communications firm to write the scientific article, and then find researchers willing to attach their names as authors of the paper after it has already been written.[26]

- The major scientific journals have turned into little more than marketing vehicles for drug companies. The leading medical journals derive their primary income from drug advertising. This advertising is not adequately reviewed by the journal, and companies often present misleading claims about drugs. Perhaps more disconcerting, the majority of clinical trial research reported in the journals is funded by drug company money, and the financial interests of the researchers involved are not fully acknowledged.[24]

In the past couple of years there have been well-publicized scandals at major medical centers that confirm these charges. In one instance, a scientist's integrity was maligned in a variety of ways by both a drug company and her university administration after she found that a drug under study had strong side effects and it lost its effectiveness.[27] In another case, a scientist speaking out about the possible side effects of antidepressants lost a job opportunity at the University of Toronto.[26] The examples go on and on.

Dr. Marcia Angell, an ex-editor of the *New England Journal of Medicine*, wrote a scathing editorial called "Is Academic Medicine for Sale?"[15]:

The ties between clinical researchers and industry include not only grant support, but also a host of other financial arrangements. Researchers serve as consultants to companies whose products they are studying, join advisory boards and speakers' bureaus, enter into patent and royalty arrangements, agree to be the listed authors of articles ghostwritten by interested companies, promote drugs and devices at company-sponsored symposiums and allow themselves to be plied with expensive gifts and trips to luxurious settings. Many also have equity interest in the companies.

Dr. Angell goes on to say that these financial associations often significantly "bias research, both the kind of work that is done and the way it is reported."

Even more dangerous than the threat of fraudulent findings is the fact that the only type of research that is funded and recognized is research on drugs. Research on the causes of disease and non-drug interventions simply doesn't occur in medical education settings. For example, academic researchers may be furiously trying to find a pill that will treat the symptoms of obesity, but not be devoting any time or money to teaching people how to live a healthier life. Dr. Angell writes[15]:

> In terms of education, medical students and house officers, under the constant tutelage of industry representatives, *learn to rely on drugs and devices more than they probably should* [my emphasis]. As the critics of medicine so often charge, *young physicians learn that for every problem, there is a pill* [my emphasis] (and a drug company representative to explain it). They also become accustomed to receiving gifts and favors from an industry that uses these courtesies to influence their continuing education. The academic medical centers, in allowing themselves to become research outposts for industry, contribute to the overemphasis on drugs and devices."

In this environment, is it possible for nutrition to be given fair and honest consideration? Despite the fact that our leading killers can be prevented and even reversed using good nutrition, will you ever hear about it from your doctor? Not as long as this environment persists in our medical schools and hospitals. Not unless your doctor has decided that standard medical practice as it is taught does not work, and decides to spend a significant amount of time educating himself or herself about good nutrition. This takes a rare individual.

The situation has gotten so bad that Dr. John McDougall said, "I don't know what to believe anymore. When I read a paper that says I should be giving my heart patients beta blockers and ACE inhibitors, two classes of heart drugs, I don't know whether it's true. *I honestly don't know if it's true because [drug research] is so tainted.*"

Do you think the following headlines are related?

"Schools report research interest conflicts" (between drug companies and researchers)[28]

"Prescription use by children multiplying, study says"[29]

"Survey: Many guidelines written by doctors with ties to companies"[30]

"Correctly Prescribed Drugs Take Heavy Toll; Millions Affected by Toxic Reactions"[31]

We pay a high price for allowing these medical biases. A recent study found that one in five new drugs will either get a "black box warning," indicating a previously unknown serious adverse reaction that may result in death or serious injury, or will be withdrawn from the market within twenty-five years.[32] Twenty percent of all new drugs have serious unknown side effects, and more than 100,000 Americans die every year from *correctly* taking their *properly prescribed* medication.[33] This is one of the leading causes of death in America!

DR. MCDOUGALL'S FATE

When Dr. John McDougall finished his formal medical education, he set up a practice on the Hawaiian island of Oahu. He began writing books about nutrition and health and established a national reputation. In the mid-1980s John was contacted by St. Helena Hospital in Napa Valley, California, and asked if he would accept a position running its health center. The hospital was a Seventh-day Adventist hospital; if you recall from chapter seven, the Seventh-day Adventists encourage followers to eat a vegetarian diet (even though they consume higher-than-average amounts of dairy products). It was an opportunity too good to pass up, and John left Hawaii and headed for California.

John had a good home at St. Helena for a number of years. He taught nutrition and used nutrition to treat sick patients, which he did with fantastic success. He treated over 2,000 very sick patients, and over the course of sixteen years, he has never been sued or even had a letter of complaint. Perhaps more importantly, John saw these patients get well. Throughout this time, he continued his publishing activity, maintaining a national reputation. But as time passed, he realized that things weren't quite the same as when he first arrived. His discontent was growing.

Of those later years he says, "I just didn't think I was going anyplace. The program had 150 or 170 people a year and that was it. Never grew. Wasn't getting any support from the hospital and we had gone through a lot of administrators."

He had small clashes with the other doctors at the hospital. At one point, the heart department objected to what John was doing with heart patients. John told them, "I'll tell you what, I'll send every one of my heart patients to you for a second opinion if you'll send yours to me." It was quite an offer, but they didn't accept it. On another occasion John had referred a patient to a cardiologist and the cardiologist incorrectly told the patient that he needed to have bypass surgery. After a couple of these incidents, John had reached the limit of his patience. Finally, after the cardiologist recommended surgery for another one of John's patients, John called him and said, "I want to talk with you and the patient about this. I would like to discuss the scientific literature that causes you to make this recommendation." The cardiologist said that he wouldn't do that, to which John responded, "Why not? You just recommended that this guy have his heart opened! And you're going to charge him 50,000 or 100,000 bucks for it. Why don't we discuss it? Don't you think that's fair to the patient?" The cardiologist declined, saying that it would just confuse the patient. That was the last time he recommended heart surgery for one of John's patients.

Meanwhile, none of the other physicians in the hospital had ever referred a patient to John. Not once. Other physicians would send their own wives and children to see him but they would never refer a patient. The reason, according to John:

> They were worried [about what would happen when] their patients would come to see me, and it happened all the time when patients would come on their own. They'd come to me with heart disease or high blood pressure or diabetes. I'd put them on the diet and they'd go back off all their pills and soon their numbers would be normal. They'd go to their doctor and say, "Why the hell didn't you tell me about this before? Why did you let me suffer, spend all this money, almost die, when all I had to do was eat oatmeal?" The doctors didn't want to hear this.

There were other moments of friction between John and the hospital, but the last straw involved the Dr. Roy Swank multiple sclerosis program mentioned in chapter nine.

John had contacted Dr. Swank when he learned that Swank was about to retire. John had known and respected Dr. Roy Swank for a long time, and he offered to take over the Swank multiple sclerosis program and merge it with his health clinic at St. Helena Hospital, preserving it in honor of Dr. Swank. Dr. Swank agreed, much to John's excitement. As John said, there were four reasons that this would be a perfect fit for St. Helena's:

- it fit in with the philosophy of the Adventists: dietary treatment of disease
- they would be helping people who desperately needed their help
- it would double their patient census, helping to grow the program
- it would cost almost nothing

In thinking back on it, John said, "Could you think of any reason not to do this? It [was] obvious!" So he took the proposal to the head of his department. After listening, she said that she didn't think the hospital wanted to do this. She said, "Well, I don't think we really want to introduce any new programs right now." John, dumbfounded, asked her, "Please tell me why. What does it mean to be a hospital? Why are we here? I thought we were here to take care of sick people."

Her response was a doozy: "Well, you know we are, but you know, MS patients are not really desirable patients. You told me yourself that most neurologists don't like to take care of MS patients." John could not believe what he had just heard. In a very tense moment, he said:

Wait a minute. I'm a doctor. This is a hospital. As far as I know our job is to relieve the suffering of the sick. These are sick people. Just because other doctors can't help them in their suffering doesn't mean that we can't. Here's the evidence that says we can. I have an effective treatment for people who need my care and this is a hospital. Will you explain to me why we don't want to take care of those kinds of patients?

He continued:

I want to talk to the head of the hospital. I want to explain to her why I need this program and why the hospital needs this program and why the patients need this program. I want you to get me an appointment.

Ultimately, though, the head of the hospital proved to be just as difficult. John reflected on the situation with his wife. He was supposed to renew his contract with the hospital in a couple of weeks, and he decided not to do it. He left on cordial terms, and to this day he does not hold personal grudges. He just explains it by saying that their directions in life were different. John would prefer to remember St. Helena for what it was: a good home to him for sixteen years, but a place nonetheless that was "just into that whole drug money thing."

Now, John runs a highly successful "lifestyle medicine" program with his family's help, writes a popular newsletter that he makes freely available (http://www.drmcdougall.com), organizes group trips with past patients and new friends and has more time to go windsurfing when the wind picks up on Bodega Bay. This is a man with a wealth of knowledge and qualifications, who could benefit the health of millions of Americans. He has never been challenged by any of his colleagues for physician "misbehavior," and yet the medical establishment does not want his services. He is reminded of this fact all the time:

> Patients will come in with rheumatoid arthritis. They'll be in wheelchairs, they can't even turn the key on their car. And I'll take care of them and three or four weeks later, they'll go back to see their doctor. They'll walk up to their doctor, grab their hand and shake it hard. Doctor will say, "Wonderful." The patient, all excited, will say, "Well, I want to tell you what I did. I went to see this Dr. McDougall, I changed my diet, and now my arthritis is gone." Their doctor simply responds, "Oh my goodness. That's great. Whatever you're doing, just keep doing it. I'll see you later." That's always the response. It's not, "Please, my god, tell me what you did so I can tell the next patient." It's, "Whatever you're doing, that's just great." If the patient starts to tell them they changed to a vegetarian diet, the doctor will cut in with, "Yeah okay, fine, you're really a strong person. Thanks a lot. See you later." Get them out of the office as quickly as they can. It's very threatening...very threatening.

ESSELSTYN'S REWARD

Back in Ohio, Dr. Esselstyn retired from active surgery in June of 2000 and assumed the position of preventive cardiology consultant in the department of general surgery at the Cleveland Clinic. He has continued to do research and to visit with patients. He holds three-hour counseling sessions in his home with new heart disease patients, gives them research evidence and provides a delicious "heart-safe" meal. In addition, he gives talks around the country and abroad.

In March of 2002, Ess and his wife Ann, whose grandfather founded the Cleveland Clinic, drafted a letter to the head of the cardiology department and the head of the hospital at the Cleveland Clinic. The letter started off by saying how proud they were of the reputation and excellence of the Clinic and the innovation of the surgical procedures, but that everyone recognized that surgery was never going to be the answer to this epidemic of heart disease. Ess formally proposed the idea that he could help set up an arrest and reversal dietary program in the department of preventive cardiology at the Cleveland Clinic. The program would mirror his own and could be administered by nurse clinicians and physician assistants. Ideally, a young physician with passion for the idea would head the program. Ultimately, every patient with heart disease at the Clinic would be offered the option of arrest and reversal therapy using dietary means, which costs very little, harbors no risks and puts the control back into the patients' hands.

You'd think that if an opportunity arose to profoundly heal sick people, and one of the most reputable people in the country was going to help you, a hospital would jump at the opportunity. But after being one of the star surgeons at the Cleveland Clinic for decades, after initiating a heart reversal study that had greater success than anything ever done at the Clinic, and after graciously offering a plan to help heal even more people, neither the head of the hospital nor the department head had the respect to even acknowledge that Ess had written to them. They didn't call. They didn't write. They completely ignored him.

Seven weeks passed, and finally Ess called the department head and the hospital head, and neither of them would take his call. Finally, after seven calls, the head of the hospital got on the phone. This man had praised Ess for years for his research and seemed excited by his results, but now he was singing a different tune. He obviously knew exactly what Ess was calling about, and told Ess that the head of the cardiology department didn't want to do it. In other words, he just passed the buck. If the head of the hospital wanted it to be done, it would be done, regardless of what the head of cardiology wanted. So Ess called the head of cardiology, who finally took his call. The man was abrasive and rude. He made it clear he had no interest in what Ess was trying to do.

Ess hasn't talked to either of these doctors since, but he still has hope that he can change their minds as more and more research supports what he has been saying. Meanwhile, many people at the Clinic are still excited about Ess's work. Many of them want to see a wider application of his program, but the powers that be will not let it happen. They get frustrated, and Ess is frustrated because the current program in preventive cardiology is a disaster:

> They still eat meat, they still eat dairy, and they don't have any cholesterol goal. It's all just so vague. Preventive cardiology takes great pride when they are able to slow the rate of progression of this disease. This isn't cancer for God's sake!

An interesting situation is now developing: just as with Dr. McDougall, many of the Clinic "bigwigs" with heart disease have themselves gone to Esselstyn for treatment and lifestyle counseling. They know it works, and they seek out the program on their own. As Ess says, this could be developing into a very interesting crisis:

> I have now treated a number of senior staff with coronary disease at the Clinic—senior staff physicians. I have also treated a number of senior staff trustees. One of the trustees knows about the frustrations that we've had trying to get this into the Clinic, and he says, "I think, if the word gets out that Esselstyn has this treatment that arrests and reverses this disease at the Cleveland Clinic, and it's been used by senior staff and he's treated senior trustees, but he's not permitted to treat the common herd, we could be open for a lawsuit."

For the time being, Ess, with his wife's help, will continue to run counseling sessions out of his own home because the institution to which he gave the greater part of his life does not want to endorse a dietary approach that competes with its standard menu of pills and procedures. This past summer Ess spent much more time than usual at his upstate New York farm, making hay. As much as Ess likes a more relaxed life, he would also love to continue to help diseased people get better with the aid of the Cleveland Clinic. *But they won't allow him to.* As far as I am concerned, this is nothing short of criminal. We, the public, turn to doctors and hospitals in times of great need. For them to provide care that is knowingly less than optimal, that doesn't protect our health, doesn't heal our disease and costs us tens of thousands of dollars is morally inexcusable. Ess sums up the situation:

The Clinic is now injecting stem cells to try to make new heart vessels grow. Wouldn't it be easier to stop the disease? It's appalling, isn't it? It's just so grippingly unbelievable to think that we're being led around by people who refuse to believe the obvious!

Both Esselstyn and McDougall have now been denied reentry into the establishment, after headline-making success at healing people with a nutritional approach. You can focus on the money—according to John and Ess, 80% of St. Helena's and 65% of the Cleveland Clinic's respective incomes were generated by traditional heart disease treatments, surgical interventions—but it's something more than just money. It may also be the intellectual threat that the patient should be in control, and not the doctor; that something as simple as food could be more powerful than all the knowledge of pills and high-tech procedures; it may be the lack of credible nutrition education in medical school; it may be the influence of the drug industry. Whatever it is, it has become clear that the medical industry in this country is not protecting our health as it should. As McDougall reaches his arms out, palms up, and scrunches his shoulders up, he simply says, "It's beyond comprehension."

18
Repeating Histories

IN 1985, when I was on sabbatical in Oxford, England, I had the opportunity to study the history of diet and disease at some of the great medical history libraries in the Western world. I made use of the famous Bodlean Library in Oxford and the London libraries of the Royal College of Surgeons and the Imperial Cancer Research Fund. In the quiet recesses of these marble-lined sanctuaries, I was thrilled to find authors who wrote eloquently on the topic of diet and cancer, among other diseases, over 150 years ago.

One such author was George Macilwain, who wrote fourteen books on medicine and health. Macilwain was born and raised in Northern Ireland. He later moved to London where he became a prominent surgeon in the early 1800s. He was to become a member, and later, an honorary fellow, of the Royal College of Surgeons. He became vegetarian at the age of forty, after identifying "grease, fat and alcohol" as being the chief causes of cancer.[1] Macilwain also popularized the theory of the "constitutional nature of disease," mostly in reference to the origins and treatment of cancer.

The constitutional nature of disease concept meant that disease is not the result of one organ, one cell or one reaction gone awry or the result of one external cause acting independently. It is the result of *multiple systems throughout the body breaking down*. Opposing this view was the local theory of disease, which said that disease is caused by a single external agent acting at a specific site in the body. At that time, a fierce fight was under way between those who believed in diet and those who

343

supported surgery and the emerging use of drugs. The "local disease" proponents argued that disease was locally caused and could be cut out or locally treated with isolated chemicals. In contrast, those who favored diet and lifestyle believed that disease was a symptom resulting from the "constitutional" characteristics of the whole body.

I was impressed that these old books contained the same ideas about diet and disease that had resurfaced in the health battles of the 1980s. As I learned more about Macilwain, I came to realize that he was a relative of mine. My paternal grandmother's maiden name was Macilwain, and that "branch" of the family had lived in the same part of Northern Ireland that George Macilwain had come from. Furthermore, there were family stories about a famous Macilwain who had left the family farm in Ireland to become a very well-known doctor in London in the early 1800s. My father, who had emigrated from Northern Ireland, had referred to an Uncle George when I was young, but I never was aware of who this man was. Through further genealogical research, I have come to the near certain conclusion that George Macilwain was my great-great uncle.

This discovery has been one of the more remarkable stories of my life. My wife Karen says, "If there's such a thing as reincarnation. . . ." I agree: if I ever lived a past life, it was as George Macilwain. He and I had similar careers; both of us became acutely aware of the importance of diet in disease, and both of us became vegetarian. Some of his ideas, written over 150 years ago, were so close to what I believed that I felt they could have come from my own mouth.

I discovered more than my family history while reading in these august, history-laden libraries. I found out that scholars have been arguing over the nature of health for centuries, even millennia. Almost 2,500 years ago, Plato wrote a dialogue between two characters, Socrates and Glaucon, in which they discuss the future of their cities. Socrates says the cities should be simple, and the citizens should subsist on barley and wheat, with "relishes" of salt, olives, cheese and "country fare of boiled onions and cabbage," with desserts of "figs, pease, beans," roasted myrtle-berries and beechnuts, and wine in moderation.[2] Socrates says, "And thus, passing their days in tranquility and sound health, they will, in all probability, live to an advanced age. . . ."

But Glaucon replies that such a diet would only be appropriate for "a community of swine," and that the citizens should live "in a civilized manner." He continues, "They ought to recline on couches . . . and have the usual dishes and dessert of a modern dinner." In other words, the citizens should have the "luxury" of eating meat. Socrates replies, "if you wish us also to contemplate a city that is suffering from inflammation.... We shall also need great quantities of all kinds of cattle for those who may wish to eat them, shall we not?"

Glaucon says, "Of course we shall." Socrates then says, "Then shall we not experience the need of medical men also to a much greater extent under this than under the former régime?" Glaucon can't deny it. "Yes, indeed," he says. Socrates goes on to say that this luxurious city will be short of land because of the extra acreage required to raise animals for food. This shortage will lead the citizens to take land from others, which could precipitate violence and war, thus a need for justice. Furthermore, Socrates writes, "when dissoluteness and diseases abound in a city, are not law courts and surgeries opened in abundance, and do not Law and Physic begin to hold their heads high, when numbers even of well-born persons devote themselves with eagerness to these professions?" In other words, in this luxurious city of sickness and disease, lawyers and doctors will become the norm.[2]

Plato, in this passage, made it perfectly clear: we shall eat animals only at our own peril. Though it is indeed remarkable that one of the greatest intellectuals in the history of the Western world condemned meat eating almost 2,500 years ago, I find it even more remarkable that few know about this history. Hardly anybody knows, for example, that the father of Western medicine, Hippocrates, advocated diet as the chief way to prevent and treat disease or that George Macilwain knew that diet was the way to prevent and treat disease or that the man instrumental in founding the American Cancer Society, Frederick L. Hoffman, knew that diet was the way to prevent and treat disease.

How did Plato predict the future so accurately? He knew that consuming animal foods would not lead to true health and prosperity. Instead, the false sense of rich luxury granted by being able to eat animals would only lead to a culture of sickness, disease, land disputes, lawyers and doctors. This is a pretty good description of some of the challenges faced by modern America!

How did Seneca, one of the great scholars 2,000 years ago, a tutor and advisor to Roman Emperor Nero, know with such certainty the trouble with consuming animals when he wrote[2]:

> An Ox is satisfied with the pasture of an acre or two: one wood suffices for several Elephants. Man alone supports himself by the

pillage of the whole earth and sea. What! Has Nature indeed given us so insatiable a stomach, while she has given us so insignificant bodies?...The slaves of the belly (as says Sallust) are to be counted in the number of the lower animals, not of men. Nay, not of them, but rather of the dead....You might inscribe on their doors, "These have anticipated death."

How did George Macilwain predict the future when he said that the local theory of disease would not lead to health? Even today, we don't have any pills or procedures that effectively prevent, eliminate or even treat the causes of any chronic diseases. The most promising preventions and treatments have now been shown to be diet and lifestyle changes, a constitutional approach to health.

How did we forget these lessons from the past? How did we go from knowing that the best athletes in the ancient Greek Olympics must consume a plant-based diet to fearing that vegetarians don't get enough protein? How did we get to a place where the healers of our society, our doctors, know little, if anything, about nutrition; where our medical institutions denigrate the subject; where using prescription drugs and going to hospitals is the third leading cause of death? How did we get to a place where advocating a plant-based diet can jeopardize a professional career, where scientists spend more time mastering nature than respecting it? How did we get to a place where the companies that profit from our sickness are the ones telling us how to be healthy; where the companies that profit from our food choices are the ones telling us what to eat; where the public's hard-earned money is being spent by the government to boost the drug industry's profits; and where there is more distrust than trust of our government's policies on foods, drugs and health? How did we get to a place where Americans are so confused about what is healthy that they no longer care?

Our country's population, which numbers almost 300 million people,[3] is sick.

- 82% of American adults have at least one risk factor for heart disease[4]
- 81% of Americans take at least one medication during any given week[5]
- 50% of Americans take at least one prescription drug during any given week[5]
- 65% of American adults are overweight[6]

- 31% of American adults are obese[6]
- Roughly one in three youths in America (ages six to nineteen) is already overweight or at risk of becoming overweight
- About 105 million American adults have dangerously high cholesterol levels[7] (defined as 200 mg/dL or higher—heart-safe cholesterol level is under 150 mg/dL)
- About 50 million Americans have high blood pressure[8]
- Over 63 million American adults have pain in the lower back (considerably related to circulation and excess body weight, both influenced by diet and aggravated by physical inactivity) during any given three-month period[9]
- Over 33 million American adults have a migraine or severe headache during any given three-month period[9]
- 23 million Americans had heart disease in 2001[9]
- At least 16 million Americans have diabetes
- Over 700,000 Americans died from heart disease in 2000
- Over 550,000 Americans died from cancer in 2000
- Over 280,000 Americans died from cerebro-vascular diseases (stroke), diabetes or Alzheimer's in 2000

At the great peril of ignoring the warnings of Plato and others, America has, in the words of Seneca, "anticipated death." Starvation, poor sanitation and communicable diseases, symbols of impoverishment, have been largely minimized in the Western world. Now we have an urgency of excess, and some of the previously less developed countries are racing to get where we are. Never before have such large percentages of the population died from diseases of "affluence." Is this the affluence that Socrates predicted 2,500 years ago—a society full of doctors and lawyers wrestling with the problems caused by people living luxuriously and eating cattle? Never before have so many people suffered such high levels of obesity and diabetes. Never before has the financial strain of health care distressed every sector of our society, from business to education to government to everyday families with inadequate insurance. If we have to decide between health insurance for our teachers and textbooks for our kids, which will we choose?

Never before have we affected the natural environment to such an extent that we are losing our topsoil, our massive North American aquifers, and our world's rainforests.[10] We are changing our climate so rapidly that many of the world's best-informed scientists fear the future. Never before have we been eliminating plant and animal species from the face of the earth as we are doing now. Never before have we introduced, on such a large scale, genetically altered varieties of plants into the environment without knowing what the repercussions will be. All of these changes in our environment are strongly affected by what we choose to eat.[11]

As the billions of people in the developing world are accumulating more wealth and adopting the Western diet and lifestyle, problems created by nutritional excess are becoming exponentially more urgent with each passing year. In 1997, the director-general of the World Health Organization, Dr. Hiroshi Nakajima, referred to the future chronic disease burden in developing countries as "a crisis of suffering on a global scale."[12]

We've fumbled around for the past 2,500 years, building up the unsustainable behemoth that we now call modern society. We certainly won't have another 2,500 years to remember the teachings of Plato, Pythagoras, Seneca and Macilwain; we won't even have 250 years. From this urgency arises great opportunity, and because of that I am filled with hope. People are beginning to sense the need for change and are beginning to question some of the most basic assumptions that we have about food and health. People are beginning to understand the conclusions of scientific literature and are changing their lives for the better.

Never before has there been such a mountain of empirical research supporting a whole foods, plant-based diet. Now, for example, we can obtain images of the arteries in the heart, and then show conclusively, as Drs. Dean Ornish and Caldwell Esselstyn, Jr., have done, that a whole foods, plant-based diet reverses heart disease.[13] We now have the knowledge to understand how this actually works. Animal protein, even more than saturated fat and dietary cholesterol, raises blood cholesterol levels in experimental animals, individual humans and entire populations. International comparisons between countries show that populations subsisting on traditional plant-based diets have far less heart disease, and studies of individuals within single populations show that those who eat more whole, plant-based foods not only have lower cholesterol levels, but have less heart disease. *We now have a deep and broad range of evidence showing that a whole foods, plant-based diet is best for the heart.*

Never before have we had such a depth of understanding of how diet affects cancer both on a cellular level as well as a population level. Published data show that animal protein promotes the growth of tumors. Animal protein increases the levels of a hormone, IGF-1, which is a risk factor for cancer, and high-casein (the main protein of cow's milk) diets allow more carcinogens into cells, which allow more dangerous carcinogen products to bind to DNA, which allow more mutagenic reactions that give rise to cancer cells, which allow more rapid growth of tumors once they are initially formed. Data show that a diet based on animal-based foods increases a female's production of reproductive hormones over her lifetime, which may lead to breast cancer. *We now have a deep and broad range of evidence showing that a whole foods, plant-based diet is best for cancer.*

Never before have we had technology to measure the biomarkers associated with diabetes, and the evidence to show that blood sugar, blood cholesterol and insulin levels improve more with a whole foods, plant-based diet than with any other treatment. Intervention studies show that Type 2 diabetics treated with a whole foods, plant-based diet may reverse their disease and go off their medications. A broad range of international studies shows that Type 1 diabetes, a serious autoimmune disease, is related to cow's milk consumption and premature weaning. We now know how our autoimmune system can attack our own bodies through a process of molecular mimicry induced by animal proteins that find their way into our bloodstream. We also have tantalizing evidence linking multiple sclerosis with animal food consumption, and especially dairy consumption. Dietary intervention studies have shown that diet can help slow, and perhaps even halt, multiple sclerosis. *We now have a deep and broad range of evidence showing that a whole foods, plant-based diet is best for diabetes and autoimmune diseases.*

Never before have we had such a broad range of evidence showing that diets containing excess animal protein can destroy our kidneys. Kidney stones arise because the consumption of animal protein creates excessive calcium and oxalate in the kidney. We know now that cataracts and age-related macular degeneration can be prevented by foods containing large amounts of antioxidants. In addition, research has shown that cognitive dysfunction, vascular dementia caused by small strokes and Alzheimer's are all related to the food we eat. Investigations of human populations show that our risk of hip fracture and osteoporosis is made worse by diets high in animal-based foods. Animal protein leeches calcium from the bones by creating an acidic environment in the blood. *We now have a deep and broad range of evidence showing that a whole foods, plant-based diet is best for our kidneys, bones, eyes and brains.*

More research can and should be done, but the idea that whole foods, plant-based diets can protect against and even treat a wide variety of chronic diseases can no longer be denied. No longer are there just a few people making claims about a plant-based diet based on their personal experience, philosophy or the occasional supporting scientific study. Now there are hundreds of detailed, comprehensive, well-done research studies that point in the same direction.

Furthermore, I have hope for the future because of our new ability to exchange information across the country and around the world. A much greater proportion of the world population is literate, and a much greater proportion of that population has the luxury of choosing what they eat from a wide variety of readily accessible foods. People can make a whole foods, plant-based diet varied, interesting, tasty and convenient. I have hope because people in small towns and in previously isolated parts of the country can now readily access cutting edge health information and put it into practice.

All of these things together create an atmosphere unlike any other, an atmosphere that demands change. Contrary to the situation in 1982, when a few colleagues tried to destroy the reputations of scientists who suggested that diet had anything to do with cancer, it is now more commonly accepted that what you eat can determine your risk of multiple cancers. I have also seen the public image of vegetarianism emerge from being considered a dangerous, passing fad to a healthful, enduring lifestyle choice. The popularity of plant-based diets has been increasing, and both the variety and availability of convenient vegetarian foods have been skyrocketing.[14] Restaurants around the country now regularly offer meat-free and dairy-free options.[15] Scientists are publishing more articles about vegetarianism and writing more about the health potential of a plant-based diet.[16] Now, over 150 years after my great-great uncle George Macilwain wrote books about diet and disease, I am writing a book about diet and disease with the help of my youngest son Tom. Tom's middle name is McIlwain (the family changed the spelling over the past couple of generations), which means that not only am I writing about many of the same ideas Macilwain wrote about, but a relative bearing his name is the co-author. History can repeat itself. This time, however, instead of the message being forgotten and confined to library stacks, I believe that the world is finally ready to accept it. More than that, I believe the world is finally ready to change. We have reached a point in our history where our bad habits can no longer be tolerated. We, as a society, are on the edge of a great precipice: we can fall to sickness, poverty and degradation, or we can embrace health, longevity and bounty. And all it takes is the courage to change. How will our grandchildren find themselves in 100 years? Only time will tell, but I hope that the history we are witnessing and the future that lies ahead will be to the benefit of us all.

APPENDIX A
Q&A: Protein Effect in Experimental Rat Studies

COULD THE DIETARY PROTEIN EFFECT
BE DUE TO OTHER NUTRIENTS IN THE RAT DIET?

Decreasing dietary protein from 20% to 5% means finding something to replace the missing 15%. We used a carbohydrate to replace the casein because it had the same energy content. As dietary protein decreased, a 1:1 mixture of starch and glucose increased by the same amount. The extra starch and glucose in the low-protein diets could not have been responsible for the lower development of foci because these carbohydrates, when tested alone, actually increase foci development.[1] If anything, a little extra carbohydrate in the low-protein diet would only increase cancer incidence and offset the low-protein effect. This makes prevention of cancer by low-protein diets even more impressive.

MIGHT THE PROTEIN EFFECT BE DUE
TO THE RATS ON A LOW-PROTEIN DIET
EATING LESS FOOD (I.E., LESS CALORIES)?

Many studies done in the 1930s, 1940s and 1950s[2] had shown that decreasing total food intake, or total calories, decreased tumor development. A review of our many experiments, however, showed that animals fed the low-protein diets did not consume less calories but, on average, actually consumed more calories.[3, 4] Again, this only reinforced the tumor-promoting effect observed for casein.

WHAT WAS THE OVERALL HEALTH OF THE RATS ON A LOW-PROTEIN DIET?

Many researchers have long assumed that animals fed diets this low in protein would not be healthy. However, the low-protein animals were healthier by every indication. They lived longer, were more physically active, were slimmer and had healthy hair coats at 100 weeks while the high-protein counterpart rats were all dead. Also, animals consuming less dietary casein not only ate more calories, but they also burned off more calories. Low-protein animals consumed more oxygen, which is required for the burning of these calories, and had higher levels of a special tissue called brown adipose tissue,[5, 6] which is especially effective in burning off calories. This occurs through a process of "thermogenesis," i.e., the expenditure of calories as body heat. This phenomenon had already been demonstrated many years before.[7-11] *Low-protein diets enhance the burning off of calories, thus leaving less calories for body weight gain and perhaps also less for tumor growth as well.*

WAS PHYSICAL ACTIVITY RELATED TO THE CONSUMPTION OF THE LOW-PROTEIN DIET?

To measure the physical activity of each group of rats, we compared how much they voluntarily operated an exercise wheel attached to their cages. A monitor recorded the number of times the animals turned the exercise wheel. The low-casein animals[12] exercised about twice as much, when measured over a two-week period! This observation seems to be very similar to how one feels after eating a high-protein meal: sluggish and sleepy. I have heard that a side effect of the protein-drenched Atkins Diet is fatigue. Have you ever noticed this feeling in yourself after a high-protein meal?

APPENDIX B
Experimental
Design of the China Study

SIXTY-FIVE COUNTIES in twenty-four different provinces (out of twenty-seven) were selected for the survey. They represented the full range of mortality rates for seven of the more common cancers. They also provided broad geographic coverage and were within four hours' travel time of a central laboratory. The survey counties represented:

- semitropical coastal areas of southeast China;
- frigid wintry areas in northeast China, near Siberia;
- areas near the Great Gobi desert and the northern steppes;
- and areas near or in the Himalaya Mountains ranging from the far northwest to the far southwest part of the country.

Except for suburban areas near Shanghai, most counties were located in rural China where people lived in the same place their entire lives and consumed locally produced food. Population densities varied widely, from 20,000 nomadic residents for the most remote county near the Great Gobi desert, to 1.3 million people for the county on the outskirts of Shanghai.

This survey is referred to as an ecological or correlation study design, meaning that we are comparing diet, lifestyle and disease characteristics of a number of sample populations, in this case the sixty-five counties. We determine how these characteristics, as county averages, correlate

353

or associate with each other. For example, how does dietary fat relate to breast cancer rates? Or how does blood cholesterol relate to coronary heart disease? How does a certain kind of fatty acid in red blood cells relate to rice consumption? We could also compare blood testosterone levels or estrogen levels with breast cancer risk. We did thousands of different comparisons of this type.

In a study of this kind, it is important to note that only the average values for county populations are being compared. Individuals are not being compared with individuals (in reality, neither does any other epidemiological study design). As ecological studies go, this study, with its sixty-five counties, was unusually large. Most such studies only have ten to twenty such population units, at most.

Each of the sixty-five counties provided 100 adults for the survey. One-half were male and one-half female, all aged thirty-five to sixty-four years. The data were collected in the following manner:

- each person volunteered a blood sample and completed a diet and lifestyle questionnaire;
- one-half of the people provided a urine sample;
- the survey teams went to 30% of the homes to carefully measure food consumed by the family over a three-day period;
- samples of food representing the typical diets at each survey site were collected at the local marketplace and were later analyzed for dietary and nutritional factors.

One of the more important questions during the early planning stages was how to survey for diet and nutrition information. Estimating consumption of food and nutrients from memory is a common method, but this is very imprecise, especially when mixed dishes are consumed. Can you remember what foods you ate last week, or even yesterday? Can you remember how much? Another even more crude method of estimating food intake is to see how much of each food is sold in the marketplace. These findings can give reasonable estimates of diet trends over time for whole populations, but they do not account for food waste or measure individual amounts of consumption.

Although each of these relatively crude methods can be useful for certain purposes, they still are subject to considerable technical error and personal bias. And the bigger the technical error, the more difficult it is to detect significant cause-effect associations.

We wanted to do better than crudely measure which foods and how much of these foods were being consumed. Thus we decided to evaluate nutritional conditions by analyzing blood and urine samples for indicators (biomarkers) of multiple nutrient intakes. These analyses would be far more objective than having people recall what they ate.

Collecting and analyzing blood, however, was not easy to arrange, at least not in the way that we preferred. The initial problem was getting *enough* blood. For cultural reasons, rural Chinese were reluctant to provide blood samples. A finger prick seemed to be the only possibility but this was not good enough. A regular vial of blood would give 100 times as much blood and allow for analyses of many more factors.

Dr. Junshi Chen of our team, at the Institute of Nutrition and Food Hygiene in the Ministry of Health, had the unenviable task of convincing these volunteers to give a regular vial of blood. He succeeded. Sir Richard Peto at the University of Oxford of our team then made the very practical suggestion of combining the individual blood samples to make a big pool of blood for each village for each sex. This strategy gave more than 1,200–1,300 times more blood when compared with the finger prick method.

Making big pools of blood had enormous implications and made possible the China Study, as it later became known. It allowed analyses of far more indicators of diet and health. This allowed us to consider relationships in a far more comprehensive manner than would have otherwise been possible. For more detail on the theoretical and practical basis for collecting and analyzing blood in this way the reader is referred to the original monograph of the study.[1]

After collecting the blood, we then had to decide who would do the many analyses that were possible. We wanted nothing but the best. While some analyses were conducted at our Cornell lab and at Dr. Chen's Beijing lab, the rest of the analyses, especially the more specialized types, were done in about two dozen laboratories located in six countries and in four continents. Laboratories were selected because of their demonstrated expertise and interest. The laboratory participants are listed in the original monograph.[1]

HOW GOOD IS THIS STUDY?

Because this survey was a one-of-a-kind opportunity, we intended that it be the best of its kind ever undertaken. It was comprehensive; it was high quality; and its uniqueness allowed new opportunities to investigate diet and disease that were never before possible. These features of comprehensiveness, quality and uniqueness greatly improved the credibility and reliability of the findings—by far. Indeed, the *New York Times*, in a lead story in its Science Section, called the study "The Grand Prix" of epidemiological studies.

COMPREHENSIVENESS OF DATA

This survey was, and still is, the most comprehensive of its kind ever undertaken. After all the blood, urine and food samples were collected, stored and analyzed, and after the final results were tabulated and evaluated for quality (a few suspect results were not included in the final publication), we were able to study 367 variables. These represented a wide variety of dietary, lifestyle and disease characteristics, now included in a dense 896-page monograph.[1] There were:

- disease mortality rates on more than forty-eight different kinds of disease[2];
- 109 nutritional, viral, hormonal and other indicators in blood;
- over twenty-four urinary factors;
- almost thirty-six food constituents (nutrients, pesticides, heavy metals);
- more than thirty-six specific nutrient and food intakes measured in the household survey;
- sixty diet and lifestyle factors obtained from questionnaires;
- and seventeen geographic and climatic factors.

The study was comprehensive, not only because of the sheer number of variables, but also because most of these variables varied over broad ranges, as with the cancer mortality rates. Broad ranges strengthened our ability to detect important previously undiscovered associations of variables.

QUALITY OF DATA

A number of features added quality to this study.

- The adults chosen for this survey were limited to those who were thirty-five to sixty-four years of age. This is the age range in which the diseases being investigated are more common. Information on death certificates of people older than sixty-four years was not included in the survey because this information was considered less reliable.

- In each of the sixty-five counties in the study, two villages were selected for the collection of the information. Having two villages in each county rather than one gives a more reliable county average. When the values of two villages are more similar to each other than to all the other counties, then this means higher-quality data.[3]

- When possible, variables were measured by more than one kind of method. For example, iron status was measured in six different ways, riboflavin (vitamin B_2) in three ways, and so forth. Also, in many cases, we could assess the quality and reliability of data by comparing variables known to have plausible biological relationships.

- The populations under study proved to be very stable. An average of 93–94% of the men in the survey were born in the county where they lived at the time of the survey; for women it was 89%. Also, according to data published by the World Bank,[4] the diets at the time of our survey were very similar to those consumed in earlier years. This was ideal because those earlier years represented the time when the diseases were initially forming.

UNIQUENESS OF DATA

One idea that makes our study unique is our use of the ecologic study design. Critics of the ecologic study design correctly assume that it is a weak design for determining cause-and-effect associations when one is interested in the effects of single causes acting on single outcomes. But this is not the way that nutrition works. Rather, nutrition causes or prevents disease by multiple nutrients and other chemicals acting together, as in foods. An ecologic study is almost ideal if we wish to learn how an array of dietary factors act together to cause disease. It is the comprehensive effects of nutrients and other factors on disease occurrence where the most important lessons are to be learned. To investigate these comprehensive causes of disease, it was therefore necessary to record as many dietary and other lifestyle factors as possible, then formulate hypotheses and interpret data that represent comprehensiveness.

Perhaps the most unique characteristic that set this study apart concerned the nutritional characteristics of the diets consumed in rural China. Virtually every other human study on diet and health, of whatever design, has involved subjects who were consuming a rich Western diet. This is true even when vegetarians are included in the study because 90% of vegetarians still consume rather large amounts of milk, cheese and eggs, while a significant number still consume some fish and poultry. As is shown in the accompanying chart (Chart B.1),[5] there is only a small difference in the nutritional properties of non-vegetarian and vegetarian diets as consumed in Western countries.

CHART B.1: VEGETARIAN AND NON-VEGETARIAN DIET COMPARISONS AMONG WESTERNERS

Nutrient	Vegetarian	Non-vegetarian
Fat (% of calories)	30–36	34–38
Cholesterol (g/day)	150–300	300–500
Carbohydrates (% of calories)	50–55	<50
Total protein (% of calories)	12–14	14–18
Animal protein (% of total protein)	40–60	60–70

A strikingly different dietary situation existed in China. In America, 15–17% of our total calories is provided by protein, and upwards of 80% of this amount is animal-based. In other words, we gorge on protein and we get most of it from meat and dairy products. But in rural China, they consume less protein overall (9–10% of total calories), and only 10% of it comes from animal-based foods. This means that there are many other major nutritional differences in the Chinese and American diets, as shown in Chart B.2.[1]

CHART B.2: CHINESE AND AMERICAN DIETARY INTAKES

Nutrient	China	United States
Calories (kcal/kg body wt./day)	40.6	30.6
Total fat (% of calories)	14.5	34–38
Dietary fiber (g/day)	33	12
Total protein (g/day)	64	91
Animal protein (% of total calories)	0.8*	10–11
Total iron (mg/day)	34	18

*Non-fish animal protein

This was the first and only large study that investigated this range of dietary experience and its health consequences. Chinese diets ranged from rich to very rich in plant-based foods. In all other studies done on Western subjects, diets ranged from rich to very rich in animal-based foods. It was this distinction that made the China Study so different from other studies.

MAKING IT HAPPEN

Organization and conduct of a study of this size, scope and quality was possible because of the exceptional skills of Dr. Junshi Chen. Survey sites were scattered across the far reaches of China. In American travel distances, they ranged from the Florida Keys to Seattle, Washington, and from San Diego, California, to Bangor, Maine. Travel between these places was more difficult than in the United States, and supplies and instructions for the survey had to be in place and standardized for all collection sites. And this was done before e-mails, fax machines and cellular phones were available.

It was important that the twenty-four provincial health teams, each comprised of twelve to fifteen health workers, be trained to carry out the blood, food and urine collections and complete the questionnaires in a systematic and standardized manner. To standardize the collection of information, Dr. Chen divided the country into regions. Each region sent trainers to Beijing for the senior training session. They, in turn, returned to their home provinces to train the provincial health teams.

Although the U.S. National Cancer Institute (NCI) of the National Institutes of Health (NIH) provided the initial funding for this project, the Chinese Ministry of Health paid the salaries of the approximately 350 health workers. It is my estimate that the Chinese contribution to the project was approximately $5–6 million. This compares with the U.S. contribution of about $2.9 million over a ten-year period. Were the U.S. government to have paid for this service in a similar project in the U.S., it would have cost at least ten times this amount, or $50–60 million.

APPENDIX C
The "Vitamin" D Connection

THE MOST IMPRESSIVE EVIDENCE favoring plant-based diets is the way that so many food factors and biological events are integrated to maximize health and minimize disease. Although the biological processes are exceptionally complex, these factors still work together as a beautifully choreographed, self-correcting network. It is exceptionally impressive, especially the coordination and control of this network.

Perhaps a couple of analogies might help to illustrate such a process. Flocks of birds in flight or schools of fish darting about are able to shift direction in a microsecond without bumping into each other. They seem to have a collective consciousness that knows where they are going and when they will rest. Colonies of ants and swarms of bees also integrate varying labor chores with great proficiency. But as amazing as these animal activities are, have you ever thought about how their behaviors are coordinated with such finesse? I see these same characteristics, and more, in the way that the countless factors of plant-based foods work their magic to create health at all levels within our body, among our organs and between our cells and among the enzymes and other sub-cellular particles within our cells.

For those unfamiliar with biomedical research laboratories, the walls of these labs are often covered with large posters showing thousands of biochemical reactions operating within our bodies. These are reactions that are known; far more remain to be discovered. The interdependence of these reactions with each other is especially informative, even awesome in its implications.

An example of a very small portion of this enormous network of re-actions is the effect of vitamin D and its metabolites on several of the diseases discussed in this book. This particular network illustrates a complex interconnection between the inner workings of our cells, the food we eat and the environment in which we live (Chart C.1). Although some of the vitamin D present in our bodies may come from food, we can usually get all that we need from a few hours of sunshine each week. In fact, it is our ability to make our vitamin D that leads to the idea that it is not a vitamin; it is a hormone (i.e., made in one part of our body but functioning in another part). The sun's UV rays make vitamin D from a precursor chemical located in our skin. Provided we get adequate sunshine, this is all the vitamin D we need.[1] We can, of course, also get vitamin D from fortified milk, certain fish oils and some vitamin supplements.

The vitamin D made in our skin then travels to our liver, where it is converted by an enzyme to a vitamin D metabolite. This metabolite's main function is to serve as the body's storage form of vitamin D (while remaining mostly in the liver but also in body fat).

The next step is the crucial one. When needed, some of the storage form of vitamin D in the liver is transported to the kidney, where another enzyme converts it into a supercharged vitamin D metabolite, which is called 1,25 D. The rate at which the storage form of vitamin D is converted to the supercharged 1,25 D is a crucial reaction in this network. The 1,25 D metabolite does most of the important work of vitamin D in our bodies.

This supercharged 1,25 D is about 1,000 times more active than the storage vitamin D. Supercharged 1,25 D only survives for six to eight hours once it is made. In contrast, our storage vitamin D survives for twenty days or more.[2, 3] This demonstrates an important principle typically found in networks like this: the far greater activity, the far shorter lifetime and the far lower amounts of the 1,25 D end product provide a very responsive system wherein the 1,25 D can quickly adjust its activity minute-by-minute and microsecond-by-microsecond as long as there is sufficient storage vitamin D to draw from. Small changes, making a big difference, can occur quickly.

The relationship between the storage form of vitamin D and the supercharged 1,25 D is like having a large tank of natural gas buried in our yard (storage vitamin D) but carefully using only a very tiny amount of gas to light the burner at our stovetop. It is critical that the amount and timing of gas (1,25 D) coming to our stovetop be carefully

CHART C.1: THE VITAMIN D NETWORK

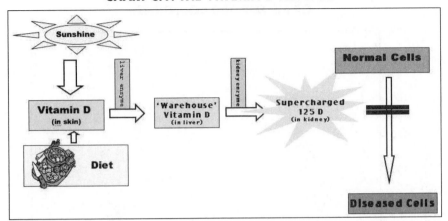

regulated, regardless of how much there may be in the tank, whether it is low or whether it is full. However, it is also useful that we maintain an adequate supply in our storage tank. In the same way, it is critical that the kidney enzyme in this reaction has a soft, sensitive touch, so to speak, as it produces the right amount of the 1,25 D at the right time for its very important work.

One of the more important things that vitamin D does, mostly through its conversion to supercharged 1,25 D, is to control the development of a wide variety of serious diseases. For the sake of simplicity, this is schematically represented by showing the inhibition of the conversion of healthy tissue to diseased tissue by 1,25 D. [4–12]

So far, we can see how adequate sunshine exposure, by ensuring enough storage form of vitamin D, helps to prevent cells from becoming diseased. This suggests that certain diseases might be more common in areas of the world where there is less sunshine, in countries nearer the North and South Poles. Indeed there is such evidence. To be more specific: *in the northern hemisphere, communities that are farther north tend to have more Type 1 diabetes, multiple sclerosis, rheumatoid arthritis, osteoporosis, breast cancer, prostate cancer and colon cancer, in addition to other diseases.*

Researchers have known for eighty years that multiple sclerosis, for example, is associated with increasing latitude.[13] As you can see in Chart C.2, there is a huge difference in MS prevalence as one goes away from the equator, being over 100 times more prevalent in the far north than at the equator.[14] Similarly, in Australia, there is less sunshine and

CHART C.2: WORLDWIDE DISTRIBUTION OF MS FOR 120 COUNTRIES

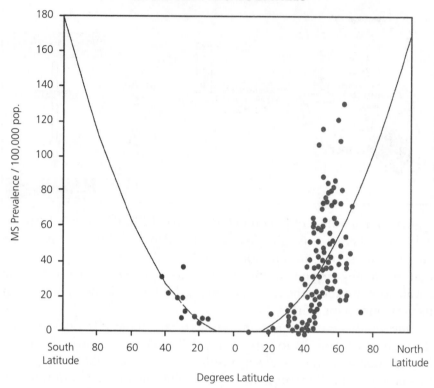

more MS as one goes farther south (r=91%).[15] MS is about sevenfold greater in southern (43°S) than in northern Australia (19°S).[16]

A lack of sunshine, however, is not the only factor related to these diseases. There is a larger context. The first thing to note is the control and coordination of these vitamin D-related reactions. Control operates at several places in this network, but, as I already said, it is the conversion of storage vitamin D into the supercharged 1,25 D in the kidneys that is especially critical. In considerable measure, this control is exercised by another complex network of reactions involving a "manager"-type hormone produced by the parathyroid gland located in our neck (Chart C.3).

When, for example, we need more 1,25 D, parathyroid hormone induces the kidney enzyme activity to produce more 1,25 D. When there is enough 1,25 D, parathyroid hormone slows down the kidney enzyme activity. Within seconds, parathyroid hormone manages how much 1,25 D there will be at each time and place. Parathyroid hormone also acts as a conductor at several other places in this network, as shown by the several arrows. By being aware of the role of each player in its "orchestra," it coordinates, controls and finely tunes these reactions as a conductor would a symphony orchestra.

Under optimal conditions, sunshine exposure alone can supply all the vitamin D that we need to produce the all-important 1,25 D at the right time. Even the elderly, who are not able to produce as much vitamin D from sunshine, have nothing to worry about if there is enough sunshine.[17] How much is "enough"? If you know how much sunshine causes a slight redness of your skin, then one-fourth of this amount, provided two to three times per week, is more than adequate to meet our vitamin D needs and to store some in our liver and body fat.[17] If your skin becomes slightly red after about thirty minutes in the sun, then ten minutes, three times per week will be enough exposure to get plenty of vitamin D.

When and if we don't get enough sunshine, it may be helpful to consume vitamin D from our diets. Almost all of the vitamin D found in our diet has been artificially added to foods like milk and breakfast cereals. Along with vitamin supplements, this amount of vitamin D can be quite significant and, under certain circumstances, there is some evidence that this practice may be beneficial.[18-21]

In this scheme, sunshine and parathyroid hormone work together in a marvelously coordinated way to keep this system running smoothly, both in filling our vitamin D tank and in helping to produce from moment to moment the exact amount of 1,25 D that we need. When it comes to getting sufficient sunshine or getting vitamin D in food, taking light from the sun makes far more sense.

THROWING WRENCHES INTO THE SYSTEM

There are several studies now showing that if 1,25 D remains at consistently low levels, the risk of several diseases increases. So then the question is: what causes low levels of 1,25 D? Animal protein-containing foods cause a significant decrease in 1,25 D.[22] These proteins create an acidic environment in the blood that blocks the kidney enzyme from producing this very important metabolite.[23]

A second factor that influences this process is calcium. Calcium in our blood is crucial for optimum muscle and nerve functioning, and it

CHART C.3: ROLE OF THE PARATHYROID HORMONE IN THE REGULATION OF SUPERCHARGED 1,25 D

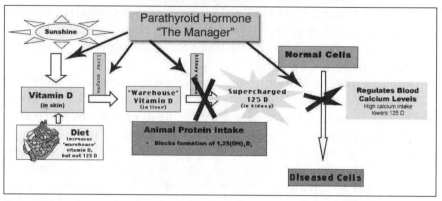

must be maintained within a fairly narrow range. The 1,25 D keeps the blood levels of calcium operating within this narrow range by monitoring and regulating how much calcium is absorbed from food being digested in the intestine, how much calcium is excreted in the urine and feces and how much is exchanged with the bone, the big supply tank for the body's calcium. For example, if there is too much calcium in the blood, 1,25 D becomes less active, less calcium is absorbed and more calcium is excreted. It is a very sensitive balancing act in our bodies. As blood calcium goes up, 1,25 D goes down, and when blood calcium goes down, 1,25 D goes up.[10, 24] Here's the kicker: if calcium consumption is unnecessarily high, it lowers the activity of the kidney enzyme and, as a consequence, the level of 1,25 D.[1, 25] In other words, routinely consuming high-calcium diets is not in our best interests.

The blood levels of 1,25 D therefore are depressed both by consuming too much animal protein and too much calcium. Animal-based food, with its protein, depresses 1,25 D. Cow's milk, however, is high both in protein and calcium. In fact, in one of the more extensive studies on MS that is associated with lower levels of 1,25 D, cow's milk was found to be as important a factor as latitude mentioned earlier.[26] For example, the association of MS with latitude and sunshine shown in Chart C.2 also is seen with animal-based foods shown in Chart C.4.[14]

One could hypothesize that diseases like MS are due, at least in part, to a lack of sunshine and lower vitamin D status. This is supported by the observation that northern people living along coastlines (e.g., Norway and Japan)[26] who consume lots of vitamin D-rich fish have less MS than people living inland. However, in these fish-eating communities with lower rates of disease, much less cow's milk is consumed. Consuming cow's milk has been shown to associate with MS[26] and Type 1 diabetes[27] independent of fish intake.

In another reaction associated with this network, increased intakes of animal protein also enhance the production of insulin-like growth factor (IGF-1, first introduced in chapter eight) and this enhances cancer cell growth.[5] In effect, there are many reactions acting in a co-ordinated and mutually consistent way to cause disease when a diet high in animal protein is consumed. When blood levels of 1,25 D are depressed, IGF-1 simultaneously becomes more active. Together, these factors increase the birth of new cells while simultaneously inhibiting the removal of old cells, both favoring the development of cancer (seven studies cited by[28]). For example, people with higher-than-normal blood levels of IGF-I have been shown to have 5.1 times the risk of

CHART C.4: WORLDWIDE DISTRIBUTION OF CALORIE CONSUMPTION FROM ANIMAL-BASED FOODS FOR 120 COUNTRIES[14]

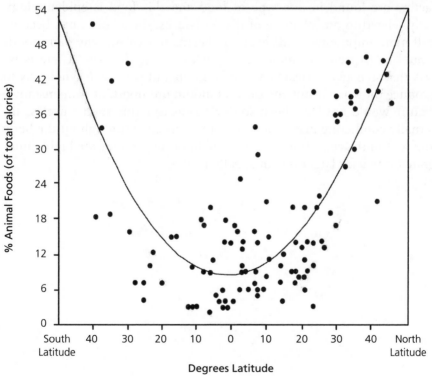

advanced-stage prostate cancer.[28] If combined with low blood levels of a protein that inactivates IGF-I[29] (i.e., more IGF-1 activity), there is *9.5 times the risk of advanced-stage prostate cancer.*[28] This level of disease risk is alarming. Fundamental to it all is the fact that animal-based foods like meat and dairy[30–32] lead to more IGF-I and less 1,25 D, both of which increase cancer risk.

These are only a few of the factors and events associated with this vitamin D network. With the right food and environment, these events and reactions cooperate in an integrated manner to produce health benefits. In contrast, when the wrong food is consumed, its adverse effects are mediated by not one, but many, of the reactions within this network. Also, many factors in such foods, even beyond the protein and calcium, participate in causing the problem. And, finally, it often is not one disease but many that are likely to occur.

What impresses me about this and other networks is the convergence of so many disease-causing factors operating through so many different reactions to produce a common result. When that common result is more than one disease, it is even more impressive. When these various factors are found in one type of food and this food is epidemiologically related to one or more of these diseases, the associations become still more impressive. This example begins to explain why dairy foods would be expected to increase the risk of these diseases. There is no way that so many intricate mechanisms, operating in such synchrony to produce the same result, are only a random unimportant happenstance. Nature would not have been so devious as to refine such a useless internally conflicting maze. Networks like this exist throughout the body and within the cells. But of even more importance, they are highly integrated into a far larger dynamic called "life."

References

PART I

Chapter 1

1. American Cancer Society. "Cancer Facts and Figures—1998." Atlanta, GA: American Cancer Society, 1998.
2. Flegal KM, Carroll MD, Ogden CL, et al. "Prevalence and trends in obesity among U.S. adults, 1999–2000." *JAMA* 288 (2002): 1723–1727.
3. National Center for Health Statistics. "Obesity still on the rise, new data show. The U.S. Department of Health and Human Services News Release." October 10, 2003. Washington, DC: 2002. Accessed at http://www.cdc.gov/nchs/releases/02news/obesityonrise.htm
4. Lin B-H, Guthrie J, and Frazao E. "Nutrient Contribution of Food Away from Home." *In:* E. Frazao (ed.), *America's Eating Habits: Changes and Consequences.* Washington, DC: Economic Research Service, USDA, 1999. Cited on p. 138 in: Information Plus. *Nutrition: a key to good health.* Wylie, TX: Information Plus, 1999.
5. Mokdad AH, Ford ES, Bowman BA, et al. "Diabetes trends in the U.S.: 1990–1998." *Diabetes Care* 23 (2000): 1278–1283.
6. Centers for Disease Control and Prevention. "National Diabetes Fact Sheet: National Estimates and General Information on Diabetes in the United States, Revised Edition." Atlanta, GA: Centers for Disease Control and Prevention, 1998.
7. American Diabetes Association. "Economic consequences of diabetes mellitus in the U.S. in 1997." *Diabetes Care* 21 (1998): 296–309. Cited In: Mokdad AH, Ford ES, Bowman BA, et al. "Diabetes trends in the U.S.: 1990–1998." *Diabetes Care* 23 (2000): 1278–1283.
8. American Heart Association. "Heart Disease and Stroke Statistics—2003 Update." Dallas, TX: American Heart Association, 2002.
9. Ornish D, Brown SE, Scherwitz LW, et al. "Can lifestyle changes reverse coronary heart disease?" *Lancet* 336 (1990): 129–133.
10. Esselstyn CB, Ellis SG, Medendorp SV, et al. "A strategy to arrest and reverse coronary artery disease: a 5-year longitudinal study of a single physician's practice." *J. Family Practice* 41 (1995): 560–568.
11. Starfield B. "Is U.S. health really the best in the world?" *JAMA* 284 (2000): 483–485.
12. Anderson RN. "Deaths: leading causes for 2000." *National Vital Statistics Reports* 50(16) (2002):
13. Phillips D, Christenfeld N, and Glynn L. "Increase in U.S. medication-error death between 1983 and 1993." *Lancet* 351 (1998): 643–644.

14. U.S. Congressional House Subcommittee Oversight Investigation. "Cost and quality of health care: unnecessary surgery." Washington, DC: 1976. Cited by: Leape, L. "Unnecessary surgery." *Ann. Rev. Publ. Health* 13 (1992): 363–383.

15. Lazarou J, Pomeranz B, and Corey PN. "Incidence of adverse drug reactions in hospitalized patients." *JAMA* 279 (1998): 1200–1205.

16. World Health Organization. Technical Report Series No. 425. "International Drug Monitoring: the Role of the Hospital." Geneva, Switzerland: World Health Organization, 1966.

17. Health Insurance Association of America. *Source Book of Health Insurance Data: 1999–2000.* Washington, DC, 1999.

18. National Center for Health Statistics. *Health, United States, 2000 with Adolescent Health Chartbook.* Hyattsville, MD: National Center for Health Statistics, 2000.

19. Starfield B. *Primary Care: Balancing Health Needs, Services, and Technology.* New York, NY: Oxford University Press, 1998.

20. World Health Organization. World Health Report 2000: Press release. "World Health Organization assesses the world's health systems." June 21, 2000. Geneva. Accessed at http://www.who.int

21. Coble YD. American Medical Association press release. "AMA decries rise in number of uninsured Americans." September 30, 2003. Chicago, IL. Accessed at http://www.ama-assn.org/ama/pub/article/1617–8064.html

22. Campbell TC. "Present day knowledge on aflatoxin." *Phil J Nutr* 20 (1967): 193–201.

23. Campbell TC, Caedo JP, Jr., Bulatao-Jayme J, et al. "Aflatoxin M_1 in human urine." *Nature* 227 (1970): 403–404.

24. This program was conducted in collaboration with the Philippine Department of Health and was funded by the United States Agency for International Development (USAID). USAID paid my full salary for six years and resulted in 110 "mother craft centers" distributed around much of the Philippines. Progress on this contract was prepared as monthly reports to USAID by Associate Dean C.W. Engel at Virginia Tech.

25. Hu J, Zhao X, Jia J, et al. "Dietary calcium and bone density among middle-aged and elderly women in China." *Am. J. Clin. Nutr.* 58 (1993): 219–227.

26. Hu J, Zhao X, Parpia B, et al. "Dietary intakes and urinary excretion of calcium and acids: a cross-sectional study of women in China." *Am. J. Clin. Nutr.* 58 (1993): 398–406.

27. Hu J, Zhao X, Parpia B, et al. "Assessment of a modified household food weighing method in a study of bone health in China." *European J. Clin. Nutr.* 48 (1994): 442–452.

28. Potischman N, McCulloch CE, Byers T, et al. "Breast cancer and dietary and plasma concentrations of carotenoids and vitamin A." *Am. J. Clin. Nutr.* 52 (1990): 909–915.

29. Potischman N, McCulloch CE, Byers T, et al. "Associations between breast cancer, triglycerides and cholesterol." *Nutr. Cancer* 15 (1991): 205–215.

30. Chen J, Campbell TC, Li J, et al. *Diet, life-style and mortality in China. A study of the characteristics of 65 Chinese counties.* Oxford, UK; Ithaca, NY; Beijing, PRC: Oxford University Press; Cornell University Press; People's Medical Publishing House, 1990.

31. Campbell TC, and Chen J. "Diet and chronic degenerative diseases:perspectives from China." *Am. J. Clin. Nutr.* 59 (Suppl.) (1994): 1153S–1161S.

32. Campbell TC. "The dietary causes of degenerative diseases: nutrients vs foods." *In:* N. J. Temple and D. P. Burkitt (eds.), *Western diseases: their dietary prevention and reversibility,* pp. 119–152. Totowa, NJ: Humana Press, 1994.

33. Campbell TC, and Chen J. "Diet and chronic degenerative diseases: a summary of results from an ecologic study in rural China." *In:* N. J. Temple and D. P. Burkitt (eds.), *Western diseases: their dietary prevention and reversibility,* pp. 67–118. Totowa, NJ: Humana Press, 1994.

34. Chittenden RH. *Physiological economy in nutrition.* New York: F.A. Stokes, 1904.

35. Chittenden RH. *The nutrition of man.* New York: F. A. Stokes, 1907.

Chapter 2

1. Stillings BR. "World supplies of animal protein." *In:* J. W. G. Porter and B. A. Rolls (eds.), *Proteins in Human Nutrition*, pp. 11–33. London: Academic Press, 1973.
2. Campbell TC, Warner RG, and Loosli JK. "Urea and biuret for ruminants." *In:* Cornell Nutrition Conference, Buffalo, NY, 1960, pp. 96–103.
3. Campbell TC, Loosli JK, Warner RG, et al. "Utilization of biuret by ruminants." *J. Animal Science* 22 (1963): 139–145.
4. Autret M. "World protein supplies and needs. Proceedings of the Sixteenth Easter School in Agricultural Science, University of Nottingham, 1969." *In:* R. A. Laurie (ed.), *Proteins in Human Food*, pp. 3–19. Westport, CT.: Avi Publishing Company, 1970.
5. Scrimshaw NS, and Young VR. "Nutritional evaluation and the utilization of protein resources." *In:* C. E. Bodwell (ed.), *Evaluation of Proteins for Humans*, pp. 1–10. Westport, CT: The Avi Publishing Co., 1976.
6. Jalil ME, and Tahir WM. "World supplies of plant proteins." *In:* J. W. G. Porter and B. A. Rolls (eds.), *Proteins in Human Nutrition*, pp. 35–46. London: Academic Press, 1973.
7. Blount WP. "Turkey "X" Disease." *Turkeys* 9 (1961): 52, 55–58, 61, 77.
8. Sargeant K, Sheridan A, O'Kelly J, et al. "Toxicity associated with certain samples of groundnuts." *Nature* 192 (1961): 1096–1097.
9. Lancaster MC, Jenkins FP, and Philp JM. "Toxicity associated with certain samples of groundnuts." *Nature* 192 (1961): 1095–1096.
10. Wogan GN, and Newberne PM. "Dose-response characteristics of aflatoxin B_1 carcinogenesis in the rat." *Cancer Res.* 27 (1967): 2370–2376.
11. Wogan GN, Paglialunga S, and Newberne PM. "Carcinogenic effects of low dietary levels of aflatoxin B_1 in rats." *Food Cosmet. Toxicol.* 12 (1974): 681–685.
12. Campbell TC, Caedo JP, Jr., Bulatao-Jayme J, et al. "Aflatoxin M_1 in human urine." *Nature* 227 (1970): 403–404.
13. Madhavan TV, and Gopalan C. "The effect of dietary protein on carcinogenesis of aflatoxin." *Arch. Path.* 85 (1968): 133–137.

Chapter 3

1. Natural Resources Defense Council. "Intolerable risk: pesticides in our children's food." New York: Natural Resources Defense Council, February 27, 1989.
2. Winter C, Craigmill A, and Stimmann M. "Food Safety Issues II. NRDC report and Alar." *UC Davis Environmental Toxicology Newsletter* 9(2) (1989): 1.
3. Lieberman AJ, and Kwon SC. "Fact versus fears: a review of the greatest unfounded health scares of recent times." New York: American Council on Science and Health, June, 1998.
4. Whelan EM, and Stare FJ. *Panic in the pantry: facts and fallacies about the food you buy*. Buffalo, NY: Prometheus Books, 1992.
5. U.S. Apple Association. "News release: synopsis of U.S. Apple Press Conference." McLean, VA: U.S. Apple Association, February 25, 1999.
6. Cassens RG. *Nitrite-cured meat: a food safety issue in perspective*. Trumbull, CT: Food and Nutrition Press, Inc., 1990.
7. Lijinsky W, and Epstein SS. "Nitrosamines as environmental carcinogens." *Nature* 225 (1970): 21–23.
8. National Toxicology Program. "Ninth report on carcinogens, revised January 2001." Washington, DC: U.S. Department of Health and Human Services, Public Health Service, January, 2001. Accessed at http://ehis.niehs.nih.gov/roc/toc9.html#viewe
9. International Agency for Cancer Research. *IARC Monographs on the Evaluation of the Carcinogenic Risk of Chemicals to Humans: Some N-Nitroso Compounds*. Vol. 17 Lyon, France: International Agency for Research on Cancer, 1978.

10. Druckrey H, Janzowski R, and Preussmann R. "Organotrope carcinogene wirkungen bei 65 verschiedenen N-nitroso-verbindungen an BD-ratten." *Z. Krebsforsch.* 69 (1967): 103–201.

11. Thomas C, and So BT. "Zur morphologie der durch N-nitroso-verbindungen erzeugten tumoren im oberen verdauungstrakt der ratte." *Arzneimittelforsch.* 19 (1969): 1077–1091.

12. Eisenbrand G, Spiegelhalder B, Janzowski C, et al. "Volatile and non-volatile N-nitroso compounds in foods and other environmental media." *IARC Sci. Publi.* 19 (1978): 311–324.

13. National Archives and Records Administration. "Code of Federal Regulations: Title 9, Animals and Animal Products, Section 319.180 (9CFR319.180)." Washington, DC: Government Printing Office, 2001.

14. Kanfer S. October 2, 1972. "The decline and fall of the American hot dog." *Time*: 86.

15. Newberne P. "Nitrite promotes lymphoma incidence in rats." *Science* 204 (1979): 1079–1081.

16. Madhavan TV, and Gopalan C. "The effect of dietary protein on carcinogenesis of aflatoxin." *Arch. Path.* 85 (1968): 133–137.

17. If this defect becomes part of the first round of daughter cells, then this will be passed on to all subsequent generations of cells, with the potential to eventually become clinically detectable cancer. However, this is an oversimplification of a very complex process. Perhaps two of the more significant omissions are the hypotheses that 1) more than one mutation may be required to initiate and promote cancer, and 2) not all genetic defects result in cancer.

18. Mgbodile MUK, and Campbell TC. "Effect of protein deprivation of male weanling rats on the kinetics of hepatic microsomal enzyme activity." *J. Nutr.* 102 (1972): 53–60.

19. Hayes JR, Mgbodile MUK, and Campbell TC. "Effect of protein deficiency on the inducibility of the hepatic microsomal drug-metabolizing enzyme system. I. Effect on substrate interaction with cytochrome P-450." *Biochem. Pharmacol.* 22 (1973): 1005–1014.

20. Mgbodile MUK, Hayes JR, and Campbell TC. "Effect of protein deficiency on the inducibility of the hepatic microsomal drug-metabolizing enzyme system. II. Effect on enzyme kinetics and electron transport system." *Biochem. Pharmacol.* 22 (1973): 1125–1132.

21. Hayes JR, and Campbell TC. "Effect of protein deficiency on the inducibility of the hepatic microsomal drug-metabolizing enzyme system. III. Effect of 3-methylcholanthrene induction on activity and binding kinetics." *Biochem. Pharmacol.* 23 (1974): 1721–1732.

22. Campbell TC. "Influence of nutrition on metabolism of carcinogens (Martha Maso Honor's Thesis)." *Adv. Nutr. Res.* 2 (1979): 29–55.

23. Preston RS, Hayes JR, and Campbell TC. "The effect of protein deficiency on the in vivo binding of aflatoxin B_1 to rat liver macromolecules." *Life Sci.* 19 (1976): 1191–1198.

24. Portman RS, Plowman KM, and Campbell TC. "On mechanisms affecting species susceptibility to aflatoxin." *Biochim. Biophys. Acta* 208 (1970): 487–495.

25. Prince LO, and Campbell TC. "Effects of sex difference and dietary protein level on the binding of aflatoxin B_1 to rat liver chromatin proteins in vivo." *Cancer Res.* 42 (1982): 5053–5059.

26. Mainigi KD, and Campbell TC. "Subcellular distribution and covalent binding of aflatoxins as functions of dietary manipulation." *J Toxicol. Eviron. Health* 6 (1980): 659–671.

27. Nerurkar LS, Hayes JR, and Campbell TC. "The reconstitution of hepatic microsomal mixed function oxidase activity with fractions derived from weanling rats fed different levels of protein." *J. Nutr.* 108 (1978): 678–686.

28. Gurtoo HL, and Campbell TC. "A kinetic approach to a study of the induction of rat liver microsomal hydroxylase after pretreatment with 3,4-benzpyrene and aflatoxin B_1." *Biochem. Pharmacol.* 19 (1970): 1729–1735.

29. Adekunle AA, Hayes JR, and Campbell TC. "Interrelationships of dietary protein level, aflatoxin B_1 metabolism, and hepatic microsomal epoxide hydrase activity." *Life Sci.* 21 (1977): 1785–1792.

30. Mainigi KD, and Campbell TC. "Effects of low dietary protein and dietary aflatoxin on hepatic glutathione levels in F-344 rats." *Toxicol. Appl. Pharmacol.* 59 (1981): 196–203.

31. Farber E, and Cameron R. "The sequential analysis of cancer development." *Adv. Cancer Res.* 31 (1980): 125–226.

32. Foci response for the various charts in this chapter mostly reflect "% of liver volume," which integrates "number of foci" and "size of foci," both of which indicate tumor-forming tendency. So that the responses from individual experiments can be compared among each other, the data are adjusted to a common scale that reflects the response produced by a standard dose of aflatoxin and by feeding a 20% protein diet.

33. Appleton BS, and Campbell TC. "Inhibition of aflatoxin-initiated preneoplastic liver lesions by low dietary protein." *Nutr. Cancer* 3 (1982): 200–206.

34. Dunaif GE, and Campbell TC. "Relative contribution of dietary protein level and Aflatoxin B₁ dose in generation of presumptive preneoplastic foci in rat liver." *J. Natl. Cancer Inst.* 78 (1987): 365–369.

35. Youngman LD, and Campbell TC. "High protein intake promotes the growth of preneoplastic foci in Fischer #344 rats: evidence that early remodeled foci retain the potential for future growth." *J. Nutr.* 121 (1991): 1454–1461.

36. Youngman LD, and Campbell TC. "Inhibition of aflatoxin B1-induced gamma-glutamyl transpeptidase positive (GGT+) hepatic preneoplastic foci and tumors by low protein diets: evidence that altered GGT+ foci indicate neoplastic potential." *Carcinogenesis* 13 (1992): 1607–1613.

37. Dunaif GE, and Campbell TC. "Dietary protein level and aflatoxin B1-induced preneoplastic hepatic lesions in the rat." *J. Nutr.* 117 (1987): 1298–1302.

38. Horio F, Youngman LD, Bell RC, et al. "Thermogenesis, low-protein diets, and decreased development of AFB1-induced preneoplastic foci in rat liver." *Nutr. Cancer* 16 (1991): 31–41.

39. About 12% dietary protein is required to maximize growth rate, according to the National Research Council of the National Academy of Sciences.

40. Subcommittee on Laboratory Animal Nutrition. *Nutrient requirements of laboratory animals. Second revised edition, number 10.* Washington, DC: National Academy Press, 1972.

41. National Research Council. *Recommended dietary allowances. Tenth edition.* Washington, DC: National Academy Press, 1989.

42. Schulsinger DA, Root MM, and Campbell TC. "Effect of dietary protein quality on development of aflatoxin B1-induced hepatic preneoplastic lesions." *J. Natl. Cancer Inst.* 81 (1989): 1241–1245.

43. Youngman LD. *The growth and development of aflatoxin B1-induced preneoplastic lesions, tumors, metastasis, and spontaneous tumors as they are influenced by dietary protein level, type, and intervention.* Ithaca, NY: Cornell University, Ph.D. Thesis, 1990.

44. Beasley RP. "Hepatitis B virus as the etiologic agent in hepatocellular carcinoma-epidemiologic considerations." *Hepatol.* 2 (1982): 21S–26S.

45. Blumberg BS, Larouze B, London WT, et al. "The relation of infection with the hepatitis B agent to primary hepatic carcinoma." *Am. J. Pathol.* 81 (1975): 669–682.

46. Chisari FV, Ferrari C, and Mondelli MU. "Hepatitis B virus structure and biology." *Microbiol. Pathol.* 6 (1989): 311–325.

47. Hu J, Cheng Z, Chisari FV, et al. "Repression of hepatitis B virus (HBV) transgene and HBV-induced liver injury by low protein diet." *Oncogene* 15 (1997): 2795–2801.

48. Cheng Z, Hu J, King J, et al. "Inhibition of hepatocellular carcinoma development in hepatitis B virus transfected mice by low dietary casein." *Hepatology* 26 (1997): 1351–1354.

49. Hawrylewicz EJ, Huang HH, Kissane JQ, et al. "Enhancement of the 7,12-dimethylbenz(a)anthracene (DMBA) mammary tumorigenesis by high dietary protein in rats." *Nutr. Reps. Int.* 26 (1982): 793–806.

50. Hawrylewicz EJ. "Fat-protein interaction, defined 2-generation studies." *In:* C. Ip, D. F. Birt, A. E. Rogers and C. Mettlin (eds.), *Dietary fat and cancer*, pp. 403–434. New York: Alan R. Liss, Inc., 1986.

51. Huang HH, Hawrylewicz EJ, Kissane JQ, et al. "Effect of protein diet on release of prolactin and ovarian steroids in female rats." *Nutr. Rpts. Int.* 26 (1982): 807–820.

52. O'Connor TP, Roebuck BD, and Campbell TC. "Dietary intervention during the post-dosing phase of L-azaserine-induced preneoplastic lesions." *J Natl Cancer Inst* 75 (1985): 955–957.

53. O'Connor TP, Roebuck BD, Peterson F, et al. "Effect of dietary intake of fish oil and fish protein on the development of L-azaserine-induced preneoplastic lesions in rat pancreas." *J Natl Cancer Inst* 75 (1985): 959–962.

54. He Y. *Effects of carotenoids and dietary carotenoid extracts on aflatoxin B₁-induced mutagenesis and hepatocarcinogenesis.* Ithaca, NY: Cornell University, PhD Thesis, 1990.

55. He Y, and Campbell TC. "Effects of carotenoids on aflatoxin B₁-induced mutagenesis in S. typhimurium TA 100 and TA 98." *Nutr. Cancer* 13 (1990): 243–253.

Chapter 4

1. Li J-Y, Liu B-Q, Li G-Y, et al. "Atlas of cancer mortality in the People's Republic of China. An aid for cancer control and research." *Int. J. Epid.* 10 (1981): 127–133.

2. Higginson J. "Present trends in cancer epidemiology." *Proc. Can. Cancer Conf.* 8 (1969): 40–75.

3. Wynder EL, and Gori GB. "Contribution of the environment to cancer incidence: an epidemiologic exercise." *J. Natl. Cancer Inst.* 58 (1977): 825–832.

4. Doll R, and Peto R. "The causes of cancer: Quantitative estimates of avoidable risks of cancer in the Unites States today." *J Natl Cancer Inst* 66 (1981): 1192–1265.

5. Fagin D. News release. "Breast cancer cause still elusive study: no clear link between pollution, breast cancer on LI." August 6, 2002. Newsday.com. Accessed at http://www.newsday.com/news/local/longisland/ny-licanc062811887aug06.story?coll=ny%2Dtop%2Dheadlines

6. There were 82 mortality rates, but about a third of these rates were duplicates of the same disease for different aged people.

7. Calorie intake in China is for a 65 kg adult male doing "light physical work." Comparable data for the American male is adjusted for a body weight of 65 kg.

8. SerVaas C. "Diets that protected against cancers in China." *The Saturday Evening Post* October 1990: 26–28.

9. All the available disease mortality rates were arranged in a matrix so that it was possible to readily determine the relationship of each rate with every other rate. Each comparison was then assigned a plus or minus, depending on whether they were directly or inversely correlated. All plus correlations were assembled in one list and all minus correlations were assembled in a second list. Each individual entry in either list was therefore positively related to entries in its own list but inversely related to diseases in the opposite list. Most, but not all, of these correlations were statistically significant.

10. Campbell TC, Chen J, Brun T, et al. "China: from diseases of poverty to diseases of affluence. Policy implications of the epidemiological transition." *Ecol. Food Nutr.* 27 (1992): 133–144.

11. Chen J, Campbell TC, Li J, et al. *Diet, life-style and mortality in China. A study of the characteristics of 65 Chinese counties.* Oxford, UK; Ithaca, NY; Beijing, PRC: Oxford University Press; Cornell University Press; People's Medical Publishing House, 1990.

12. Lipid Research Clinics Program Epidemiology Committee. "Plasma lipid distributions in selected North American Population. The Lipid Research Clinics Program Prevalence Study." *Circulation* 60 (1979): 427–439.

13. Campbell TC, Parpia B, and Chen J. "Diet, lifestyle, and the etiology of coronary artery disease: The Cornell China Study." *Am. J. Cardiol.* 82 (1998): 18T-21T.

14. These data are for villages SA, LC and RA for women and SA, QC and NB for men, as seen in the monograph (Chen, et al. 1990)

15. Sirtori CR, Noseda G, and Descovich GC. "Studies on the use of a soybean protein diet for the management of human hyperlipoproteinemias." *In:* M. J. Gibney and D. Kritchevsky (eds.), *Current Topics in Nutrition and Disease, Volume 8: Animal and Vegetable Proteins in Lipid Metabolism and Atherosclerosis.*, pp. 135–148. New York, NY: Alan R. Liss, Inc., 1983.

16. Carroll KK. "Dietary proteins and amino acids—their effects on cholesterol metabolism." *In:* M. J. Gibney and D. Kritchevsky (eds.), *Animal and Vegetable Proteins in Lipid Metabolism and Atherosclerosis,* pp. 9–17. New York, NY: Alan R. Liss, Inc., 1983.

17. Terpstra AHM, Hermus RJJ, and West CE. "Dietary protein and cholesterol metabolism in rabbits and rats." *In:* M. J. Gibney and D. Kritchevsky (eds.), *Animal and Vegetable Proteins in Lipid Metabolism and Athersclerosis,* pp. 19–49. New York: Alan R. Liss, Inc., 1983.

18. Kritchevsky D, Tepper SA, Czarnecki SK, et al. "Atherogenicity of animal and vegetable protein. Influence of the lysine to arginine ratio." *Atherosclerosis* 41 (1982): 429–431.

19. Dietary fat can be expressed as percent of total weight of the diet or as percent of total calories. Most commentators and researchers express fat as percent of total calories because we primarily consume food to satisfy our need for calories, not our need for weight. I will do the same throughout this book.

20. National Research Council. *Diet, Nutrition and Cancer.* Washington, DC: National Academy Press, 1982.

21. United States Department of Health and Human Services. *The Surgeon General's Report on Nutrition and Health.* Washington, DC: Superintendant of Documents, U.S. Government Printing Office, 1988.

22. National Research Council, and Committee on Diet and Health. *Diet and health: implications for reducing chronic disease risk.* Washington, DC: National Academy Press, 1989.

23. Expert Panel. *Food, nutrition and the prevention of cancer, a global perspective.* Washington, DC: American Institute for Cancer Research/World Cancer Research Fund, 1997.

24. Exceptions include those foods artificially stripped of their fat, such as non-fat milk.

25. Armstrong D, and Doll R. "Environmental factors and cancer incidence and mortality in different countries, with special reference to dietary practices." *Int. J. Cancer* 15 (1975): 617–631.

26. U.S. Senate. "Dietary goals for the United States, 2nd Edition." Washington, DC: U.S. Government Printing Office, 1977.

27. Committee on Diet Nutrition and Cancer. *Diet, nutrition and cancer: directions for research.* Washington, DC: National Academy Press, 1983.

28. There also were a number of other policy statements and large human studies that were begun at about this time that were to receive much public discussion and that were founded and/or interpreted in relation to dietary fat and these diseases. These included the initiation of the U.S. Dietary Guidelines report series begun in 1980, the Harvard Nurses' Health Study in 1984, the initial reports of the Framingham Heart Study in the 1960s, the Seven Countries Study of Ancel Keys, the Multiple Risk Factor Intervention Trial (MRFIT) and others.

29. Carroll KK, Braden LM, Bell JA, et al. "Fat and cancer." *Cancer* 58 (1986): 1818–1825.

30. Drasar BS, and Irving D. "Environmental factors and cancer of the colon and breast." *Br. J. Cancer* 27 (1973): 167–172.

31. Haenszel W, and Kurihara M. "Studies of Japanese Migrants: mortality from cancer and other disease among Japanese and the United States." *J Natl Cancer Inst* 40 (1968): 43–68.

32. Higginson J, and Muir CS. "Epidemiology in Cancer." *In:* J. F. Holland and E. Frei (eds.), *Cancer Medicine,* pp. 241–306. Philadelphia, PA: Lea and Febiger, 1973.

33. The correlation of fat intake with animal protein intake is 84% for grams of fat consumed and 70% for fat as a percent of calories.

34. Kelsey JL, Gammon MD, and Esther MJ. "Reproductive factors and breast cancer." *Epidemiol. Revs.* 15 (1993): 36–47.

35. de Stavola BL, Wang DY, Allen DS, et al. "The association of height, weight, menstrual and reproductive events with breast cancer: results from two prospective studies on the island of Guernsey (United Kingdom)." *Cancer Causes and Control* 4 (1993): 331–340.

36. Rautalahti M, Albanes D, Virtamo J, et al. "Lifetime menstrual activity—indicator of breast cancer risk." (1993): 17–25

37. It was not possible to statistically detect an association of blood hormone levels with breast cancer risk within this group of women because their blood samples were taken at random times of their menstrual cycles and breast cancer rates were so low, thus minimizing the ability to detect such an association, even when real.

38. Key TJA, Chen J, Wang DY, et al. "Sex hormones in women in rural China and in Britain." *Brit. J. Cancer* 62 (1990): 631–636.

39. These biomarkers include plasma copper, urea nitrogen, estradiol, prolactin, testosterone and, inversely, sex hormone binding globulin, each of which has been known to be associated with animal protein intake from previous studies.

40. For the total dietary fiber (TDF), the averages for China and the U.S. were 33.3 and 11.1 grams per day, respectively. The range of the county averages are 7.7–77.6 grams per day in China, compared with a range of 2.4–26.6 grams per day for the middle 90% of American males.

41. The correlation for plant protein was +0.53*** and for animal protein was +0.12.

42. In principle, using "cancer prevalence within families" as the outcome measurement more effectively controls for the various causes of cancer that associate with different kinds of cancer, thus permitting study of an isolated effect of the dietary factor.

43. Guo W, Li J, Blot WJ, et al. "Correlations of dietary intake and blood nutrient levels with esophageal cancer mortality in China." *Nutr. Cancer* 13 (1990): 121–127.

44. The full effects of these fat-soluble antioxidants can be demonstrated only when antioxidant concentrations are adjusted for the levels of LDL for individual subjects. This was not known at the time of the survey, thus provisions were not made for this adjustment.

45. Kneller RW, Guo W, Hsing AW, et al. "Risk factors for stomach cancer in sixty-five Chinese counties." *Cancer Epi. Biomarkers Prev.* 1 (1992): 113–118.

46. Information Plus. *Nutrition: a key to good health.* Wylie, TX: Information Plus, 1999.

47. Westman EC, Yancy WS, Edman JS, et al. "Carbohydrate Diet Program." *Am. J. Med.* 113 (2002): 30–36.

48. Atkins RC. *Dr. Atkins' New Diet Revolution.* New York, NY: Avon Books, 1999.

49. Wright JD, Kennedy-Stephenson J, Wang CY, et al. "Trends in Intake of Energy and Macronutrients—United States, 1971–2000." *Morbidity and mortality weekly report* 53 (February 6, 2004): 80–82.

50. Noakes M, and Clifton PM. "Weight loss and plasma lipids." *Curr. Opin. Lipidol.* 11 (2000): 65–70.

51. Bilsborough SA, and Crowe TC. "Low-carbohydrate diets: what are the potential short- and long-term health implications?" *Asia Pac. J. Clin. Nutr.* 12 (2003): 396–404.

52. Stevens A, Robinson DP, Turpin J, et al. "Sudden cardiac death of an adolescent during dieting." *South. Med. J.* 95 (2002): 1047–1049.

53. Patty A. "Low-carb fad claims teen's life - Star diet blamed in death." *The Daily Telegraph (Sidney, Australia)* November 2, 2002: 10.

54. Atkins, 1999. Page 275.

55. Atkins claims that an antioxidant cocktail can protect against heart disease, cancer and aging, a claim refuted by several large trials recently completed (see chapter 11).

56. Atkins, 1999. Page 103.

57. Bone J. "Diet doctor Atkins 'obese', had heart problems: coroner: Widow angrily denies that opponents' claims that heart condition caused by controverial diet." *Ottawa Citizen* February 11, 2004: A11.

58. Campbell TC. "Energy balance: interpretation of data from rural China." *Toxicological Sciences* 52 (1999): 87–94.

59. Horio F, Youngman LD, Bell RC, et al. "Thermogenesis, low-protein diets, and decreased development of AFB1-induced preneoplastic foci in rat liver." *Nutr. Cancer* 16 (1991): 31–41.

60. Krieger E, Youngman LD, and Campbell TC. "The modulation of aflatoxin(AFB1) induced preneoplastic lesions by dietary protein and voluntary exercise in Fischer 344 rats." *FASEB J.* 2 (1988): 3304 Abs.

61. The cited associations of total animal and plant protein intakes are taken from manuscript under review.

62. Campbell TC, Chen J, Liu C, et al. "Non-association of aflatoxin with primary liver cancer in a cross-sectional ecologic survey in the People's Republic of China." *Cancer Res.* 50 (1990): 6882–6893.

PART II

Chapter 5

1. Adams CF. "How many times does your heart beat per year?" Accessed October 20, 2003. Accessed at http://www.straightdope.com/classics/a1_088a.html

2. National Heart, Lung, and Blood Institute. "Morbidity and Mortality: 2002 Chart Book on Cardiovascular, Lung, and Blood Diseases." Bethesda, MD: National Institutes of Health, 2002.

3. American Heart Association. "Heart Disease and Stroke Statistics-2003 Update." Dallas, TX: American Heart Association, 2002.

4. Braunwald E. "Shattuck lecture-cardiovascular medicine at the turn of the millenium: triumphs, concerns and opportunities." *New Engl. J. Med.* 337 (1997): 1360–1369.

5. American Cancer Society. "Cancer Facts and Figures-1998." Atlanta, GA: American Cancer Society, 1998.

6. Anderson RN. "Deaths: leading causes for 2000." *National Vital Statistics Reports* 50(16) (2002):

7. Enos WF, Holmes RH, and Beyer J. "Coronary disease among United States soldiers killed in action in Korea." *JAMA* 152 (1953): 1090–1093.

8. Esselstyn CJ. "Resolving the coronary artery disease epidemic through plant-based nutrition." *Prev. Cardiol.* 4 (2001): 171–177.

9. Antman EM, and Braunwald E. "Acute myocardial infarction." *In:* E. Braunwald (ed.), *Heart disease, a textbook of cardiovascular disease*, Vol. II (Fifth Edition), pp. 1184–1288. Philadelphia: W.B. Saunders Company, 1997.

10. Esselstyn CJ. "Lecture: Reversing heart disease." December 5, 2002. Ithaca, NY: Cornell University, 2002.

11. Ambrose JA, and Fuster V. "Can we predict future acute coronary events in patients with stable coronary artery disease?" *JAMA* 277 (1997): 343–344.

12. Forrester JS, and Shah PK. "Lipid lowering versus revascularization: an idea whose time (for testing) has come." *Circulation* 96 (1997): 1360–1362.

13. Now named the National Heart, Lung, and Blood Institute of the National Institutes of Health in Bethesda, Maryland.

14. Gofman JW, Lindgren F, Elliot H, et al. "The role of lipids and lipoproteins in atherosclerosis." *Science* 111 (1950): 166.

15. Kannel WB, Dawber TR, Kagan A, et al. "Factors of risk in the development of coronary heart disease—six-year follow-up experience." *Ann. Internal Medi.* 55 (1961): 33–50.

16. Jolliffe N, and Archer M. "Statistical associations between international coronary heart disease death rates and certain environmental factors." *J. Chronic Dis.* 9 (1959): 636–652.
17. Scrimgeour EM, McCall MG, Smith DE, et al. "Levels of serum cholesterol, triglyceride, HDL cholesterol, apolipoproteins A-1 and B, and plasma glucose, and prevalence of diastolic hypertension and cigarette smoking in Papua New Guinea Highlanders." *Pathology* 21 (1989): 46–50.
18. Campbell TC, Parpia B, and Chen J. "Diet, lifestyle, and the etiology of coronary artery disease: The Cornell China Study." *Am. J. Cardiol.* 82 (1998): 18T–21T.
19. Kagan A, Harris BR, Winkelstein W, et al. "Epidemiologic studies of coronary heart disease and stroke in Japanese men living in Japan, Hawaii and California." *J. Chronic Dis.* 27 (1974): 345–364.
20. Kato H, Tillotson J, Nichaman MZ, et al. "Epidemiologic studies of coronary heart disease and stroke in Japanese men living in Japan, Hawaii and California: serum lipids and diet." *Am. J. Epidemiol.* 97 (1973): 372–385.
21. Morrison LM. "Arteriosclerosis." *JAMA* 145 (1951): 1232–1236.
22. Morrison LM. "Diet in coronary atherosclerosis." *JAMA* 173 (1960): 884–888.
23. Lyon TP, Yankley A, Gofman JW, et al. "Lipoproteins and diet in coronary heart disease." *California Med.* 84 (1956): 325–328.
24. Gibney MJ, and Kritchevsky D, eds. *Current Topics in Nutrition and Disease, Volume 8: Animal and Vegetable Proteins in Lipid Metabolism and Atherosclerosis.* New York, NY: Alan R. Liss, Inc., 1983.
25. Sirtori CR, Noseda G, and Descovich GC. "Studies on the use of a soybean protein diet for the management of human hyperlipoproteinemias." *In:* M. J. Gibney and D. Kritchevsky (eds.), *Current Topics in Nutrition and Disease, Volume 8: Animal and Vegetable Proteins in Lipid Metabolism and Atherosclerosis.*, pp. 135–148. New York, NY: Alan R. Liss, Inc., 1983.
26. G.S. Myers, personal communication, cited by Groom, D. "Population studies of atherosclerosis." Ann. Internal Med. 55(1961):51–62.
27. Centers for Disease Control. "Smoking and Health: a national status report." *Morbidity and Mortality Weekly Report* 35 (1986): 709–711.
28. Centers for Disease Control. "Cigarette smoking among adults—United States, 2000." *Morbidity and Mortality Weekly Report* 51 (2002): 642–645.
29. Age-adjusted, ages 25–74.
30. Marwick C. "Coronary bypass grafting economics, including rehabilitation. Commentary." *Curr. Opin. Cardiol.* 9 (1994): 635–640.
31. Page 1319 in Gersh BJ, Braunwald E, and Rutherford JD. "Chronic coronary artery disease." In: E. Braunwald (ed.), Heart Disease: A Textbook of cardiovascular medicine, Vol. 2(Fifth Edition), pp. 1289–1365. Philadelphia, PA: W.B. Saunders, 1997.
32. Ornish D. "Avoiding revascularization with lifestyle changes: the Multicenter Lifestyle Demonstration Project." *Am. J. Cardiol.* 82 (1998): 72T–76T.
33. Shaw PJ, Bates D, Cartlidge NEF, et al. "Early intellectual dysfunction following coronary bypass surgery." *Quarterly J. Med.* 58 (1986): 59–68.
34. Cameron AAC, Davis KB, and Rogers WJ. "Recurrence of angina after coronary artery bypass surgery. Predictors and prognosis (CASS registry)." *J. Am. Coll. Cardiol.* 26 (1995): 895–899.
35. Page 1320 in Gersh BJ, Braunwald E, and Rutherford JD. "Chronic coronary artery disease." In: E. Braunwald (ed.), Heart Disease: A Textbook of cardiovascular medicine, Vol. 2(Fifth Edition), pp. 1289–1365. Philadelphia, PA: W.B. Saunders, 1997.
36. Kirklin JW, Naftel DC, Blackstone EH, et al. "Summary of a consensus concerning death and ischemic events after coronary artery bypass grafting." *Circulation* 79(Suppl 1) (1989): I81–I91.
37. Page 1368–9 in Lincoff AM, and Topol EJ. "Interventional catherization techniques." In: E.

Braunwald (ed.), Heart Disease: A Textbook of Cardiovascular Medicine, pp. 1366–1391. Philadelphia, PA: W.B. Saunders, 1997.

38. Hirshfeld JW, Schwartz JS, Jugo R, et al. "Restenosis after coronary angioplasty: a multivariate statistical model to relate lesion and procedure variables to restenosis." *J. Am. Coll. Cardiol.* 18 (1991): 647–656.

39. Information Plus. *Nutrition: a key to good health.* Wylie, TX: Information Plus, 1999.

40. Naifeh SW. *The Best Doctors in America, 1994–1995.* Aiken, S.C.: Woodward & White, 1994.

41. Esselstyn CB, Jr. "Foreward: changing the treatment paradigm for coronary artery disease." *Am. J. Cardiol.* 82 (1998): 2T-4T.

42. Esselstyn CB, Ellis SG, Medendorp SV, et al. "A strategy to arrest and reverse coronary artery disease: a 5-year longitudinal study of a single physician's practice." *J. Family Practice* 41 (1995): 560–568.

43. Esselstyn CJ. "Introduction:more than coronary artery disease." *Am. J. Cardiol.* 82 (1998): 5T-9T.

44. The flow of blood is related to the fourth power of the radius. Thus, a reduction of seven percent is approximately related to a 30% greater blood flow, although it is not possible to obtain by calculation a more precise determination of this number.

45. Personal communication with Dr. Esselstyn, 9/15/03.

46. Ornish D, Brown SE, Scherwitz LW, et al. "Can lifestyle changes reverse coronary heart disease?" *Lancet* 336 (1990): 129–133.

47. Ratliff NB. "Of rice, grain, and zeal: lessons from Drs. Kempner and Esselstyn." *Cleveland Clin. J. Med.* 67 (2000): 565–566.

48. American Heart Association. "AHA Dietary Guidelines. Revision 2000: A Statement for Healthcare Professionals from the Nutrition Committee of the American Heart Association." *Circulation* 102 (2000): 2296–2311.

49. National Cholesterol Education Program. "Third report of the National Cholesterol Education Program (NCEP) expert panel on detection, evaluation and treatment of high blood cholesterol in adult (adult treatment panel III): executive summary." Bethesda, MD: National Institutes of Health, 2001.

50. Castelli W. "Take this letter to your doctor." *Prevention* 48 (1996): 61–64.

51. Schuler G, Hambrecht R, Schlierf G, et al. "Regular physical exercise and low-fat diet." *Circulation* 86 (1992): 1–11.

Chapter 6

1. Flegal KM, Carroll MD, Ogden CL, et al. "Prevalence and trends in obesity among U.S. adults, 1999–2000." *JAMA* 288 (2002): 1723–1727.

2. Ogden CL, Flegal KM, Carroll MD, et al. "Prevalence and trends in overweight among U.S. children and adolescents." *JAMA* 288 (2002): 1728–1732.

3. Dietz WH. "Health consequences of obesity in youth: childhood predictors of adult disease." *Pediatrics* 101 (1998): 518–525.

4. Fontaine KR, and Barofsky I. "Obesity and health-related quality of life." *Obesity Rev.* 2 (2001): 173–182.

5. Colditz GA. "Economic costs of obesity and inactivity." *Med. Sci. Sports Exerc.* 31 (1999): S663–S667.

6. Adcox S. "New state law seeks to cut down obesity." *Ithaca Journal* Sept. 21, 2002: 5A.

7. Ellis FR, and Montegriffo VME. "Veganism, clinical findings and investigations." *Am. J. Clin. Nutr.* 23 (1970): 249–255.

8. Berenson, G., Srinivasan, S., Bao, W., Newman, W. P. r., Tracy, R. E., and Wattigney, W. A. "Association between multiple cardiovascular risk factors and atherosclerosis to children and young adults. The Bogalusa Heart Study." *New Engl. J. Med.*, 338: 1650–1656, 1998.

9. Key TJ, Fraser GE, Thorogood M, et al. "Mortality in vegetarians and nonvegetarians: detailed findings from a collaborative analysis of 5 prospective studies." *Am. J. Clin. Nutri.* 70(Suppl.) (1999): 516S–524S.

10. Bergan JG, and Brown PT. "Nutritional status of "new" vegetarians." *J. Am. Diet. Assoc.* 76 (1980): 151–155.

11. Appleby PN, Thorogood M, Mann J, et al. "Low body mass index in non-meat eaters: the possible roles of animal fat, dietary fibre, and alcohol." *Int J. Obes.* 22 (1998): 454–460.

12. Dwyer JT. "Health aspects of vegetarian diets." *Am. J. Clin. Nutr.* 48 (1988): 712–738.

13. Key TJ, and Davey G. "Prevalence of obesity is low in people who do not eat meat." *Brit. Med. Journ.* 313 (1996): 816–817.

14. Shintani TT, Hughes CK, Beckham S, et al. "Obesity and cardiovascular risk intervention through the ad libitum feeding of traditional Hawaiian diet." *Am. J. Clin. Nutr.* 53 (1991): 1647S–1651S.

15. Barnard RJ. "Effects of life-style modification on serum lipids." *Arch. Intern. Med.* 151 (1991): 1389–1394.

16. McDougall J, Litzau K, Haver E, et al. "Rapid reduction of serum cholesterol and blood pressure by a twelve-day, very low fat, strictly vegetarian diet." *J. Am. Coll. Nutr.* 14 (1995): 491–496.

17. Ornish D, Scherwitz LW, Doody RS, et al. "Effects of stress management training and dietary changes in treating ischemic heart disease." *JAMA* 249 (1983): 54–59.

18. Shintani TT, Beckham S, Brown AC, et al. "The Hawaii diet: ad libitum high carbohydrate, low fat multi-cultural diet for the reduction of chronic disease risk factors: obesity, hypertension, hypercholesterolemia, and hyperglycemia." *Hawaii Med. Journ.* 60 (2001): 69–73.

19. Nicholson AS, Sklar M, Barnard ND, et al. "Toward improved management of NIDDM: a randomized, controlled, pilot intervention using a lowfat, vegetarian diet." *Prev. Med.* 29 (1999): 87–91.

20. Ornish D, Scherwitz LW, Billings JH, et al. "Intensive lifestyle changes for reversal of coronary heart disease." *JAMA* 280 (1998): 2001–2007.

21. Astrup A, Toubro S, Raben A, et al. "The role of low-fat diets and fat substitutes in body weight management: what have we learned from clinical studies?" *J. Am. Diet. Assoc.* 97(suppl) (1997): S82–S87.

22. Duncan KH, Bacon JA, and Weinsier RL. "The effects of high and low energy density diets on satiety, energy intake, and eating time of obese and nonobese subjects." *Am. J. Clin. Nutr.* 37 (1983): 763–767.

23. Heaton KW. "Food fibre as an obstacle to energy intake." *Lancet* (1973): 1418–1421.

24. Levin N, Rattan J, and Gilat T. "Energy intake and body weight in ovo-lacto vegetarians." *J. Clin. Gastroenterol.* 8 (1986): 451–453.

25. Campbell TC. "Energy balance: interpretation of data from rural China." *Toxicological Sciences* 52 (1999): 87–94.

26. Poehlman ET, Arciero PJ, Melby CL, et al. "Resting metabolic rate and postprandial thermogenesis in vegetarians and nonvegetarians." *Am. J. Clin. Nutr.* 48 (1988): 209–213.

27. The study by Poehlman et al. showed high oxygen consumption and higher resting metabolic rate but was badly misinterpreted by the authors. We had very similar results with experimental rats.

28. Fogelholm M, and Kukkonen-Harjula K. "Does physical activity prevent weight gain—a systematic review." *Obesity Rev.* 1 (2000): 95–111.

29. Ravussin E, Lillioja S, Anderson TE, et al. "Determinants of 24-hour energy expenditure in man. Methods and results using a respiratory chamber." *J. Clin. Invest.* 78 (1986): 1568–1578.

30. Thorburn AW, and Proietto J. "Biological determinants of spontaneous physical activity." *Obesity Rev.* 1 (2000): 87–94.

31. Krieger E, Youngman LD, and Campbell TC. "The modulation of aflatoxin(AFB1) induced preneoplastic lesions by dietary protein and voluntary exercise in Fischer 344 rats." *FASEB J.* 2 (1988): 3304 Abs.

32. Heshka S, and Allison DB. "Is obesity a disease?" *Int. J. Obesity Rel. Dis.* 25 (2001): 1401–1404.

33. Kopelman PG, and Finer N. "Reply: is obesity a disease?" *Int J. Obes.* 25 (2001): 1405–1406.

34. Campbell TC. "Are your genes hazardous to your health?" *Nutrition Advocate* 1 (1995): 1–2, 8.

35. Campbell TC. "Genetic seeds of disease. How to beat the odds." *Nutrition Advocate* 1 (1995): 1–2, 8.

36. Campbell TC. "The 'Fat Gene' dream machine." *Nutrition Advocate* 2 (1996): 1–2.

Chapter 7

1. Mokdad AH, Ford ES, Bowman BA, et al. "Diabetes trends in the U.S.: 1990–1998." *Diabetes Care* 23 (2000): 1278–1283.

2. Centers for Disease Control and Prevention. "National Diabetes Fact Sheet: General Information and National Estimates on Diabetes in the United States, 2000." Atlanta, GA: Centers for Disease Control and Prevention.

3. Griffin KL. "New lifestyles: new lifestyles, hope for kids with diabetes." *Milwaukee Journal Sentinel* 22 July 2002: 1G.

4. American Diabetes Association. "Type 2 diabetes in children and adolescents." *Diabetes Care* 23 (2000): 381–389.

5. Himsworth HP. "Diet and the incidence of diabetes mellitus." *Clin. Sci.* 2 (1935): 117–148.

6. West KM, and Kalbfleisch JM. "Glucose tolerance, nutrition, and diabetes in Uruguay, Venezuela, Malaya, and East Pakistan." *Diabetes* 15 (1966): 9–18.

7. West KM, and Kalbfleisch JM. "Influence of nutritional factors on prevalence of diabetes." *Diabetes* 20 (1971): 99–108.

8. Fraser GE. "Associations between diet and cancer, ischemic heart disease, and all-cause mortality in non-Hispanic white California Seventh-day Adventists." *Am. J. Clin. Nutr.* 70(Suppl.) (1999): 532S–538S.

9. Snowdon DA, and Phillips RL. "Does a vegetarian diet reduce the occurrence of diabetes?" *Am. J. Publ. Health* 75 (1985): 507–512.

10. Tsunehara CH, Leonetti DL, and Fujimoto WY. "Diet of second generation Japanese-American men with and without non-insulin-dependent diabetes." *Am. J. Clin. Nutri.* 52 (1990): 731–738.

11. Marshall J, Hamman RF, and Baxter J. "High-fat, low-carbohydrate diet and the etiology of non-insulin-dependent diabetes mellitus: the San Luis Valley Study." *Am. J. Epidemiol.* 134 (1991): 590–603.

12. Kittagawa T, Owada M, Urakami T, et al. "Increased incidence of non-insulin-dependent diabetes mellitus among Japanese schoolchildren correlates with an increased intake of animal protein and fat." *Clin. Pediatr.* 37 (1998): 111–116.

13. Trowell H. "Diabetes mellitus death-rates in England and Wales 1920–1970 and food supplies." *Lancet* 2 (1974): 998–1002.

14. Meyer KA, Kushi LH, Jacobs DR, Jr., et al. "Carbohydrates, dietary fiber, and incident Type 2 diabetes in older women." *Am. J. Clin. Nutri.* 71 (2000): 921–930.

15. Anderson JW. "Dietary fiber in nutrition management of diabetes." *In:* G. Vahouny, V. and D. Kritchevsky (eds.), *Dietary Fiber: Basic and Clinical Aspects,* pp. 343–360. New York: Plenum Press, 1986.

16. Anderson JW, Chen WL, and Sieling B. "Hypolipidemic effects of high-carbohydrate, high-fiber diets." *Metabolism* 29 (1980): 551–558.

17. Story L, Anderson JW, Chen WL, et al. "Adherence to high-carbohydrate, high-fiber diets: long-term studies of non-obese diabetic men." *Journ. Am. Diet. Assoc.* 85 (1985): 1105–1110.

18. Barnard RJ, Lattimore L, Holly RG, et al. "Response of non-insulin-dependent diabetic patients to an intensive program of diet and exercise." *Diabetes Care* 5 (1982): 370–374.

19. Barnard RJ, Massey MR, Cherny S, et al. "Long-term use of a high-complex-carbohydrate, high-fiber, low-fat diet and exercise in the treatment of NIDDM patients." *Diabetes Care* 6 (1983): 268–273.

20. Anderson JW, Gustafson NJ, Bryant CA, et al. "Dietary fiber and diabetes: a comprehensive review and practical application." *J. Am. Diet. Assoc.* 87 (1987): 1189–1197.

21. Jenkins DJA, Wolever TMS, Bacon S, et al. "Diabetic diets: high carbohydrate combined with high fiber." *Am. J. Clin. Nutri.* 33 (1980): 1729–1733.

22. Diabetes Prevention Program Research Group. "Reduction in the incidence of Type 2 diabetes with lifestyle intervention or Metformin." *New Engl. J. Med.* 346 (2002): 393–403.

23. Tuomilehto J, Lindstrom J, Eriksson JG, et al. "Prevention of Type 2 diabetes mellitus by changes in lifestyle among subjects with impaired glucose tolerance." *New Engl. J. Med.* 344 (2001): 1343–1350.

Chapter 8

1. Estrogen present in its free, unbound form.

2. Estrogen activity is due to more than one analogue, but usually refers to estradiol. I will use the general term "estrogen" to include all steroid and related female hormones whose effects parallel estradiol activity. A small amount of testosterone in women also shows the same effect.

3. Wu AH, Pike MC, and Stram DO. "Meta-analysis: dietary fat intake, serum estrogen levels, and the risk of breast cancer." *J. Nat. Cancer Inst.* 91 (1999): 529–534.

4. Bernstein L, and Ross RK. "Endogenous hormones and breast cancer risk." *Epidemiol. Revs.* 15 (1993): 48–65.

5. Pike MC, Spicer DV, Dahmoush L, et al. "Estrogens, progestogens, normal breast cell proliferation, and breast cancer risk." *Epidemiol. Revs.* 15 (1993): 17–35.

6. Bocchinfuso WP, Lindzey JK, Hewitt SC, et al. "Induction of mammary gland development in estrogen receptor-alpha knockout mice." *Endocrinology* 141 (2000): 2982–2994.

7. Atwood CS, Hovey RC, Glover JP, et al. "Progesterone induces side-branching of the ductal epithelium in the mammary glands of peripubertal mice." *J. Endocrinol.* 167 (2000): 39–52.

8. Rose DP, and Pruitt BT. "Plasma prolactin levels in patients with breast cancer." *Cancer* 48 (1981): 2687–2691.

9. Dorgan JF, Longcope C, Stephenson HE, Jr., et al. "Relation of prediagnostic serum estrogen and androgen levels to breast cancer risk." *Cancer Epidemiol Biomarkers Prev* 5 (1996): 533–539.

10. Dorgan JF, Stanczyk FZ, Longcope C, et al. "Relationship of serum dehydroepiandrosterone (DHEA), DHEA sulfate, and 5-androstene-3 beta, 17 beta-diol to risk of breast cancer in postmenopausal women." *Cancer Epidemiol Biomarkers Prev* 6 (1997):

11. Thomas HV, Key TJ, Allen DS, et al. "A prospective study of endogenous serum hormone concentrations and breast cancer risk in post-menopausal women on the island of Guernsey." *Brit. J. Cancer* 76 (1997): 410–405.

12. Hankinson SE, Willett W, Manson JE, et al. "Plasma sex steroid hormone levels and risk of breast cancer in postmenopausal women." *J. Nat. Cancer Inst.* 90 (1998): 1292–1299.

13. Rosenthal MB, Barnard RJ, Rose DP, et al. "Effects of a high-complex-carbohydrate, low-fat, low-cholesterol diet on levels of serum lipids and estradiol." *Am. J. Med.* 78 (1985): 23–27.

14. Adlercreutz H. "Western diet and Western diseases: some hormonal and biochemical mechanisms and associations." *Scand. J. Clin. Lab. Invest.* 50(Suppl.201) (1990): 3–23.

15. Heber D, Ashley JM, Leaf DA, et al. "Reduction of serum estradiol in postmenopausal women given free access to low-fat high-carbohydrate diet." *Nutrition* 7 (1991): 137–139.
16. Rose DP, Goldman M, Connolly JM, et al. "High-fiber diet reduces serum estrogen concentrations in premenopausal women." *Am. J. Clin. Nutr.* 54 (1991): 520–525.
17. Rose DP, Lubin M, and Connolly JM. "Efects of diet supplementation with wheat bran on serum estrogen levels in the follicular and luteal phases of the menstrual cycle." *Nutrition* 13 (1997): 535–539.
18. Tymchuk CN, Tessler SB, and Barnard RJ. "Changes in sex hormone-binding globulin, insulin, and serum lipids in postmenopausal women on a low-fat, high-fiber diet combined with exercise." *Nutr. Cancer* 38 (2000): 158–162.
19. Key TJA, Chen J, Wang DY, et al. "Sex hormones in women in rural China and in Britain." *Brit. J. Cancer* 62 (1990): 631–636.
20. Prentice R, Thompson D, Clifford C, et al. "Dietary fat reduction and plasma estradiol concentration in healthy postmenopausal women." *J. Natl. Cancer Inst.* 82 (1990): 129–134.
21. Boyar AP, Rose DP, and Wynder EL. "Recommendations for the prevention of chronic disease: the application for breast disease." *Am. J. Clin. Nutr.* 48(3 Suppl) (1988): 896–900.
22. Nandi S, Guzman RC, and Yang J. "Hormones and mammary carcinogenesis in mice, rats and humans: a unifying hypothesis." *Proc. National Acad. Sci* 92 (1995): 3650–3657.
23. Peto J, Easton DF, Matthews FE, et al. "Cancer mortality in relatives of women with breast cancer, the OPCS study." *Int. J. Cancer* 65 (1996): 275–283.
24. Colditz GA, Willett W, Hunter DJ, et al. "Family history, age, and risk of breast cancer. Prospective data from the Nurses' Health Study." *JAMA* 270 (1993): 338–343.
25. National Human Genome Research Institute. "Learning About Breast Cancer." Accessed at http://www.genome.gov/10000507#ql
26. Futreal PA, Liu Q, Shattuck-Eidens D, et al. "BRCA1 mutations in primary breast and ovarian carcinomas." *Science* 266 (1994): 120–122.
27. Miki Y, Swensen J, Shatttuck-Eidens D, et al. "A strong candidate for the breast and ovarian cancer susceptibility gene BRCA1." *Science* 266 (1994): 66–71.
28. Wooster R, Bignell G, Lancaster J, et al. "Identification of the breast cancer susceptibility gene BRCA2." *Nature* 378 (1995): 789–792.
29. Tavtigian SV, Simard J, Rommens J, et al. "The complete BRCA2 gene and mutations in chromosome 13q-linked kindreds." *Nat. Genet.* 12 (1996): 333–337.
30. Ford D, Easton D, Bishop DT, et al. "Risks of cancer in BRCA1 mutation carriers." *Lancet* 343 (1994): 692–695.
31. Antoniou A, Pharoah PDP, Narod S, et al. "Average risks of breast and ovarian cancer associated with BRCA1 or BRCA2 mutations detected in case series unselected for family history: a combined analysis of 22 studies." *Am. J. Hum. Genet.* 72 (2003): 1117–1130.
32. Newman B, Mu H, Butler LM, et al. "Frequency of breast cancer attributable to BRCA1 in a population-based series of American women." *JAMA* 279 (1998): 915–921.
33. Peto J, Collins N, Barfoot R, et al. "Prevalence of BRCA1 and BRCA2 gene mutations in patients with early-onset breast cancer." *J. Nat. Cancer Inst.* 91 (1999): 943–949.
34. Tabar L, Fagerberg G, Chen HH, et al. "Efficacy of breast cancer screening by age. New results from the Swedish Two-County Trial." *Cancer* 75 (1995): 2507–2517.
35. Bjurstram N, Bjorneld L, Duffy SW, et al. "The Gothenburg Breast Cancer Screening Trial: first results on mortality, incidence, and mode of detection for women ages 39–49 years at randomization." *Cancer* 80 (1997): 2091–2099.
36. Frisell J, Lidbrink E, Hellstrom L, et al. "Follow-up after 11 years: update of mortality results in the Stockholm mammographic screening trial." *Breast Cancer Res. Treat 1997* 45 (1997): 263–270.
37. Greenlee RT, Hill-Harmon MB, Murray T, et al. "Cancer statistics, 2001." *CA Cancer J. Clin.* 51 (2001): 15–36.

38. Cairns J. "The treatment of diseases and the War against Cancer." *Sci. Am.* 253 (1985): 31–39.

39. Cuzick J, and Baum M. "Tamoxifen and contralateral breast cancer." *Lancet* 2 (1985): 282.

40. Cuzick J, Wang DY, and Bulbrook RD. "The prevention of breast cancer." *Lancet* 1 (1986): 83–86.

41. Fisher B, Costantino JP, Wickerham DL, et al. "Tamoxifen for prevention of breast cancer: report of the National Surgical Adjuvant Breast and Bowel Project P-1 Study." *J. Nat. Cancer Inst.* 90 (1998): 1371–1388.

42. Freedman AN, Graubard BI, Rao SR, et al. "Estimates of the number of U.S. women who could benefit from tamoxifen for breast cancer chemoprevention." *J. Nat. Cancer Inst.* 95 (2003): 526–532.

43. Powles T, Eeles R, Ashley S, et al. "Interim analysis of the incidence of breast cancer in the Royal Marsden Hospital tamoxifen randomised chemoprevention trial." *Lancet* 352 (1998): 98–101.

44. Veronesi U, Maisonneuve P, Costa A, et al. "Prevention of breast cancer with tamoxifen: preliminary findings from the Italian randomised trial among hysterectomised women." *Lancet* 352 (1998): 93–97.

45. Cuzick J. "A brief review of the current breast cancer prevention trials and proposals for future trials." *Eur J Cancer* 36 (2000): 1298–1302.

46. Cummings SR, Eckert S, Krueger KA, et al. "The effect of raloxifene on risk of breast cancer in postmenopausal women: results from the MORE randomized trial." *JAMA* 281 (1999): 2189–2197.

47. Dorgan JF, Hunsberger S, A., McMahon RP, et al. "Diet and sex hormones in girls: findings from a randomized controlled clinical trial." *J. Nat. Cancer Inst.* 95 (2003): 132–141.

48. Ornish D, Scherwitz LW, Billings JH, et al. "Intensive lifestyle changes for reversal of coronary heart disease." *JAMA* 280 (1998): 2001–2007.

49. Esselstyn CB, Ellis SG, Medendorp SV, et al. "A strategy to arrest and reverse coronary artery disease: a 5-year longitudinal study of a single physician's practice." *J. Family Practice* 41 (1995): 560–568.

50. Hildenbrand GLG, Hildenbrand LC, Bradford K, et al. "Five-year survival rates of melanoma patients treated by diet therapy after the manner of Gerson: a retrospective review." *Alternative Therapies in Health and Medicine* 1 (1995): 29–37.

51. Youngman LD, and Campbell TC. "Inhibition of aflatoxin B1-induced gamma-glutamyl transpeptidase positive (GGT+) hepatic preneoplastic foci and tumors by low protein diets: evidence that altered GGT+ foci indicate neoplastic potential." *Carcinogenesis* 13 (1992): 1607–1613.

52. Ronai Z, Gradia S, El-Bayoumy K, et al. "Contrasting incidence of ras mutations in rat mammary and mouse skin tumors induced by anti-benzo[c]phenanthrene-3,4-diol-1,2-epoxide." *Carcinogensis* 15 (1994): 2113–2116.

53. Jeffy BD, Schultz EU, Selmin O, et al. "Inhibition of BRCA-1 expression by benzo[a]pyrene and diol epoxide." *Mol. Carcinogenesis* 26 (1999): 100–118.

54. Gammon MD, Santella RM, Neugut AI, et al. "Environmental toxins and breast cancer on Long Island. I. Polycyclic aromatic hydrocarbon DNA adducts." *Cancer Epidemiol Biomarkers Prev* 11 (2002): 677–685.

55. Gammon MD, Wolff MS, Neugut AI, et al. "Environmental toxins and breast cancer on Long Island. II. Organchlorine compound levels in blood." *Cancer Epidemiol Biomarkers Prev* 11 (2002): 686–697.

56. Humphries KH, and Gill S. "Risks and benefits of hormone replacement therapy: the evidence speaks." *Canadian Med. Assoc. Journ.* 168 (2003): 1001–1010.

57. Writing Group for the Women's Health Initiative Investigators. "Risks and benefits of estro-

gen plus progestin in healthy postmenopausal women: principal results from the Women's Health Initiative Randomized Controlled Trial." *JAMA* 288 (2002): 321–333.

58. Hulley S, Grady D, Bush T, et al. "Randomized trial of estrogen plus progestin for secondary prevention of coronary heart disease in postmenopausal women. Heart and Estrogen/progestin Replacement Study (HERS) Research Group." *JAMA* 280 (1998): 605–613.

59. While this finding is not statistically significant, its consistency with the WHI finding is striking.

60. International Agency for Cancer Research. "Globocan" (accessed 18 October 2002), http://www-dep.iarc/globocan.html."

61. Kinzler KW, and Vogelstein B. "Lessons from Heredity. Colorectal Cancer." *Cell* 87 (1996): 159–170.

62. Ferlay J, Bray F, Pisani P, et al. *GLOBOCAN 2000: Cancer Incidence, mortality and prevalence worldwide, Version 1.0.* Lyon, France: IARCPress, 2001.

63. Limited version of Ferlay et al. document available at http://www.dep.iarc.fr/globocan/globocan.htm, last updated on 03/02/2001.

64. Expert Panel. *Food, nutrition and the prevention of cancer, a global perspective.* Washington, DC: American Institute for Cancer Research/World Cancer Research Fund, 1997.

65. Armstrong D, and Doll R. "Environmental factors and cancer incidence and mortality in different countries, with special reference to dietary practices." *Int. J. Cancer* 15 (1975): 617–631.

66. Burkitt DP. "Epidemiology of cancer of the colon and the rectum." *Cancer* 28 (1971): 3–13.

67. Jansen MCJF, Bueno-de-Mesquita HB, Buzina R, et al. "Dietary fiber and plant foods in relation to colorectal cancer mortality: The Seven Countries Study." *Int. J. Cancer* 81 (1999): 174–179.

68. Whiteley LO, and Klurfeld DM. "Are dietary fiber-induced alterations in colonic epithelial cell proliferation predictive of fiber's effect on colon cancer?" *Nutr. Cancer* 36 (2000): 131–149.

69. Most of these associations were not statistically significant, but the consistency of the inverse association between fiber and colorectal cancer was impressive.

70. Campbell TC, Wang G, Chen J, et al. "Dietary fiber intake and colon cancer mortality in The People's Republic of China." In: D. Kritchevsky, C. Bonfield and J. W. Anderson (eds.), *Dietary Fiber*, pp. 473–480. New York, NY: Plenum Publishing Corporation, 1990.

71. Trock B, Lanza E, and Greenwald P. "Dietary fiber, vegetables, and colon cancer: critical review and meta-analysis of the epidemiologic evidence." *J. Nat. Cancer Inst.* 82 (1990): 650–661.

72. Howe GR, Benito E, Castelleto R, et al. "Dietary intake of fiber and decreased risk of cancers of the colon and rectum: evidence from the combined analysis of 13 case-control studies." *J. Nat. Cancer Inst.* 84 (1992): 1887–1896.

73. Bingham SA, Day NE, Luben R, et al. "Dietary fibre in food and protection against colorectal cancer in the European Prospective Investigation into Cancer and Nutrition (EPIC): an observational study." *Lancet* 361 (2003): 1496–1501.

74. O'Keefe SJD, Ndaba N, and Woodward A. "Relationship between nutritional status, dietary intake patterns and plasma lipoprotein concentrations in rural black South Africans." *Hum. Nutr. Clin. Nutr.* 39 (1985): 335–341.

75. Sitas F. "Histologically diagnosed cancers in South Africa, 1988." *S. African Med. J.* 84 (1994): 344–348.

76. O'Keefe SJD, Kidd M, Espitalier-Noel G, et al. "Rarity of colon cancer in Africans is associated with low animal product consumption, not fiber." *Am. J. Gastroenterology* 94 (1999): 1373–1380.

77. McKeown-Eyssen G. "Epidemiology of colorectal cancer revisited: are serum triglycerides

and/or plasma glucose associated with risk?" *Cancer Epidemiol Biomarkers Prev* 3 (1994): 687–695.

78. Giovannucci E. "Insulin and colon cancer." *Cancer Causes and Control* 6 (1995): 164–179.

79. Bruce WR, Giacca A, and Medline A. "Possible mechanisms relating diet and risk of colon cancer." *Cancer Epidemiol Biomarkers Prev* 9 (2000): 1271–1279.

80. Kono S, Honjo S, Todoroki I, et al. "Glucose intolerance and adenomas of the sigmoid colon in Japanese men (Japan)." *Cancer Causes and Control* 9 (1998): 441–446.

81. Schoen RE, Tangen CM, Kuller LH, et al. "Increased blood glucose and insulin, body size, and incident colorectal cancer." *J. Nat. Cancer Inst.* 91 (1999): 1147–1154.

82. Bruce WR, Wolever TMS, and Giacca A. "Mechanisms linking diet and colorectal cancer: the possible role of insulin resistance." *Nutr. Cancer* 37 (2000): 19–26.

83. Lipkin M, and Newmark H. "Development of clinical chemoprevention trials." *J. Nat. Cancer Inst.* 87 (1995): 1275–1277.

84. Holt PR, Atillasoy EO, Gilman J, et al. "Modulation of abnormal colonic epithelial cell proliferation and differentiation by low-fat dairy foods. A randomized trial." *JAMA* 280 (1998): 1074–1079.

85. Mobarhan S. "Calcium and the colon: recent findings." *Nutr. Revs.* 57 (1999): 124–126.

86. Alberts DS, Ritenbuagh C, Story JA, et al. "Randomized, double-blinded, placebo-controlled study of effect of wheat bran fiber and calcium on fecal bile acids in patients with resected adenomatous colon polyps." *J. Nat. Cancer Inst.* 88 (1996): 81–92.

87. Chen J, Campbell TC, Li J, et al. *Diet, life-style and mortality in China. A study of the characteristics of 65 Chinese counties.* Oxford, UK; Ithaca, NY; Beijing, PRC: Oxford University Press; Cornell University Press; People's Medical Publishing House, 1990.

88. Jass JR. "Colon cancer: the shape of things to come." *Gut* 45 (1999): 794–795.

89. Burt RW. "Colon cancer screening." *Gastroenterology* 119 (2000): 837–853.

90. Winawer SJ, Zauber AG, Ho MN, et al. "Prevention of colorectal cancer by colonoscopic polypectomy." *New Engl. J. Med.* 329 (1993): 1977–1981.

91. Pignone M, Rich M, Teutsch SM, et al. "Screening for colorectal cancer in adults at average risk: a summary of the evidence for the U.S. Preventive Services Task Force." *Ann. Internal Med.* 137 (2002): 132–141.

92. Scott RJ, and Sobol HH. "Prognostic implications of cancer susceptibility genes: Any news?" *Recent Results in Cancer Research* 151 (1999): 71–84.

93. Lee ML, Wang R-T, Hsing AW, et al. "Case-control study of diet and prostate cancer in China." *Cancer Causes and Control* 9 (1998): 545–552.

94. Villers A, Soulie M, Haillot O, et al. "Prostate cancer screening (III): risk factors, natural history, course without treatment." *Progr. Urol.* 7 (1997): 655–661.

95. Stanford JL. "Prostate cancer trends 1973–1995." Bethesda, MD: SEER Program, National Cancer Institute, 1998.

96. Chan JM, and Giovannucci EL. "Dairy products, calcium, and vitamin D and risk of prostate cancer." *Epidemiol. Revs.* 23 (2001): 87–92.

97. Giovannucci E. "Dietary influences of 1,25 (OH)$_2$ vitamin D in relation to prostate cancer: a hypothesis." *Cancer Causes and Control* 9 (1998): 567–582.

98. Chan JM, Stampfer MJ, Ma J, et al. "Insulin-like growth factor-I (IGF-I) and IGF binding protein-3 as predictors of advanced-stage prostate cancer." *J Natl Cancer Inst* 94 (2002): 1099–1109.

99. Doi SQ, Rasaiah S, Tack I, et al. "Low-protein diet suppresses serum insulin-like growth factor-1 and decelerates the progresseion of growth hormone-induced glomerulosclerosis." *Am. J. Nephrol.* 21 (2001): 331–339.

100. Heaney RP, McCarron DA, Dawson-Hughes B, et al. "Dietary changes favorably affect bond remodeling in older adults." *J. Am. Diet. Assoc.* 99 (1999): 1228–1233.

101. Allen NE, Appleby PN, Davey GK, et al. "Hormones and diet: low insulin-like growth factor-I but normal bioavailable androgens in vegan men." *Brit. J. Cancer* 83 (2000): 95–97.

102. Cohen P, Peehl DM, and Rosenfeld RG. "The IGF axis in the prostate." *Horm. Metab. res.* 26 (1994): 81–84.

Chapter 9

1. Mackay IR. "Tolerance and immunity." *Brit. Med. Journ.* 321 (2000): 93–96.

2. Jacobson DL, Gange SJ, Rose NR, et al. "Short analytical review. Epidemiology and estimated population burden of selected autoimmune diseases in the United States." *Clin. Immunol. Immunopath.* 84 (1997): 223–243.

3. Davidson A, and Diamond B. "Autoimmune diseases." *New Engl. J. Med.* 345 (2001): 340–350.

4. Aranda R, Sydora BC, McAllister PL, et al. "Analysis of intestinal lymphocytes in mouse colitis mediated by transfer of CD4+, CD45RB^high T cells to SCID recipients." *J. Immunol.* 158 (1997): 3464–3473.

5. Folgar S, Gatto EM, Raina G, et al. "Parkinsonism as a manifestation of multiple sclerosis." *Movement Disorders* 18 (2003): 108–113.

6. Cantorna MT. "Vitamin D and autoimmunity: is vitamin D status an environmental factor affecting autoimmune disease prevalence?" *Proc. Soc. Exp. Biol. Med.* 223 (2000): 230–233.

7. DeLuca HF, and Cantorna MT. "Vitamin D: its role and uses in immunology." *FASEB J.* 15 (2001): 2579–2585.

8. Winer S, Astsaturov I, Cheung RK, et al. "T cells of multiple sclerosis patients target a common environmental peptide that causes encephalitis in mice." *J. Immunol.* 166 (2001): 4751–4756.

9. Davenport CB. "Multiple sclerosis from the standpoint of geographic distribution and race." *Arch. Neurol. Pschiatry* 8 (1922): 51–58.

10. Alter M, Yamoor M, and Harshe M. "Multiple sclerosis and nutrition." *Arch. Neurol.* 31 (1974): 267–272.

11. Carroll M. "Innate immunity in the etiopathology of autoimmunity." *Nature Immunol.* 2 (2001): 1089–1090.

12. Karjalainen J, Martin JM, Knip M, et al. "A bovine albumin peptide as a possible trigger of insulin-dependent Diabetes Mellitus." *New Engl. Journ. Med.* 327 (1992): 302–307.

13. Akerblom HK, and Knip M. "Putative environmental factors and Type 1 diabetes." *Diabetes/Metabolism Revs.* 14 (1998): 31–67.

14. Naik RG, and Palmer JP. "Preservation of beta-cell function in Type 1 diabetes." *Diabetes Rev.* 7 (1999): 154–182.

15. Virtanen SM, Rasanen L, Aro A, et al. "Infant feeding in Finnish children less than 7 yr of age with newly diagnosed IDDM. Childhood diabetes in Finland Study Group." *Diabetes Care* 14 (1991): 415–417.

16. Savilahti E, Akerblom HK, Tainio V-M, et al. "Children with newly diagnosed insulin dependent diabetes mellitus have increased levels of cow's milk antibodies." *Diabetes Res.* 7 (1988): 137–140.

17. Yakota A, Yamaguchi T, Ueda T, et al. "Comparison of islet cell antibodies, islet cell surface antibodies and anti-bovine serum albumin antibodies in Type 1 diabetes." *Diabetes Res. Clin. Pract.* 9 (1990): 211–217.

18. Hammond-McKibben D, and Dosch H-M. "Cow's milk, bovine serum albumin, and IDDM: can we settle the controversies?" *Diabetes Care* 20 (1997): 897–901.

19. Akerblom HK, Vaarala O, Hyoty H, et al. "Environmental factors in the etiology of Type 1 diabetes." *Am. J. Med. Genet. (Semin. Med. Genet.)* 115 (2002): 18–29.

20. Gottlieb MS, and Root HF. "Diabetes mellitus in twins." *Diabetes* 17 (1968): 693–704.

21. Barnett AH, Eff C, Leslie RDG, et al. "Diabetes in identical twins: a study of 200 pairs." *Diabetologia* 20 (1981): 87–93.
22. Borch-Johnsen K, Joner G, Mandrup-Poulsen T, et al. "Relation between breast feeding and incidence rates of insulin-dependent diabetes mellitus: a hypothesis." *Lancet* 2 (1984): 1083–1086.
23. Perez-Bravo F, Carrasco E, Gutierrez-Lopez MD, et al. "Genetic predisposition and environmental factors leading to the development of insulin-dependent diabetes mellitus in Chilean children." *J. Mol. Med.* 74 (1996): 105–109.
24. Kostraba JN, Cruickshanks KJ, Lawler-Heavner J, et al. "Early exposure to cow's milk and solid foods in infancy, genetic predisposition, and risk of IDDM." *Diabetes* 42 (1993): 288–295.
25. Pyke DA. "The genetic perspective: putting research into practice." *In:* Diabetes 1988, Amsterdam, 1989, pp. 1227–1230.
26. Kaprio J, Tuomilehto J, Koskenvuo M, et al. "Concordance for Type 1 (insulin-dependent) and Type 2 (non-insulin-dependent) diabetes mellitus in a population-based cohort of twins in Finland." *Diabetologia* 35 (1992): 1060–1067.
27. Dahl-Jorgensen K, Joner G, and Hanssen KF. "Relationship between cow's milk consumption and incidence of IDDM in childhood." *Diabetes Care* 14 (1991): 1081–1083.
28. The proportion of Type 1 diabetes due to the consumption of cow's milk, the r2 value, is 96%.
29. LaPorte RE, Tajima N, Akerblom HK, et al. "Geographic differences in the risk of insulin-dependent diabetes mellitus: the importance of registries." *Diabetes Care* 8(Suppl. 1) (1985): 101–107.
30. Bodansky HJ, Staines A, Stephenson C, et al. "Evidence for an environmental effect in the aetiology of insulin dependent diabetes in a transmigratory population." *Brit. Med. Journ.* 304 (1992): 1020–1022.
31. Burden AC, Samanta A, and Chaunduri KH. "The prevalence and incidence of insulin-dependent diabetes in white and Indian children in Leicester city (UK)." *Int. J. Diabetes Dev. Countries* 10 (1990): 8–10.
32. Elliott R, and Ong TJ. "Nutritional genomics." *Brit. Med. Journ.* 324 (2002): 1438–1442.
33. Onkamo P, Vaananen S, Karvonen M, et al. "Worldwide increase in incidence of Type 1 diabetes—the analysis of the data on published incidence trends." *Diabetologia* 42 (1999): 1395–1403.
34. Gerstein HC. "Cow's milk exposure and Type 1 diabetes mellitus: a critical overview of the clinical literature." *Diabetes Care* 17 (1994): 13–19.
35. Kimpimaki T, Erkkola M, Korhonen S, et al. "Short-term exclusive breastfeeding predisposes young children with increased genetic risk of Type 1 diabetes to progressive beta-cell autoimmunity." *Diabetologia* 44 (2001): 63–69.
36. Virtanen SM, Laara E, Hypponen E, et al. "Cow's milk consumption, HLA-DQB1 genotype, and Type 1 diabetes." *Diabetes* 49 (2000): 912–917.
37. Monetini L, Cavallo MG, Stefanini L, et al. "Bovine beta-casein antibodies in breast- and bottle-fed infants: their relevance in Type 1 diabetes." *Diabetes Metab. Res. Rev.* 17 (2001): 51–54.
38. Norris JM, and Pietropaolo M. "Review article. Controversial topics series: milk proteins and diabetes." *J. Endocrinol. Invest.* 22 (1999): 568–580.
39. Reingold SC. "Research Directions in Multiple Sclerosis." National Multiple Sclerosis Society, November 25, 2003. Accessed at http://www.nationalmssociety.org/%5CBrochures-Research.asp
40. Ackermann A. "Die multiple sklerose in der Schweiz." *Schweiz. med. Wchnschr.* 61 (1931): 1245–1250.
41. Swank RL. "Multiple sclerosis: correlation of its incidence with dietary fat." *Am. J. Med. Sci.* 220 (1950): 421–430.

42. Dip JB. "The distribution of multiple sclerosis in relation to the dairy industry and milk consumption." *New Zealand Med. J.* 83 (1976): 427–430.

43. McDougall JM. 2002. *Multiple sclerosis stopped by McDougall/Swank Program.* http://www.nealhendrickson.com/McDougall/McDnewannouncementSwank021112.htm. Accessed Nov. 16, 2002.

44. McLeod JG, Hammond SR, and Hallpike JF. "Epidemiology of multiple sclerosis in Australia. With NSW and SA survey results." *Med. J. Austr* 160 (1994): 117–122.

45. Lawrence JS, Behrend T, Bennett PH, et al. "Geographical studies of rheumatoid arthritis." *Ann. Rheum. Dis.* 25 (1966): 425–432.

46. Keen H, and Ekoe JM. "The geography of diabetes mellitus." *Brit. Med. Journ.* 40 (1984): 359–365.

47. Swank RL. "Effect of low saturated fat diet in early and late cases of multiple sclerosis." *Lancet* 336 (1990): 37–39.

48. Swank RL. "Treatment of multiple sclerosis with low fat diet." *A.M.A. Arch. Neurol. Psychiatry* 69 (1953): 91–103.

49. Swank RL, and Bourdillon RB. "Multiple sclerosis: assessment of treatment with modified low fat diet." *J. Nerv. Ment. Dis.* 131 (1960): 468–488.

50. Swank RL. "Multiple sclerosis: twenty years on low fat diet." *Arch. Neurol.* 23 (1970): 460–474.

51. Agranoff BW, and Goldberg D. "Diet and the geographical distribution of multiple sclerosis." *Lancet* 2(7888) (November 2 1974): 1061–1066.

52. Malosse D, Perron H, Sasco A, et al. "Correlation between milk and dairy product consumption and multiple sclerosis prevalence: a worldwide study." *Neuroepidemiology* 11 (1992): 304–312.

53. Malosse D, and Perron H. "Correlation analysis between bovine populations, other farm animals, house pets, and multiple sclerosis prevalence." *Neuroepidemiology* 12 (1993): 15–27.

54. Lauer K. "Diet and multiple sclerosis." *Neurology* 49(suppl 2) (1997): S55–S61.

55. Swank RL, Lerstad O, Strom A, et al. "Multiple sclerosis in rural Norway. Its geographic distribution and occupational incidence in relation to nutrition." *New Engl. J. Med.* 246 (1952): 721–728.

56. Dalgleish AG. "Viruses and multiple sclerosis." *Acta Neurol. Scand.* Suppl. 169 (1997): 8–15.

57. McAlpine D, Lumsden CE, and Acheson ED. *Multiple sclerosis: a reappraisal.* Edinburgh and London: E&S Livingston, 1965.

58. Alter M, Liebowitz U, and Speer J. "Risk of multiple sclerosis related to age at immigration to Israel." *Arch. Neurol.* 15 (1966): 234–237.

59. Kurtzke JF, Beebe GW, and Norman JE, Jr. "Epidemiology of multiple sclerosis in U.S. veterans: 1. Race, sex, and geographic distribution." *Neurology* 29 (1979): 1228–1235.

60. Ebers GC, Bulman DE, Sadovnick AD, et al. "A population-based study of multiple sclerosis in twins." *New Engl. J. Med.* 315 (1986): 1638–1642.

61. Acheson ED, Bachrach CA, and Wright FM. "Some comments on the relationship of the distribution of multiple sclerosis to latitude solar radiation and other variables." *Acta Psychiatrica Neurologica Scand.* 35 (Suppl.147) (1960): 132–147.

62. Warren S, and Warren KG. "Multiple sclerosis and associated diseases: a relationship to diabetes mellitus." *J. Canadian Sci. Neurol.* 8 (1981): 35–39.

63. Wertman E, Zilber N, and Abransky O. "An association between multiple sclerosis and Type 1 diabetes mellitus." *J. Neurol.* 239 (1992): 43–45.

64. Marrosu MG, Cocco E, Lai M, et al. "Patients with multiple sclerosis and risk of Type 1 diabetes mellitus in Sardinia, Italy: a cohort study." *Lancet* 359 (2002): 1461–1465.

65. Buzzetti R, Pozzilli P, Di Mario U, et al. "Multiple sclerosis and Type 1 diabetes." *Diabetologia* 45 (2002): 1735–1736.

66. Lux WE, and Kurtzke JF. "Is Parkinson's disease acquired? Evidence from a geographic comparison with multiple sclerosis." *Neurology* 37 (1987): 467–471.

67. Prahalad S, Shear ES, Thompson SD, et al. "Increased Prevalence of Familial Autoimmunity in Simplex and Multiplex Families with Juvenile Rheumatoid Arthritis." *Arthritis Rheumatism* 46 (2002): 1851–1856.

68. Cantorna MT, Munsick C, Bemiss C, et al. "1,25-Dihydroxycholecalciferol Prevents and Ameliorates Symptoms of Experimental Murine Inflammatory Bowel Disease." *J. Nutr.* 130 (2000): 2648–2652.

69. Cantorna MT, Woodward WD, Hayes CE, et al. "1,25-Dihydroxyvitamin D_3 is a positive regulator for the two anti-encephalitogenic cytokines TGF-B1 and IL-4." *J Immunol.* 160 (1998): 5314–5319.

70. Cantorna MT, Humpal-Winter J, and DeLuca HF. "Dietary calcium is a major factor in 1,25-dihydroxycholecalciferol suppression of experimental autoimmune encephalomyelitis in mice." *J. Nutr.* 129 (1999): 1966–1971.

71. Multiple Sclerosis International Federation. "Alternative Therapies." November 25, 2003. Accessed at http://www.msif.org/en/symptoms_treatments/treatment_overview/alternative.html

Chapter 10

1. Frassetto LA, Todd KM, Morris C, Jr., et al. "Worldwide incidence of hip fracture in elderly women: relation to consumption of animal and vegetable foods." *J. Gerontology* 55 (2000): M585–M592.

2. Abelow BJ, Holford TR, and Insogna KL. "Cross-cultural association between dietary animal protein and hip fracture: a hypothesis." *Calcif. Tissue Int.* 50 (1992): 14–18.

3. Wachsman A, and Bernstein DS. "Diet and osteoporosis." *Lancet* May 4, 1968 (1968): 958–959.

4. Barzel U.S.. "Acid loading and osteoporosis." *J. Am. Geriatr. Soc.* 30 (1982): 613.

5. Sherman HC. "Calcium requirement for maintenance in man." *J. Biol. Chem.* 39 (1920): 21–27.

6. Animal protein includes more of the sulphur-containing amino acids. When digested and metabolized, these amino acids produce the acid-forming sulphate ion, which must be excreted by the kidney. A recent report showed a remarkable 84% correlation between animal protein consumption and urinary acid excretion of sulphate.

7. Brosnan JT, and Brosnan ME. "Dietary protein, metabolic acidosis, and calcium balance." *In:* H. H. Draper (ed.), *Advances in Nutritional Research*, pp. 77–105. New York: Plenum Press, 1982.

8. Frassetto LA, Todd KM, Morris RC, Jr., et al. "Estimation of net endogenous noncarbonic acid production in humans from diet potassium and protein contents." *Am. J. Clin. Nutri.* 68 (1998): 576–583.

9. Margen S, Chu J-Y, Kaufmann NA, et al. "Studies in calcium metabolism. I. The calciuretic effect of dietary protein." *Am. J. Clin. Nutr.* 27 (1974): 584–589.

10. Hegsted M, Schuette SA, Zemel MB, et al. "Urinary calcium and calcium balance in young men as affected by level of protein and phosphorus intake." *J. Nutr.* 111 (1981): 553–562.

11. Kerstetter JE, and Allen LH. "Dietary protein increases urinary calcium." *J. Nutr.* 120 (1990): 134–136.

12. Westman EC, Yancy WS, Edman JS, et al. "Carbohydrate Diet Program." *Am. J. Med.* 113 (2002): 30–36.

13. Sellmeyer DE, Stone KL, Sebastian A, et al. "A high ratio of dietary animal to vegetable protein increases the rate of bone loss and the risk of fracture in postmenopausal women." *Am. J. Clin. Nutr.* 73 (2001): 118–122.

14. Hegsted DM. "Calcium and osteoporosis." *J. Nutr.* 116 (1986): 2316–2319.
15. Heaney RP. "Protein intake and bone health: the influence of belief systems on the conduct of nutritional science." *Am. J. Clin. Nutr.* 73 (2001): 5–6.
16. Cummings SR, and Black D. "Bone mass measurements and risk of fracture in Caucasian women: a review of findings for prospective studies." *Am. J. Med.* 98(Suppl 2A) (1995): 2S–24S.
17. Marshall D, Johnell O, and Wedel H. "Meta-analysis of how well measures of bone mineral density predict occurrence of osteoporotic fractures." *Brit. Med. Journ.* 312 (1996): 1254–1259.
18. Lips P. "Epidemiology and predictors of fractures associated with osteoporosis." *Am. J. Med.* 103(2A) (1997): 3S–11S.
19. Lane NE, and Nevitt MC. "Osteoarthritis, bone mass, and fractures: how are they related?" *Arthritis Rheumatism* 46 (2002): 1–4.
20. Lucas FL, Cauley JA, Stone RA, et al. "Bone mineral density and risk of breast cancer: differences by family history of breast cancer." *Am. J. Epidemiol.* 148 (1998): 22–29.
21. Cauley JA, Lucas FL, Kuller LH, et al. "Bone mineral density and risk of breast cancer in older women: the study of osteoporotic fractures." *JAMA* 276 (1996): 1404–1408.
22. Mincey BA. "Osteoporosis in women with breast cancer." *Curr. Oncol. Rpts.* 5 (2003): 53–57.
23. Riis BJ. "The role of bone loss." *Am. J. Med.* 98(Suppl 2A) (1995): 2S–29S.
24. Ho SC. "Body measurements, bone mass, and fractures: does the East differ from the West?" *Clin. Orthopaed. Related Res.* 323 (1996): 75–80.
25. Aspray TJ, Prentice A, Cole TJ, et al. "Low bone mineral content is common but osteoporotic fractures are rare in elderly rural Gambian women." *J. Bone Min. Res.* 11 (1996): 1019–1025.
26. Tsai K-S. "Osteoporotic fracture rate, bone mineral density, and bone metabolism in Taiwan." *J. Formosan Med. Assoc.* 96 (1997): 802–805.
27. Wu AH, Pike MC, and Stram DO. "Meta-analysis: dietary fat intake, serum estrogen levels, and the risk of breast cancer." *J. Nat. Cancer Inst.* 91 (1999): 529–534.
28. UCLA Kidney Stone Treatment Center. "Kidney Stones—Index." March, 1997. Accessed at http://www.radsci.ucla.edu:8000/gu/stones/kidneystone.html
29. Stamatelou KK, Francis ME, Jones CA, et al. "Time trends in reported prevalence of kidney stones." *Kidney Int.* 63 (2003): 1817–1823.
30. This genetically rare type of kidney stone results from an inability of the kidney to reabsorb cysteine, an amino acid.
31. Ramello A, Vitale C, and Marangella M. "Epidemiology of nephrolothiasis." *J. Nephrol.* 13(Suppl 3) (2000): S65–S70.
32. Robertson WG, Peacock M, and Hodgkinson A. "Dietary changes and the incidence of urinary calculi in the U.K. between 1958 and 1976." *Chron. Dis.* 32 (1979): 469–476.
33. Robertson WG, Peacock M, Heyburn PJ, et al. "Risk factors in calcium stone disease of the urinary tract." *Brit. J. Urology* 50 (1978): 449–454.
34. Robertson WG. "Epidemiological risk factors in calcium stone disease." *Scand. J. Urol. Nephrol. Suppl.* 53 (1980): 15–30.
35. Robertson WG, Peacock M, Heyburn PJ, et al. "Should recurrent calcium oxalate stone formers become vegetarians?" *Brit. J. Urology* 51 (1979): 427–431.
36. This information was shown in Dr. Robertson's seminar in Toronto.
37. Robertson WG. "Diet and calcium stones." *Miner Electrolyte Metab.* 13 (1987): 228–234.
38. Cao LC, Boeve ER, de Bruijn WC, et al. "A review of new concepts in renal stone research." *Scanning Microscopy* 7 (1993): 1049–1065.
39. Friedman DS, Congdon N, Kempen J, et al. "Vision problems in the U.S.: prevalence of adult

vision impairment and age-related eye disease in America." Bethesda, MD: Prevent Blindness in America. National Eye Institute, 2002.

40. Foote CS. *Photosensitized oxidation and singlet oxygen: consequences in biological systems.* Vol. 2 New York: Academic Press, 1976.

41. Seddon JM, Ajani UA, Sperduto RD, et al. "Dietary carotenoids, vitamins A, C, and E, and advanced age-related macular degeneration." *JAMA* 272 (1994): 1413–1420.

42. Eye Disease Case-Control Study Group. "Antioxidant status and neovascular age-related macular degeneration." *Arch. Ophthalmol.* 111 (1993): 104–109.

43. The other four food groups were broccoli, carrot, sweet potato, and winter squash, showing disease reductions of 53%, 28%, 33% and 44%, respectively. Each reduction was only approaching or was marginally statistically significant.

44. Berman ER. *Biochemistry of the eye. (Perspectives in vision research).* New York, N.Y.: Plenum Publishing Corporation, 1991.

45. Lyle BJ, Mares-Perlman JA, Klein BEK, et al. "Antioxidant Intake and Risk of Incident Age-related Nuclear Cataracts in the Beaver Dam Eye Study." *Am. J. Epidemiol.* 149 (1999): 801–809.

46. Bates CJ, Chen SJ, Macdonald A, et al. "Quantitation of vitamin E and a carotenoid pigment in cataracterous human lenses, and the effect of a dietary supplement." *Int. J. Vitam. Nutr. Res.* 66 (1996): 316–321.

47. Varma SD, Beachy NA, and Richards RD. "Photoperoxidation of lens lipids: prevention by vitamin E." *Photochem. Photobiol.* 36 (1982): 623–626.

48. Talan J. "Alzheimer's diagnoses can be two years late." *Ithaca Journal*: 8A.

49. Petersen RC, Smith GE, Waring SC, et al. "Mild cognitive impairment." *Arch. Neurol.* 56 (1999): 303–308.

50. Kivipelto M, Helkala E-L, Hanninen T, et al. "Midlife vascular risk factors and late-life mild cognitive impairment. A population based study." *Neurology* 56 (2001): 1683–1689.

51. Breteler MMB, Claus JJ, Grobbee DE, et al. "Cardiovascular disease and distribution of cognitive function in elderly people: the Rotterdam Study." *Brit. Med. Journ.* 308 (1994): 1604–1608.

52. Haan MN, Shemanski L, Jagust WJ, et al. "The role of APOE e4 in modulating effects of other risk factors for cognitive decline in elderly persons." *JAMA* 282 (1999): 40–46.

53. Sparks DL, Martin TA, Gross DR, et al. "Link between heart disease, cholesterol, and Alzheimer's Disease: a review." *Microscopy Res. Tech.* 50 (2000): 287–290.

54. Slooter AJ, Tang MX, van Duijn CM, et al. "Apolipoprotein E e4 and risk of dementia with stroke. A population based investigation." *JAMA* 277 (1997): 818–821.

55. Messier C, and Gagnon M. "Glucose regulation and cognitive functions: relation to Alzheimer's disease and diabetes." *Behav. Brain Res.* 75 (1996): 1–11.

56. Ott A, Stolk RP, Hofman A, et al. "Association of diabetes mellitus and dementia: the Rotterdam Study." *Diabetologia* 39 (1996): 1392–1397.

57. Kannel WB, Wolf PA, Verter J, et al. "Epidemiologic assessment of the role of blood pressure in stroke." *JAMA* 214 (1970): 301–310.

58. Launer LJ, Masaki K, Petrovitch H, et al. "The association between midlife blood pressure levels and late-life cognitive function." *JAMA* 274 (1995): 1846–1851.

59. White, L., Petrovitch, H., Ross, G. W., Masaki, K. H., Abbott, R. D., Teng, E. L., Rodriquez, B. L., Blanchette, P. L., Havlik, R., Wergowske, G., Chiu, D., Foley, D. J., Murdaugh, C., and Curb, J. D. "Prevalence of dementia in older Japanese-American men in Hawaii. The Honolulu-Asia Aging Study." *JAMA*, 276: 955–960, 1996.

60. Hendrie HC, Ogunniyi A, Hall KS, et al. "Incidence of dementia and Alzheimer Disease in 2 communities: Yoruba residing in Ibadan, Nigeria and African Americans residing in Indianapolis, Indiana." *JAMA* 285 (2001): 739–747.

61. Chandra V, Pandav R, Dodge HH, et al. "Incidence of Alzheimer's disease in a rural community in India: the Indo-U.S. Study." *Neurology* 57 (2001): 985–989.

62. Grant WB. "Dietary links to Alzheimer's Disease: 1999 Update." *J. Alzheimer's Dis* 1 (1999): 197–201.

63. Grant WB. "Incidence of dementia and Alzheimer disease in Nigeria and the United States." *JAMA* 285 (2001): 2448.

64. This recently published study is more interesting than the others because vitamin E was measured in a way that is more discriminating by considering the fact that vitamin E is carried in the blood fat. That is, a high level of blood vitamin E may, at times, be due to high levels of blood fat. (*Am. J. Epidemiol.* 150 (1999); 37–44)

65. The effects of vitamin C and selenium in a study by Perkins (*Am. J. Epidemiol.* 150 (1999): 37–44) were not statistically significant in a logistic regression model, according to the authors. I disagree with their conclusion because the inverse "dose-response" trend (high antioxidant blood levels, less memory loss) was impressive and clearly significant. The authors failed to address this finding in their analysis.

66. Ortega RM, Requejo AM, Andres P, et al. "Dietary intake and cognitive function in a group of elderly people." *Am. J. Clin. Nutr.* 66 (1997): 803–809.

67. Perrig WJ, Perrig P, and Stahelin HB. "The relation between antioxidants and memory performance in the old and very old." *J. Am. Geriatr. Soc.* 45 (1997): 718–724.

68. Gale CR, Martyn CN, and Cooper C. "Cognitive impairment and mortality in a cohort of elderly people." *Brit. Med. Journ.* 312 (1996): 608–611.

69. Goodwin JS, Goodwin JM, and Garry PJ. "Association between nutritional status and cognitive functioning in a healthy elderly population." *JAMA* 249 (1983): 2917–2921.

70. Jama JW, Launer LJ, Witteman JCM, et al. "Dietary antioxidants and cognitive function in a population-based sample of older persons: the Rotterdam Study." *Am. J. Epidemiol.* 144 (1996): 275–280.

71. Martin A, Prior R, Shukitt-Hale B, et al. "Effect of fruits, vegetables or vitamin E-rich diet on vitamins E and C distribution in peripheral and brain tissues: implications for brain function." *J. Gerontology* 55A (2000): B144–B151.

72. Joseph JA, Shukitt-Hale B, Denisova NA, et al. "Reversals of age-related declines in neuronal signal transduction, cognitive, and motor behavioral deficits with blueberry, spinach, or strawberry dietary supplementation." *J. Neurosci.* 19 (1999): 8114–8121.

73. Gillman MW, Cupples LA, Gagnon D, et al. "Protective effect of fruits and vegetables on development of stroke in men." *JAMA* 273 (1995): 1113–1117.

74. Kalmijn S, Launer LJ, Ott A, et al. "Dietary fat intake and the risk of incident dementia in the Rotterdam Study." *Ann. Neurol.* 42 (1997): 776–782.

75. Alzheimer's trend was not statistically significant, perhaps due to the small number of disease cases.

76. Clarke R, Smith D, Jobst KA, et al. "Folate, vitamin B12, and serum total homocysteine levels in confirmed Alzheimer disease." *Arch. Neurol.* 55 (1998): 1449–1455.

77. McCully KS. "Homocysteine theory of arteriosclerosis: development and current status." *In:* A. M. Gotto, Jr. and R. Paoletti (eds.), *Athersclerosis reviews*, Vol. 11, pp. 157–246. New York: Raven Press, 1983.

78. There is a potential snag in this logic, however. Homocysteine levels are regulated in part by B vitamins, most notably folic acid and vitamin B_{12}, and people who are deficient in these vitamins may have higher homocysteine levels. People who do not consume animal-based foods are at risk for having low B_{12} levels, and thus high homocysteine levels. However, as described in chapter eleven, this has more to do with our separation from nature, and not a deficiency of plant-based diets.

PART III

1. http://www.southbeachdiet.com, accessed 4/26/04

Chapter 11

1. Atkins RC. *Dr. Atkins' New Diet Revolution*. New York, NY: Avon Books, 1999.
2. The Alpha-Tocopherol Beta Carotene Cancer Prevention Study Group. "The effect of vitamin E and beta carotene on the incidence of lung cancer and other cancers in male smokers." *New Engl. J. Med.* 330 (1994): 1029–1035.
3. Omenn GS, Goodman GE, Thornquist MD, et al. "Effects of a combination of beta carotene and vitamin A on lung cancer and cardiovascular disease." *New Engl. J. Med.* 334 (1996): 1150–1155.
4. U.S. Preventive Services Task Force. "Routine vitamin supplementation to prevent cancer and cardiovascular disease: recommendations and rationale." *Ann. Internal Med.* 139 (2003): 51–55.
5. Morris CD, and Carson S. "Routine vitamin supplementation to prevent cardiovascular disease: a summary of the evidence for the U.S. Preventive Services Task Force." *Ann. Internal Med.* 139 (2003): 56–70.
6. Kolata G. "Vitamins: more may be too many (Science Section)." The *New York Times* April 29, 2003: 1, 6.
7. U.S. Department of Agriculture. "USDA Nutrient Database for Standard Reference." Washington, DC: U.S. Department of Agriculture, Agriculture Research Service, 2002. Accessed at http://www.nal.USDA.gov/fnic/foodcomp
8. Holden JM, Eldridge AL, Beecher GR, et al. "Carotenoid content of U.S. foods: an update of the database." *J. Food Comp. Anal.* 12 (1999): 169–196.
9. The exact food listings in the database were: Ground Beef, 80% lean meat/20% fat, raw; Pork, fresh, ground, raw; Chicken, broilers or fryers, meat and skin, raw; Milk, dry, whole; Spinach, raw; Tomatoes, red, ripe, raw, year-round average; Lima Beans, large, mature seeds, raw; Peas, green, raw; Potatoes, russet, flesh and skin, raw.
10. Mozafar A. "Enrichment of some B-vitamins in plants with application of organic fertilizers." *Plant and Soil* 167 (1994): 305–311.
11. Brand D, and Segelken R. "Largest scientific effort in Cornell's history announced." *Cornell Chronicle* May 9, 2002
12. Ashrafi K, Chang FY, Watts JL, et al. "Genome-wide RNAi analysis of Caenorhabitis elegans fat regulatory genes." *Nature* 421 (2003): 268–272.
13. Shermer M. "Skeptical sayings. Wit and wisdom from skeptics past and present." *Skeptic* 9 (2002): 28.
14. I've never really liked putting such specific cutoff points on initiation, promotion and progression of chronic disease, because these cutoff points for each stage of chronic disease are completely arbitrary. What's important to know is that a chronic disease can be with us for most of our lives, and if it progresses, it will do so in a very fluid, continuous manner.
15. Hildenbrand GLG, Hildenbrand LC, Bradford K, et al. "Five-year survival rates of melanoma patients treated by diet therapy after the manner of Gerson: a retrospective review." *Alternative Therapies in Health and Medicine* 1 (1995): 29–37.
16. McDougall JA. *McDougall's Medicine, A Challenging Second Opinion*. Piscataway, NJ: New Century Publishers, Inc., 1985.
17. Swank RL. "Multiple sclerosis: twenty years on low fat diet." *Arch. Neurol.* 23 (1970): 460–474.

18. Swank RL. "Effect of low saturated fat diet in early and late cases of multiple sclerosis." *Lancet* 336 (1990): 37–39.

PART IV

Chapter 13

1. Colen BD. "To die in Tijuana; a story of faith, hope and laetrile." The *Washington Post Magazine*, September 4, 1977: 10.
2. Burros M. "The sting? America's supplements appetite; scientists are dubious, but America's appetite for food supplements keeps growing." The *Washington Post* August 2, 1979: E1.
3. Hilgartner S. *Science on Stage. Expert advice as public drama.* Stanford, CA: Stanford University Press, 2000.
4. National Research Council. *Diet, Nutrition and Cancer.* Washington, DC: National Academy Press, 1982.
5. U.S. Senate. "Dietary goals for the United States, 2nd Edition." Washington, DC: U.S. Government Printing Office, 1977.
6. American Council of Science and Health. 01/08/04. Accessed at http://www.achs.org/about/index.html
7. Mindfully.org. 01/08/2004. Accessed at http://www.mindfully.org/Pesticide/ACSH-koop.htm
8. American Society for Nutritional Sciences. 01/08/04. Accessed at http://www.asns.org

Chapter 14

1. National Research Council. *Diet, Nutrition and Cancer.* Washington, DC: National Academy Press, 1982.
2. United States Federal Trade Commission. "Complaint counsel's proposed findings of fact, conclusions of law and proposed order (Docket No. 9175)." Washington, DC: United States Federal Trade Commission, December 27, 1985.
3. Associated Press. "Company news; General Nutrition settles complaint." The *New York Times* June 14, 1988: D5.
4. Willett W. "Diet and cancer: one view at the start of the millennium." *Cancer Epi. Biom. Prev.* 10 (2001): 3–8.
5. Belanger CF, Hennekens CH, Rosner B, et al. "The Nurses' Health Study." *Am. J. Nursing* (1978): 1039–1040.
6. Marchione M. "Taking the long view; for 25 years, Harvard's Nurses' Health Study has sought answers to women's health questions." *Milwaukee Journal-Sentinel* July 16, 2001: 01G.
7. Carroll KK. "Experimental evidence of dietary factors and hormone-dependent cancers." *Cancer Res.* 35 (1975): 3374–3383.
8. Chen J, Campbell TC, Li J, et al. *Diet, life-style and mortality in China. A study of the characteristics of 65 Chinese counties.* Oxford, UK; Ithaca, NY; Beijing, PRC: Oxford University Press; Cornell University Press; People's Medical Publishing House, 1990.
9. Hu FB, Stampfer MJ, Manson JE, et al. "Dietary protein and risk of ischemic heart disease in women." *Am. Journ. Clin. Nutr.* 70 (1999): 221–227.
10. Holmes MD, Hunter DJ, Colditz GA, et al. "Association of dietary intake of fat and fatty acids with risk of breast cancer." *JAMA* 281 (1999): 914–920.
11. U.S. Department of Agriculture. "Agriculture Fact Book." Washington, DC: U.S. Department of Agriculture, 1998. cited in: Information Plus *Nutrition: a key to good health.* Wylie, TX: Information Plus, 1999.
12. While the average percentage of calories derived from fat has gone down slightly, average daily fat intake, in grams, has stayed the same or has gone up.
13. Information Plus. *Nutrition: a key to good health.* Wylie, TX: Information Plus, 1999.

14. Wegmans.com. 01/19/04. Accessed at http://www.wegmans.com/recipes

15. Mardiweb.com. "Cheesecake." 01/19/04. Accessed at http://mardiweb.com/lowfat/dessert.ht m#Recipe000857

16. Anonymous. "Center to Coordinate Women's Health Study." *Chicago Sun-Times* October 12, 1992: 14N.

17. Prentice RL, Kakar F, Hursting S, et al. "Aspects of the rationale for the Women's Health Trial." *J. Natl. Cancer Inst.* 80 (1988): 802–814.

18. Henderson MM, Kushi LH, Thompson DJ, et al. "Feasibility of a randomized trial of a low-fat diet for the prevention of breast cancer: dietary compliance in the Women's Health Trail Vanguard Study." *Prev. Med.* 19 (1990): 115–133.

19. Self S, Prentice R, Iverson D, et al. "Statistical design of the Women's Health Trial." *Controlled Clin. Trials* 9 (1988): 119–136.

20. Armstrong D, and Doll R. "Environmental factors and cancer incidence and mortality in different countries, with special reference to dietary practices." *Int. J. Cancer* 15 (1975): 617–631.

21. Campbell TC. "The dietary causes of degenerative diseases: nutrients vs foods." *In:* N. J. Temple and D. P. Burkitt (eds.), *Western diseases: their dietary prevention and reversibility*, pp. 119–152. Totowa, NJ: Humana Press, 1994.

22. White E, Shattuck AL, Kristal AR, et al. "Maintenance of a low-fat diet: follow-up of the Women's Health Trial." *Cancer Epi. Biom. Prev.* 1 (1992): 315–323.

23. Willett WC, Hunter DJ, Stampfer MJ, et al. "Dietary fat and fiber in relation to risk of breast cancer. An 8-year follow-up." *J. Am. Med. Assoc.* 268 (1992): 2037–2044.

24. Willett W. "Dietary fat and breast cancer." *Toxicol. Sci.* 52[Suppl] (1999): 127–146.

25. Hunter DJ, Spiegelman D, Adami H-O, et al. "Cohort studies of fat intake and the risk of breast cancer—a pooled analysis." *New Engl. J. Med.* 334 (1996): 356–361.

26. Missmer SA, Smith-Warner SA, Spiegelman D, et al. "Meat and dairy consumption and breast cancer: a pooled analysis of cohort studies." *Int. J. Epidemiol.* 31 (2002): 78–85.

27. Rockhill B, Willett WC, Hunter DJ, et al. "Physical activity and breast cancer risk in a cohort of young women." *J. Nat. Cancer Inst.* 90 (1998): 1155–1160.

28. Smith-Warner SA, Spiegelman D, Adami H-O, et al. "Types of dietary fat and breast cancer: a pooled analysis of cohort studies." *Int. J. Cancer* 92 (2001): 767–774.

29. Hunter DJ, Morris JS, Stampfer MJ, et al. "A prospective study of selenium status and breast cancer risk." *JAMA* 264 (1990): 1128–1131.

30. Smith-Warner SA, Spiegelman D, Yaun S-S, et al. "Intake of fruits and vegetables and risk of breast cancer: a pooled analysis of cohort studies." *JAMA* 285 (2001): 769–776.

31. Mukamal KJ, Conigrave KM, Mittleman MA, et al. "Roles of drinking pattern and type of alcohol consumed in coronary heart disease in men." *New Engl. J. Med.* 348 (2003): 109–118.

32. Tanasescu M, Hu FB, Willett WC, et al. "Alcohol consumption and risk of coronary heart disease among men with Type 2 diabetes mellitus." *J. Am. Coll. Cardiol.* 38 (2001): 1836–1842.

33. Smith-Warner SA, Spiegelman D, Yaun S-S, et al. "Alcohol and breast cancer in women. A pooled analysis of cohort studies." *JAMA* 279 (1998): 535–540.

34. He K, Rimm EB, Merchant A, et al. "Fish consumption and risk of stroke in men." *JAMA* 288 (2002): 3130–3136.

35. Albert CM, Hennekens CH, O'Donnell CJ, et al. "Fish consumption and risk of sudden cardiac death." *JAMA* 279 (1998): 23–28.

36. U.S. Department of Agriculture. "USDA Nutrient Database for Standard Reference." Washington, DC: U.S. Department of Agriculture, Agriculture Research Service, 2002. Accessed at http://www.nal.usda.gov/fnic/foodcomp

37. Hu FB, Stampfer MJ, Rimm EB, et al. "A prospective study of egg consumption and risk of cardiovascular disease in men and women." *JAMA* 281 (1999): 1387–1394.

38. Hu FB, Manson JE, and Willett WC. "Types of dietary fat and risk of coronary heart disease: a critical review." *J. Am. Coll. Nutr.* 20 (2001): 5–19.
39. Mitchell S. "Eggs might reduce breast cancer risk." *United Press International* Feb. 21, 2003
40. Steinmetz, K. A. and Potter, J. D. "Egg consumption and cancer of the colon and rectum." *Eur. J. Cancer Prev.*, 3: 237–245, 1994.
41. Giovannucci E, Rimm EB, Stampfer MJ, et al. "Intake of fat, meat, and fiber in relation to risk of colon cancer in men." *Cancer Res.* 54 (1994): 2390–2397.
42. Fuchs CS, Giovannucci E, Colditz GA, et al. "Dietary fiber and the risk of colorectal cancer and adenoma in women." *New Engl. J. Med.* 340 (1999): 169–176.
43. Higginson J. "Present trends in cancer epidemiology." *Proc. Can. Cancer Conf.* 8 (1969): 40–75.
44. Burkitt DP. "Epidemiology of cancer of the colon and the rectum." *Cancer* 28 (1971): 3–13.
45. Trowell HC, and Burkitt DP. *Western diseases: their emergence and prevention.* London: Butler & Tanner, Ltd., 1981.
46. Boyd NF, Martin LJ, Noffel M, et al. "A meta-analysis of studies of dietary-fat and breast cancer risk." *Brit. J. Cancer* 68 (1993): 627–636.
47. Campbell TC. "Animal protein and ischemic heart disease." *Am. J. Clin. Nutr.* 71 (2000): 849–850.
48. Hu FB, and Willett W. "Reply to TC Campbell." *Am. J. Clin. Nutr.* 71 (2000): 850.
49. Morris CD, and Carson S. "Routine vitamin supplementation to prevent cardiovascular disease: a summary of the evidence for the U.S. Preventive Services Task Force." *Ann. Internal Med.* 139 (2003): 56–70.
50. U.S. Preventive Services Task Force. "Routine vitamin supplementation to prevent cancer and cardiovascular disease: recommendations and rationale." *Ann. Internal Med.* 139 (2003): 51–55.

Chapter 15

1. Putman JJ, and Allshouse JE. "Food Consumption, Prices, and Expenditures, 1970–95." Washington, DC: United States Department of Agriculture, 1997. Cited in: Information Plus. *Nutrition: a key to good health.* Wylie, TX: Information Plus, 1999.
2. National Dairy Council. July 15, 2003. Accessed at http://www.nationaldairycouncil.org/aboutus.asp
3. Dairy Management Inc. "What is Dairy Management Inc.?" February 12, 2004. Accessed at http://www.dairycheckoff.com/whatisdmi.htm
4. Dairy Management Inc. Press release. "Dairy checkoff 2003 unified marketing plan budget geared to help increase demand in domestic and international markets." Rosemont, IL: January 24, 2003. Accessed at http://www.dairycheckoff.com/news/release-012403.asp
5. National Watermelon Promotion Board. January 12, 2004. Accessed at http://www.watermelon.org
6. Dairy Management Inc. "2001 Annual Report." Dairy Management, Inc., 2001. Accessed at http://www.dairycheckoff.com/annualreport.htm/
7. United States Department of Agriculture. "Report to Congress on the National Dairy Promotion and Research Program and the National Fluid Milk Processor Promotion Program." 2000. Accessed at http://www.ams.usda.gov/dairy/prb_intro.htm.IN
8. United States Department of Agriculture. "Report to Congress on the National Dairy Promotion and Research Program and the National Fluid Milk Processor Promotion Program." 2003. Accessed at http://www.ams.usda.gov/dairy/prb/prb_rept_2003.htm
9. Nutrition Explorations. July, 2003. Accessed at http://www.nutritionexplorations.com
10. Powell A. "School of Public Health hosts food fight: McDonald's, dairy industry, dietary reformers face off at symposium." *Harvard Gazette*: 24 October 2002. Accessed at http://www.news.harvard.edu/gazette/2002/10.24/09-food.html
11. Ha YL, Grimm NK, and Pariza MW. "Anticarcinogens from fried ground beef: heat-altered derivatives of linoleic acid." *Carcinogensis* 8 (1987): 1881–1887.

12. Ha YL, Storkson J, and Pariza MW. "Inhibition of benzo(a)pyrene-induced mouse forestomach neoplasia by conjugated denoic derivatives of linoleic acid." *Cancer Res.* 50 (1990): 1097–1101.
13. Aydin R, Pariza MW, and Cook ME. "Olive oil prevents the adverse effects of dietary conjugated linoleic acid on chick hatchability and egg quality." *J. Nutr.* 131 (2001): 800–806.
14. Peters JM, Park Y, Gonzalez FJ, et al. "Influence of conjugated linoleic acid on body composition and target gene expression in peroxisome proliferator-activated receptor alpha-null mice." *Biochim. Biophys. Acta* 1533 (2001): 233–242.
15. Ntambi JM, Choi Y, Park Y, et al. "Effect of conjugated linoleic acid (CLA) on immune responses, body composition and stearoyl-CoA desaturase." *Can. J. Appl. Physiol.* 27 (2002): 617–627.
16. Ip C, Chin SF, Scimeca JA, et al. "Mammary cancer prevention by conjugated dienoic derivative of linoleic acid." *Cancer Res.* 51 (1991): 6118–6124.
17. Ip C, Cheng J, Thompson HJ, et al. "Retention of conjugated linoleic acid in the mammary gland is associated with tumor inhibition during the post-initiation phase of carcinogenesis." *Carcinogensis* 18 (1997): 755–759.
18. Yaukey J. "Changing cows' diets elevates milks' cancer-fighting." *Ithaca Journal* November 12, 1996: 1.
19. Belury MA. "Inhibition of carcinogenesis by conjugated linoleic acid: potential mechanisms of action." *J. Nutr.* 132 (2002): 2995–2998.
20. Ip C, Banni S, Angioni E, et al. "Conjugated linoleic acid-enriched butter fat alters mammary gland morphogenesis and reduces cancer risk in rats." *J. Nutr.* 129 (1999): 2135–2142.
21. Griinari JM, Corl BA, Lacy SH, et al. "Conjugated linoleic acid is synthesized endogenously in lactating dairy cows by D⁹-desaturase." *J. Nutr.* 130 (2000): 2285–2291.
22. Ip C, Dong Y, Thompson HJ, et al. "Control of rat mammary epithelium proliferation by conjugated linoleic acid." *Nutr. Cancer* 39 (2001): 233–238.
23. Ip C, Dong Y, Ip MM, et al. "Conjugated linoleic acid isomers and mammary cancer prevention." *Nutr. Cancer* 43 (2002): 52–58.
24. Giovannucci E. "Insulin and colon cancer." *Cancer Causes and Control* 6 (1995): 164–179.
25. Mills PK, Beeson WL, Phillips RL, et al. "Cohort study of diet, lifestyle, and prostate cancer." *Cancer* 64 (1989): 598–604.
26. Search for keyword "lycopene" at http://www.ncbi.nlm.nih.gov
27. Christian MS, Schulte S, and Hellwig J. "Developmental (embryo-fetal toxicity/teratogenecity) toxicity studies of synthetic crystalline lycopene in rats and rabbits." *Food Chem. Toxicol.* 41 (2003): 773–783.
28. Giovannucci E, Rimm E, Liu Y, et al. "A prospective study of tomato products, lycopene, and prostate cancer risk." *J. Nat. Cancer Inst.* 94 (2002): 391–398.
29. Gann PH, and Khachik F. "Tomatoes or lycopene versus prostate cancer: is evolution anti-reductionist?" *J. Nat. Cancer Inst.* 95 (2003): 1563–1565.
30. Tucker G. "Nutritional enhancement of plants." *Curr. Opin.* 14 (2003): 221–225.
31. He Y. *Effects of carotenoids and dietary carotenoid extracts on aflatoxin B₁-induced mutagenesis and hepatocarcinogenesis.* Ithaca, NY: Cornell University, PhD Thesis, 1990.
32. He Y, and Campbell TC. "Effects of carotenoids on aflatoxin B₁-induced mutagenesis in S. typhimurium TA 100 and TA 98." *Nutr. Cancer* 13 (1990): 243–253.
33. Giovannucci E, Ascherio A, Rimm EB, et al. "Intake of carotenoids and retinol in relation to risk of prostate cancer." *J. Nat. Cancer Inst.* 87 (1995): 1767–1776.
34. U.S. Department of Agriculture. "USDA Nutrient Database for Standard Reference." Washington, DC: U.S. Department of Agriculture, Agriculture Research Service, 2002. Accessed at http://www.nal.usda.gov/fnic/foodcomp
35. Eberhardt MV, Lee CY, and Liu RH. "Antioxidant activity of fresh apples." *Nature* 405 (2000): 903–904.

Chapter 16

1. Food and Nutrition Board, and Institute of Medicine. "Dietary reference intakes for energy, carbohydrates, fiber, fat, fatty acids, cholesterol, protein, and amino acids (macronutrients)." Washington, DC: The National Academy Press, 2002. Accessed at http://www.nap.edu/catalog/10490.html?onpi_newsdoc090502

2. National Academy of Sciences. Press Release. "Report offers new eating and physical activity targets to reduce chronic disease risk." Sept. 5, 2002. Washington, DC: National Research Council, Institute of Medicine. Accessed at http://www4.nationalacademies.org/news.nsf/isbn/0309085373?OpenDocument

3. Wegmans Company. *Recipe and nutrient facts*. Accessed 2003. Available from http://www.wegmans.com.

4. U.S. Department of Agriculture. "USDA Nutrient Database for Standard Reference." Washington, DC: U.S. Department of Agriculture, Agriculture Research Service, 2002. Accessed at http://www.nal.usda.gov/fnic/foodcomp

5. The RDA has been expressed as a singular quantity of protein, as 0.8 grams of protein per kilogram of body weight. Assuming a daily intake of 2,200 calories for a 70 kg person, this 0.8 grams is equivalent to about 10–11% of total calories: 70 kg X 0.8 gm/kg X 4 cal/gm X 1/2200 cal X 100 = 10.2%

6. Wright JD, Kennedy-Stephenson J, Wang CY, et al. "Trends in Intake of Energy and Macronutrients - United States, 1971–2000." *Morbidity and mortality weekly report* 53 (February 6, 2004): 80–82.

7. Boseley S. "Sugar industry threatens to scupper WHO." *The Guardian* April 21, 2003

8. Brundtland GH. "Sweet and sour; The WHO is accused by the sugar industry of giving unscientific nutrition advice. But its recommendations are based on solid evidence, says Gro Harlem Brundtland." *New Scientist*, May 03, 2003: 23.

9. International Life Sciences Institute. *ILSI North America*. Accessed February 13, 2004. Available from http://www.ilsina.org.

10. Kursban M. *Commentary: conflicted panel makes for unfit guidelines*. Physicians Committee for Responsible Medicine. Accessed June, 2003. Available from http://www.pcrm.org/health/commentary/commentary0004.html.

11. Chaitowitz S. *Court rules against USDA's secrecy and failure to disclose conflict of interest in setting nutrition policies*. Physicians Committee for Responsible Medicine. Accessed January 27, 2004. Available from http://www.pcrm.org/news/health001002.html.

12. I have been for several years on the science advisory board of PCRM.

13. National Academy of Sciences, and Institute of Medicine. "Dietary Reference Intakes for Energy, Carbohydrates, Fiber, Fat, Fatty Acids, Cholesterol, Protein, and Amino Acids [summary statement]." Washington, DC: National Academy Press, September, 2002.

14. National Institutes of Health. February 2004. Accessed at http://www.nih.gov

15. National Institutes of Health. "National Institutes of Health. Summary of the FY 2005 President's Budget." February 2, 2004. Accessed at http://www.nih.gov/news

16. National Institutes of Health. *NIH Disease Funding Table: Special Areas of Interest*. Accessed August 18, 2003. Available from http://www.nih.gov/news/findingresearchareas.htm.

17. Calculated from NIH Disease Funding Table: Special Areas of Interest. See previous reference.

18. National Cancer Institute. "FY 1999 Questions and Answers provided for the record for the FY 1999 House Appropriations Subcommitee." July 15, 2003. Accessed at http://www3.cancer.gov/admin/fmb/1999QAs.htm

19. National Cancer Institute. *FY 2001 Congressional Justification*. Accessed March 2, 2004. Available from http://www3.cancer.gov/admin/fmb/index.html.

20. Angell M. "The pharmaceutical industry—to whom is it accountable?" *New Engl. J. Med.* 342 (2000): 1902–1904.

21. National Cancer Institute. *FY 2004 Congressional Justification*. Accessed 2003. Available from http://www3.cancer.gov/admin/fmb/index/html.

22. Demas A. *Food Education in the Elementary Classroom as a Means of Gaining Acceptance of Diverse Low Fat Foods in the School Lunch Program* [PhD Dissertation]. Ithaca, NY: Cornell University, 1995:325pp.

Chapter 17

1. Austoker J. "The 'treatment of choice': breast cancer surgery 1860–1985." *Soc. Soc. Hist. Med. Bull.(London)* 37 (1985): 100–107.

2. Naifeh SW. *The Best Doctors in America, 1994–1995*. Aiken, S.C.: Woodward & White, 1994.

3. McDougall JA, and McDougall MA. *The McDougall Plan*. Clinton, NJ: New Win Publishing, Inc., 1983.

4. Committee on Nutrition in Medical Education. "Nutrition Education in U.S. Medical Schools." Washington, DC: National Academy of Sciences, 1985.

5. White PL, Johnson OC, and Kibler MJ. "Council on Foods and Nutrition, American Medical Association—its relation to physicians." *Postgraduate Med.* 30 (1961): 502–507.

6. Lo C. "Integrating nutrition as a theme throughout the medical school curriculum." *Am. J. Clin. Nutr.* 72(Suppl) (2000): 882S–889S.

7. Pearson TA, Stone EJ, Grundy SM, et al. "Translation of nutrition science into medical education: the Nutrition Academic Award Program." *Am. J. Clin. Nutr.* 74 (2001): 164–170.

8. Kassler WJ. "Appendix F: Testimony of the American Medical Student Association." Washington, DC: National Academy of Sciences, 1985.

9. Zeisel SH, and Plaisted CS. "CD-ROMs for Nutrition Education." *J. Am. Coll. Nutr.* 18 (1999): 287.

10. Two or three reputable agencies have also sponsored this program, but I suspect that the administrators of these agencies felt it necessary to associate with a project in medical education for their own purposes, regardless of the dubious list of other organizations.

11. http://www.med.unc.edu/nutr/nim/FAQ.htm#anchor197343

12. Weinsier RL, Boker JR, Brooks CM, et al. "Nutrition training in graduate medical (residency) education: a survey of selected training programs." *Am. J. Clin. Nutr.* 54 (1991): 957–962.

13. Young EA. "National Dairy Council Award for Excellence in Medical/Dental Nutrition Education Lecture, 1992: perspectives on nutrition in medical education." *Am. J. Clin. Nutr.* 56 (1992): 745–751.

14. Kushner RF. "Will there be a tipping point in medical nutrition education?" *Am. J. Clin. Nutr.* 77 (2003): 288–291.

15. Angell M. "Is academic medicine for sale?" *New Engl. J. Med.* 342 (2000): 1516–1518.

16. Moynihan R. "Who pays for the pizza? Redefining the relationships between doctors and drug companies 1: Entanglement." *Brit. Med. Journ.* 326 (2003): 1189–1192.

17. Moynihan R. "Who pays for the pizza? Redefining the relationships between doctors and drug companies. 2. Disentanglement." *Brit. Med. Journ.* 326 (2003): 1193–1196.

18. Avorn J, Chen M, and Hartley R. "Scientific versus commercial sources of influence on the prescribing behavior of physicians." *Am. J. Med.* 73 (1982): 4–8.

19. Lurie N, Rich EC, Simpson DE, et al. "Pharmaceutical representatives in academic medical centers: interaction with faculty and housestaff." *J. Gen. Intern. Med.* 5 (1990): 240–243.

20. Steinman MA, Shlipak MG, and McPhee SJ. "Of principles and pens: attitudes and practices of medicine housestaff toward pharmaceutical industry promotions." *Am. J. Med.* 110 (2001): 551–557.

21. Lexchin J. "Interactions between physicians and the pharmaceutical industry: what does the literature say?" *Can.. Med. Assoc. J.* 149 (1993): 1401–1407.

22. Lexchin J. "What information do physicians receive from pharmaceutical representatives?" *Can. Fam. Physician* 43 (1997): 941–945.

23. Baird P. "Getting it right: industry sponsorship and medical research." *Can. Med. Assoc. Journ.* 168 (2003): 1267–1269.

24. Smith R. "Medical journals and pharmaceutical companies: uneasy bedfellows." *Brit. Med. Journ.* 326 (2003): 1202–1205.

25. Chopra SS. "Industry funding of clinical trials: benefit or bias?" *JAMA* 290 (2003): 113–114.

26. Healy D. "In the grip of the python: conficts at the university-industry interface." *Sci. Engineering Ethics* 9 (2003): 59–71.

27. Olivieri NF. "Patients' health or company profits? The commericalization of academic research." *Sci. Engineering Ethics* 9 (2003): 29–41.

28. Johnson L. "Schools report research interest conflicts." The *Ithaca Journal* October 24, 2002: 3A.

29. Agovino T. "Prescription use by children multiplying, study says." The *Ithaca Journal* Sept. 19, 2002: 1A.

30. Associated Press. "Survey: many guidelines written by doctors with ties to companies." The *Ithaca Journal* Feb. 12, 2002

31. Weiss R. "Correctly prescribed drugs take heavy toll; millions affected by toxic reactions." The *Washington Post* Apr. 15, 1998: A01.

32. Lasser KE, Allen PD, Woolhandler SJ, et al. "Timing of new black box warnings and withdrawals for prescription medications." *JAMA* 287 (2002): 2215–2220.

33. Lazarou J, Pomeranz B, and Corey PN. "Incidence of adverse drug reactions in hospitalized patients." *JAMA* 279 (1998): 1200–1205.

Chapter 18

1. Macilwain G. *The General Nature and Treatment of Tumors.* London, UK: John Churchill, 1845.

2. Williams H. *The Ethics of Diet. A Catena of Authorities Deprecatory of the Practice of Flesh-Eating.* London: F. Pitman, 1883.

3. U.S. Census Bureau. "U.S. Popclock Projection." March, 2004. Accessed at http://www.census.gov/cgi-bin/popclock

4. Centers for Disease Control. "Prevalence of adults with no known risk factors for coronary heart disease-behavioral risk factor surveillance system, 1992." *Morbidity and mortality weekly report* 43 (February 4, 1994): 61–63,69.

5. Kaufman DW, Kelly JP, Rosenberg L, et al. "Recent patterns of medication use in the ambulatory adult population of the United States: the Slone survey." *J. Am. Med. Assoc.* 287 (2002): 337–344.

6. Flegal KM, Carroll MD, Ogden CL, et al. "Prevalence and trends in obesity among U.S. adults, 1999–2000." *JAMA* 288 (2002): 1723–1727.

7. American Heart Association. "High blood cholesterol and other lipids—statistics." March, 2004. Accessed at http://www.americanheart.org/presenter.jhtml?identifier=2016

8. Wolz M, Cutler J, Roccella EJ, et al. "Statement from the National High Blood Pressure Education Program: prevalence of hypertension." *Am. J. Hypertens.* 13 (2000): 103–104.

9. Lucas JW, Schiller JS, and Benson V. "Summary health statistics for U.S. Adults: National Health Interview Survey, 2001." National Center for Health Statistics. Vital Health Stat. 10(218). 2004

10. Robbins J. *The Food Revolution.* Berkeley, California: Conari Press, 2001.

11. I strongly recommend reading John Robbins' "The Food Revolution," which convincingly details the connection between your diet and the environment.

12. World Health Organization. "The World Health Report 1997: Press Release. Human and social costs of chronic diseases will rise unless confronted now, WHO Director-General says." Geneva, Switzerland: World Health Organization, 1997. Accessed at http://www.who.int/whr2001/2001/archives/1997/presse.htm

13. Ornish, D., Brown, S. E., Scherwitz, L. W., Billings, J. H., Armstrong, W. T., Ports, T. A., McLanahan, S. M., Kirkeeide, R. L., Brand, R. J., and Gould, K. L. "Can lifestyle changes reverse coronary heart disease?" *Lancet*, 336: 129–133, 1990.

Esselstyn, C. B., Ellis, S. G., Medendorp, S. V., and Crowe, T. D. "A strategy to arrest and reverse coronary artery disease: a 5-year longitudinal study of a single physician's practice." *J. Family Practice*, 41: 560–568, 1995.

14. Vegetarian Resource Group. "How Many Vegetarians Are There?" March, 2004. Accessed at http://www.vrg.org/journal/vj2003issue3/vj2003issue3poll.htm

15. Herman-Cohen V. "Vegan revolution." *Ithaca Journal (reprinted from LA Times)* Aug 11, 2003: 12A.

16. Sabate J, Duk A, and Lee CL. "Publication trends of vegetarian nutrition articles in biomedical literature, 1966–1995." *Am. J. Clin. Nutr.* 70(Suppl) (1999): 601S–607S.

Appendix A

1. Boyd JN, Misslbeck N, Parker RS, et al. "Sucrose enhanced emergence of aflatoxin B$_1$ (AFB$_1$)-induced GGt positive rat hepatic cell foci." *Fed. Proc.* 41 (1982): 356 Abst.

2. Tannenbaum A, and Silverstone H. "Nutrition in relation to cancer." *Adv. Cancer Res.* 1 (1953): 451–501.

3. Youngman LD. *The growth and development of aflatoxin B1-induced preneoplastic lesions, tumors, metastasis, and spontaneous tumors as they are influenced by dietary protein level, type, and intervention.* Ithaca, NY: Cornell University, Ph.D. Thesis, 1990.

4. Youngman LD, and Campbell TC. "Inhibition of aflatoxin B1-induced gamma-glutamyl transpeptidase positive (GGT+) hepatic preneoplastic foci and tumors by low protein diets: evidence that altered GGT+ foci indicate neoplastic potential." *Carcinogenesis* 13 (1992): 1607–1613.

5. Horio F, Youngman LD, Bell RC, et al. "Thermogenesis, low-protein diets, and decreased development of AFB1-induced preneoplastic foci in rat liver." *Nutr. Cancer* 16 (1991): 31–41.

6. Bell RC, Levitsky DA, and Campbell TC. "Enhanced thermogenesis and reduced growth rates do not inhibit GGT+ hepatic preneoplastic foci development." *FASEB J.* 6 (1992): 1395 Abs.

7. Miller DS, and Payne PR. "Weight maintenance and food intake." *J. Nutr.* 78 (1962): 255–262.

8. Stirling JL, and Stock MJ. "Metabolic origins of thermogenesis by diet." *Nature* 220 (1968): 801–801.

9. Donald P, Pitts GC, and Pohl SL. "Body weight and composition in laboratory rats: effects of diets with high or low protein concentrations." *Science* 211 (1981): 185–186.

10. Rothwell NJ, Stock MJ, and Tyzbir RS. "Mechanisms of thermogenesis induced by low protein diets." *Metabolism* 32 (1983): 257–261.

11. Rothwell NJ, and Stock MJ. "Influence of carbohydrate and fat intake on diet-induced thermogenesis and brown fat activity in rats fed low protein diets." *J Nutr* 117 (1987): 1721–1726.

12. Krieger E, Youngman LD, and Campbell TC. "The modulation of aflatoxin(AFB1) induced preneoplastic lesions by dietary protein and voluntary exercise in Fischer 344 rats." *FASEB J.* 2 (1988): 3304 Abs.

Appendix B

1. Chen J, Campbell TC, Li J, et al. *Diet, life-style and mortality in China. A study of the characteristics of 65 Chinese counties.* Oxford, UK; Ithaca, NY; Beijing, PRC: Oxford University Press; Cornell University Press; People's Medical Publishing House, 1990.

2. There were eight-two mortality rates, but about a third of these rates were duplicates of the same disease for people of different ages.

3. This also means that very little or no useful information is obtained by including the values of all the individuals in the county. There is only one disease rate for each county; thus it is only necessary to have one number for any of the variables being compared with the disease rate.
4. Piazza A. *Food consumption and nutritional status in the People's Republic of China.* London: Westview Press, 1986.
5. Messina M, and Messina V. *The Dietitian's Guide to Vegetarian Diets. Issues and Applications.* Gaithersburg, MD: Aspen Publishers, Inc., 1996.

Appendix C

1. Holick MF. *In:* M. E. Shils, J. A. Olson, M. Shike and e. al (eds.), *Modern nutrition in health and disease, 9th ed.*, pp. 329–345. Baltimore, MD: Williams and Wilkins, 1999.
2. Barger-Lux MJ, Heaney R, Dowell S, et al. "Vitamin D and its major metabolites: serum levels after graded oral dosing in healthy men." *Osteoporosis Int.* 8 (1998): 222–230.
3. The biological half-life of storage vitamin D is 10–19 days, the time it takes for half of it to disappear.
4. Colston KW, Berger U, and Coombes RC. "Possible role for vitamin D in controlling breast cancer cell proliferation." *Lancet* 1 (1989): 188–191.
5. Nieves J, Cosman F, Herbert J, et al. "High prevalence of vitamin D deficiency and reduced bone mass in multiple sclerosis." *Neurology* 44 (1994): 1687–1692.
6. Al-Qadreh A, Voskaki I, Kassiou C, et al. "Treatment of osteopenia in children with insulin-dependent diabetes mellitus: the effect of 1-alpha hydroxyvitamin D3." *Eur. J. Pediatr.* 155 (1996): 15–17.
7. Cantorna MT, Hayes CE, and DeLuca HF. "1,25-Dihydroxyvitamin D_3 reversibly blocks the progression of relapsing encephalomyelitis, a model of multiple sclerosis." *Proc. National Acad. Sci* 93 (1996): 7861–7864.
8. Rozen F, Yang X-F, Huynh H, et al. "Antiproliferative action of vitamin D-related compounds and insulin-like growth factor-binding protein 5 accumulation." *J. Nat. Cancer Inst.* 89 (1997): 652–656.
9. Cosman F, Nieves J, Komar L, et al. "Fracture history and bone loss in patients with MS." *Neurology* 51 (1998): 1161–1165.
10. Giovannucci E, Rimm E, Wolk A, et al. "Calcium and fructose intake in relation to risk of prostate cancer." *Cancer Res.* 58 (1998): 442–447.
11. Peehl DM, Krishnan AV, and Feldman D. "Pathways mediating the growth-inhibitory action of vitamin D in prostate cancer." *J. Nutr.* 133(Suppl) (2003): 2461S–2469S.
12. Zella JB, McCary LC, and DeLuca HF. "Oral administration of 1,25-dihydroxyvitamin D_3 completely protects NOD mice from insulin-dependent diabetes mellitus." *Arch. Biochem Biophys.* 417 (2003): 77–80.
13. Davenport CB. "Multiple sclerosis from the standpoint of geographic distribution and race." *Arch. Neurol. Pschiatry* 8 (1922): 51–58.
14. Alter M, Yamoor M, and Harshe M. "Multiple sclerosis and nutrition." *Arch. Neurol.* 31 (1974): 267–272.
15. Van der Mei IA, Ponsonby AL, Blizzard L, et al. "Regional variation in multiple sclerosis prevalence in Australia and its association with ambivalent ultraviolet radiaion." *Neuroepidemiology* 20 (2001): 168–174.
16. McLeod JG, Hammond SR, and Hallpike JF. "Epidemiology of multiple sclerosis in Australia. With NSW and SA survey results." *Med. J. Austr* 160 (1994): 117–122.
17. Holick MF. "Vitamin D: a millenium perspective." *J. Cell. Biochem.* 88 (2003): 296–307.
18. MacLaughlin JA, Gange W, Taylor D, et al. "Cultured psoriatic fibroblasts from involved and uninvolved sites have a partial, but not absolute resistance to the proliferation-inhibtion activity of 1,25-dihydroxyvitamin D_s." *Proc. National Acad. Sci* 52 (1985): 5409–5412.

19. Goldberg P, Fleming MC, and Picard EH. "Multiple sclerosis: decreased relapse rate through dietary supplementation with calcium, magnesium and vitamin D." *Med. Hypoth.* 21 (1986): 193–200.

20. Andjelkovic Z, Vojinovic J, Pejnovic N, et al. "Disease modifying and immunomodulatory effects of high dose 1a(OH)D$_3$ in rheumatoid arthritis patients." *Clin. Exp. Rheumatol.* 17 (1999): 453–456.

21. Hypponen E, Laara E, Reunanen A, et al. "Intake of vitamin D and risk of Type 1 diabetes: a birth-cohort study." *Lancet* 358 (2001): 1500–1503.

22. Breslau NA, Brinkley L, Hill KD, et al. "Relationship of animal protein-rich diet to kidney stone formation and calcium metabolism." *J. Clin. Endocrinol. Metab.* 66 (1988): 140–146.

23. Langman CB. "Calcitriol metabolism during chronic metabolic acidosis." *Semin. Nephrol.* 9 (1989): 65–71.

24. Chan JM, Giovannucci EL, Andersson S-O, et al. "Dairy products, calcium, phosphorus, vitamin D, and risk of prostate cancer (Sweden)." *Cancer Causes and Control* 9 (1998): 559–566.

25. Byrne PM, Freaney R, and McKenna MJ. "Vitamin D supplementation in the elderly: review of safety and effectiveness of different regimes." *Calcified Tissue Int.* 56 (1995): 518–520.

26. Agranoff BW, and Goldberg D. "Diet and the geographical distribution of multiple sclerosis." *Lancet* 2(7888) (November 2 1974): 1061–1066.

27. Akerblom HK, Vaarala O, Hyoty H, et al. "Environmental factors in the etiology of Type 1 diabetes." *Am. J. Med. Genet. (Semin. Med. Genet.)* 115 (2002): 18–29.

28. Chan JM, Stampfer MJ, Ma J, et al. "Insulin-like growth factor-I (IGF-I) and IGF binding protein-3 as predictors of advanced-stage prostate cancer." *J Natl Cancer Inst* 94 (2002): 1099–1109.

29. Cohen P, Peehl DM, and Rosenfeld RG. "The IGF axis in the prostate." *Horm. Metab. res.* 26 (1994): 81–84.

30. Doi SQ, Rasaiah S, Tack I, et al. "Low-protein diet suppresses serum insulin-like growth factor-1 and decelerates the progresseion of growth hormone-induced glomerulosclerosis." *Am. J. Nephrol.* 21 (2001): 331–339.

31. Heaney RP, McCarron DA, Dawson-Hughes B, et al. "Dietary changes favorably affect bond remodeling in older adults." *J. Am. Diet. Assoc.* 99 (1999): 1228–1233.

32. Allen NE, Appleby PN, Davey GK, et al. "Hormones and diet: low insulin-like growth factor-I but normal bioavailable androgens in vegan men." *Brit. J. Cancer* 83 (2000): 95–97.

Index

About the Authors

For more than forty years, **DR. T. COLIN CAMPBELL** has been at the forefront of nutrition research. His legacy, the China Study, is the most comprehensive study of health and nutrition ever conducted. Dr. Campbell is Jacob Gould Schurman Professor Emeritus of Nutritional Biochemisty at Cornell University. He has received more than seventy grant-years of peer-reviewed research funding and authored more than 300 research papers. The China Study was the culmination of a twenty-year partnership of Cornell University, Oxford University and the Chinese Academy of Preventive Medicine.

A 1999 graduate of Cornell University, **THOMAS CAMPBELL** is currently pursuing a career in medicine. In addition, he is a writer, actor and three-time marathon runner. Born and raised in Ithaca, NY, he has appeared on stage in London, Chicago and most of the states east of the Mississippi River. Mr. Campbell enjoys playing soccer, skiing and hiking.

Ready to take the next step?

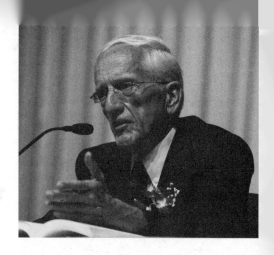

For more information:
1-866-eCornell (1-866-326-7635)
info@ecornell.com
www.ecornell.com/online/tcc

CERTIFICATE IN PLANT-BASED NUTRITION

The *Certificate in Plant-Based Nutrition,* a series of 3 online courses offered by the T. Colin Campbell Foundation and eCornell, trains students to understand the connection between diet and disease. Each course is approximately 6 hours of learning and covers studies published in the very best scientific journals. The program was created by one of Cornell University's most distinguished researchers, Dr. T. Colin Campbell, PhD and features renowned guest lecturers, including:

Antonia Demas, PhD - **Nutrition in the Public Schools**
Caldwell Esselstyn, MD - **Reversing Heart Disease**
Doug Lisle, PhD - **Obesity and The Pleasure Trap**
John McDougall, MD - **Nutrition in the Medical Clinic**
Bruce Monger, PhD - **Coastal Eutrophication and Overfishing**
Jeff Novick, MS, RD, LD, LN - **Food Labeling**
David Pimentel, PhD - **Environmental Impact of Our Diet**
Pamela Popper, ND, PhD - **Nutrition and Corporate Wellness**

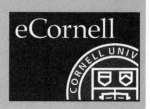

BE PART OF THE SOLUTION

Health Education at its Best

Let's solve the healthcare crisis one student at a time. Help us create more science-based, educational tools and programs with your tax-exempt donation. Be a part of the most effective prevention there is for degenerative disease, and provide much needed support to the organization working to make it happen. Our future is in our hands.

**Donate online at www.tcolincampbell.org/courses-resources/donate/
  or email meg@tcolincampbell.org**